Healthy Heart Sourcebook for Women

Heart Diseases & Disorders Sourcebook, 2nd Edition

Household Safety Sourcebook

Immune System Disorders Sourcebook

Infant & Toddler Health Sourcebook

Infectious Diseases Sourcebook

Injury & Trauma Sourcebook

Kidney & Urinary Tract Diseases & Disorders Sourcebook

Learning Disabilities Sourcebook, 2nd Edition

Leukemia Sourcebook

Liver Disorders Sourcebook

Lung Disorders Sourcebook

Medical Tests Sourcebook, 2nd Edition

Men's Health Concerns Sourcebook, 2nd Edition

Mental Health Disorders Sourcebook, 2nd Edition

Mental Retardation Sourcebook

Movement Disorders Sourcebook

Obesity Sourcebook

Osteoporosis Sourcebook

Pain Sourcebook, 2nd Edition

Pediatric Cancer Sourcebook

Physical & Mental Issues in Aging Sourcebook

Podiatry Sourcebook

Pregnancy & Birth Sourcebook, 2nd Edition

Prostate Cancer

Public Health Sourcebook

Reconstructive & Cosmetic Surgery Sourcebook

Rehabilitation Sourcebook

Respiratory Diseases & Disorders Sourcebook

Sexually Transmitted Diseases Sourcebook, 2nd Edition

Skin D...

Sleep ...

Sports ...

Stress ...

Stroke Source...

Substance Abuse Sourcebook

Surgery Sourcebook

Transplantation Sourcebook

Traveler's Health Sourcebook

Vegetarian Sourcebook

Women's Health Concerns Sourcebook, 2nd Edition

Workplace Health & Safety Sourcebook

Worldwide Health Sourcebook

Teen Health Series

Cancer Information for Teens

Diet Information for Teens

Drug Information for Teens

Fitness Information for Teens

Mental Health Information for Teens

Sexual Health Information for Teens

Skin Health Information for Teens

Sports Injuries Information for Teens

Infectious
Diseases
SOURCEBOOK

Health Reference Series

First Edition **WITHDRAWN**

Infectious Diseases SOURCEBOOK

*Basic Consumer Health Information about
Non-Contagious Bacterial, Viral, Prion, Fungal, and
Parasitic Diseases Spread by Food and Water, Insects and
Animals, or Environmental Contact, Including Botulism,
E. Coli, Encephalitis, Legionnaires' Disease, Lyme Disease,
Malaria, Plague, Rabies, Salmonella, Tetanus, and Others,
and Facts about Newly Emerging Diseases, Such as
Hantavirus, Mad Cow Disease, Monkeypox, and
West Nile Virus*

*Along with Information about Preventing Disease
Transmission, the Threat of Bioterrorism, and Current
Research Initiatives, with a Glossary and Directory of
Resources for More Information*

Edited by
Karen Bellenir

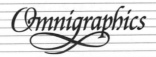

Omnigraphics

615 Griswold Street • Detroit, MI 48226

Bibliographic Note

Because this page cannot legibly accommodate all the copyright notices, the Bibliographic Note portion of the Preface constitutes an extension of the copyright notice.

Edited by Karen Bellenir

Health Reference Series

Karen Bellenir, *Managing Editor*
David A. Cooke, M.D., *Medical Consultant*
Elizabeth Barbour, *Permissions Associate*
Dawn Matthews, *Verification Assistant*
Laura Pleva Nielsen, *Index Editor*
EdIndex, Services for Publishers, *Indexers*

* * *

Omnigraphics, Inc.

Matthew P. Barbour, *Senior Vice President*
Kay Gill, *Vice President—Directories*
Kevin Hayes, *Operations Manager*
Leif Gruenberg, *Development Manager*
David P. Bianco, *Marketing Director*

* * *

Peter E. Ruffner, *Publisher*

Frederick G. Ruffner, Jr., *Chairman*

Copyright © 2004 Omnigraphics, Inc.

ISBN 0-7808-0675-1

Library of Congress Cataloging-in-Publication Data

Infectious diseases sourcebook : basic consumer health information about non-contagious bacterial, viral, prion, fungal, and parasitic diseases spread by food and water, insects and animals, or environmental contact, including botulism, E. coli, encephalitis, Legionnaires' disease, Lyme disease, malaria, plague, rabies, salmonella, tetanus, and others, and facts about newly emerging diseases, such as hantavirus, mad cow disease, monkeypox, and West Nile virus, along with information about preventing disease transmission, the threat of bioterrorism, and current research initiatives, with a glossary and directory of resources for more information / edited by Karen Bellenir.-- 1st ed.
    p. ; cm. -- (Health reference series)
  Includes bibliographical references and index.
  ISBN 0-7808-0675-1 (hard cover : alk. paper)
  1. Communicable diseases--Popular works.
  [DNLM: 1. Communicable Diseases--Popular Works. 2. Communicable Diseases--Resource Guides. WC 39 I438 2004] I. Bellenir, Karen. II. Health reference series (Unnumbered)
  RA643.I6545 2004
  616.9--dc22

                                                    2004004726

The information in this publication was compiled from the sources cited and from other sources considered reliable. While every possible effort has been made to ensure reliability, the publisher will not assume liability for damages caused by inaccuracies in the data, and makes no warranty, express or implied, on the accuracy of the information contained herein.

∞

This book is printed on acid-free paper meeting the ANSI Z39.48 Standard. The infinity symbol that appears above indicates that the paper in this book meets that standard.

Printed in the United States

Table of Contents

Part III: Insect and Animal Borne Diseases

Part IV: Environmental Contamination and Microbe Overgrowth

Part V: The Threat of Bioterrorism

Part VI: Infectious Disease Research

Part VII: Additional Help and Information

Preface

About This Book

Infectious diseases are illnesses caused by bacteria, viruses, and other microbes. Combined, they represent the leading cause of death worldwide and the third leading cause of death in the United States— where the annual cost of medical care for treating them is estimated at $120 billion. In the last century, the development of antibiotics and vaccines led to a hope that infectious diseases could be overcome; however, microbes have proven themselves to be persistent and tenacious opponents. Newly emerging diseases are a growing concern and new microbe strains that are resistant to the drugs previously used to stop them are a serious public health threat. In addition, the possibility of biological terrorism presents a challenge that medical researchers are working to address.

This book provides information about non-contagious infectious diseases that can be spread through contaminated food and drinking water, by insects and animals, or by contact with microorganisms in the environment. These include botulism, *E. coli*, various forms of encephalitis, hantavirus, Legionnaires' disease, Lyme disease, mad cow disease, malaria, monkeypox, plague, rabies, *Salmonella*, tetanus, and many others. Individual chapters provide details about the organisms responsible for the diseases, how they are spread, their symptoms, and treatments. Special sections focus on bioterrorism and current research initiatives. A glossary, directory of resources, and suggestions for further reading are also included.

ix

Readers seeking information about contagious infectious diseases (those that are spread by person-to-person contact) may wish to consult *Contagious Diseases Sourcebook,* a separate volume in the *Health Reference Series.*

How to Use This Book

This book is divided into parts and chapters. Parts focus on broad areas of interest. Chapters are devoted to single topics within a part.

Part I: Understanding Infectious Diseases describes various types of infectious diseases and the microbes that cause them. It offers general suggestions for avoiding infectious diseases and explains how the body's immune system works to fend off attacks from invading bacteria, viruses, and other disease-causing agents.

Part II: Diseases Acquired from Food and Drinking Water provides information about illnesses that are contracted from eating and drinking contaminated food or water. These include botulism, *Campylobacter* infections, *E. coli,* giardiasis, *Salmonella* infections, traveler's diarrhea, vibrio diseases, and many others.

Part III: Insect and Animal Borne Diseases provides information about diseases that are acquired as a result of contact with mosquitos, ticks, fleas, rodents, other wild animals, and pets. Cat scratch disease, hantavirus, Lyme disease, malaria, rabies, and West Nile virus are among the nearly two dozen diseases addressed in this part.

Part IV: Environmental Contamination and Microbe Overgrowth describes illnesses caused by coming into contact with microbes in the environment. These include amoeba infections, various types of parasitic worms, fungal infections, swimmers itch, and tetanus. Diseases associated with the overgrowth of microbes that normally exist in the human body, such as candidiasis, are also included.

Part V: The Threat of Bioterrorism discusses the possible terrorist use of biological weapons and the steps that can be taken to ensure preparedness. Agents of special concern include anthrax, *botulinum* toxin, glanders, melioidosis, Q fever, plague, smallpox, tularemia, and viral hemorrhagic fevers. Related topics, including radiation hazards and toxic chemical agents, are also discussed because of their potential inclusion in the terrorist arsenal.

Part VI: Infectious Disease Research reports on recent studies and ongoing initiatives to better understand microbes and reduce the burden caused by the diseases associated with them.

Part VII: Additional Help and Information includes a glossary, a directory of resources, and a list of suggestions for further reading.

Bibliographic Note

This volume contains documents and excerpts from publications issued by the National Institutes of Health (NIH) and its subagencies, including: National Digestive Diseases Information Clearinghouse, National Eye Institute, National Institute of Allergy and Infectious Diseases, National Institute of Diabetes and Digestive and Kidney Diseases, National Institute of Neurological Disorders and Stroke, and the National Kidney and Urologic Diseases Information Clearinghouse; by the Centers for Disease Control and Prevention (CDC) and its subagencies, including: Division of Bacterial and Mycotic Diseases, Division of Healthcare Quality Promotion, Division of Parasitic Diseases, Division of Vector-Borne Infectious Diseases, National Center for Health Statistics, National Center for Infectious Diseases, Public Health Emergency Preparedness and Response, Public Health Image Library, Respiratory and Enteric Viruses Branch, Special Pathogens Branch, and Viral and Rickettsial Zoonoses Branch; and by these other U.S. government agencies: U.S. Department of Agriculture, U.S. Department of Homeland Security, U.S. Federal Trade Commission, and the U.S. Food and Drug Administration.

In addition, this volume contains copyrighted documents from the following organizations and individuals: A.D.A.M., Inc.; American Academy of Family Physicians; American Lyme Disease Foundation, Inc.; American Society for Microbiology; Association for Professionals in Infection Control and Epidemiology, Inc.; Association of State and Territorial Directors of Health Promotion and Public Health Education; Bowling Green State University Center for Algal Microscopy and Image Digitization; Center for Biosecurity (University of Pittsburgh Medical Center); Caroline Harwood, PhD; Infectious Diseases Society of America; Dennis Kunkel Microscopy, Inc.; John's Hopkins University, Division of Infectious Diseases; National Foundation for Infectious Diseases; Nemours Center for Children's Health Media, a division of The Nemours Foundation; Jean Yves Sgro, University of Wisconsin; Wisconsin Department of Health and Family Services; and the World Health Organization.

Acknowledgements

In addition to the organizations, agencies, and individuals listed above, special thanks go to many others who have worked hard to help bring this book to fruition. They include editorial assistant Michael Bellenir, permissions associate Liz Barbour, and indexer Edward J. Prucha.

Note from the Editor

This book is part of Omnigraphics' *Health Reference Series*. The *Series* provides basic information about a broad range of medical concerns. It is not intended to serve as a tool for diagnosing illness, in prescribing treatments, or as a substitute for the physician/patient relationship. All persons concerned about medical symptoms or the possibility of disease are encouraged to seek professional care from an appropriate health care provider.

Our Advisory Board

The *Health Reference Series* is reviewed by an Advisory Board comprised of librarians from public, academic, and medical libraries. We would like to thank the following board members for providing guidance to the development of this series:

Dr. Lynda Baker,
Associate Professor of Library and Information Science,
Wayne State University, Detroit, MI

Nancy Bulgarelli,
William Beaumont Hospital Library, Royal Oak, MI

Karen Imarisio,
Bloomfield Township Public Library, Bloomfield Township, MI

Karen Morgan,
Mardigian Library, University of Michigan-Dearborn,
Dearborn, MI

Rosemary Orlando,
St. Clair Shores Public Library, St. Clair Shores, MI

Medical Consultant

Medical consultation services are provided to the *Health Reference Series* editors by David A. Cooke, M.D. Dr. Cooke is a graduate of

Brandeis University, and he received his M.D. degree from the University of Michigan. He completed residency training at the University of Wisconsin Hospital and Clinics. He is board-certified in Internal Medicine. Dr. Cooke currently works as part of the University of Michigan Health System and practices in Brighton, MI. In his free time, he enjoys writing, science fiction, and spending time with his family.

Health Reference Series *Update Policy*

The inaugural book in the *Health Reference Series* was the first edition of *Cancer Sourcebook* published in 1989. Since then, the *Series* has been enthusiastically received by librarians and in the medical community. In order to maintain the standard of providing high-quality health information for the layperson the editorial staff at Omnigraphics felt it was necessary to implement a policy of updating volumes when warranted.

Medical researchers have been making tremendous strides, and it is the purpose of the *Health Reference Series* to stay current with the most recent advances. Each decision to update a volume will be made on an individual basis. Some of the considerations will include how much new information is available and the feedback we receive from people who use the books. If there is a topic you would like to see added to the update list, or an area of medical concern you feel has not been adequately addressed, please write to:

Editor
Health Reference Series
Omnigraphics, Inc.
615 Griswold Street
Detroit, MI 48226
E-mail: editorial@omnigraphics.com

Part One

Understanding
Infectious Diseases

Chapter 1

What Are Infectious Diseases?

Addressing Infectious Disease Threats

Infectious diseases are human illnesses caused by viruses, bacteria, parasites, fungi, and other microbes. They may be spread by direct contact with an infected person or animal, by ingesting contaminated food or water, by insects like mosquitos or ticks (disease vectors), or by contact with contaminated surroundings like animal droppings or even contaminated air.

A Problem That Won't Go Away

With the advent of antibiotics 50 years ago, scientists made sweeping predictions heralding the end of death and suffering from infectious diseases. During the past 25 years, however, microbes have demonstrated their tremendous ability to adapt, survive, and challenge us anew.

This chapter includes "Addressing Infectious Disease Threats," excerpted from *Model Emergency Response Communications Planning for Infectious Disease Outbreaks and Bioterrorist Events, Second Edition*, October 2001. © 2001 Association of State and Territorial Directors of Health Promotion and Public Health Education. All rights reserved. Developed with funding from the Centers for Disease Control and Prevention (CDC) through cooperative agreement #U50/CCU012359 to the Directors of Health Promotion and Education. And, "How Do Microbes Make Us Sick?" excerpted from "Microbes in Sickness and in Health," National Institute of Allergy and Infectious Diseases, February 2001, updated July 2002.

Once thought almost eliminated as a public health problem, infectious diseases remain the leading cause of death worldwide. In 1996, infectious diseases killed about one-third of the more than 52 million people who died that year. In the United States, two of the ten leading causes of death are infectious diseases (HIV and pneumonia/influenza). The Centers for Disease Control and Prevention (CDC) reports that 160,000 Americans die each year with an infectious disease as the underlying cause of death.

Ranging from childhood ear infections to measles to sexually transmitted diseases (STDs), infectious illnesses account for 25% of all physician visits each year, and antimicrobial agents are second only to pain relievers as the most frequently prescribed class of drugs.

Anticipating and coping with these microbial threats requires vigilance. We must maintain global surveillance and a strong public health infrastructure with state-of-the-art laboratories and solid partnerships with colleagues in medical, scientific, and policy arenas. Research and creativity are crucial, as is targeted public education at all levels of society to ensure a well-informed public. Knowing that local threats can balloon into national or global problems, partnerships must be formed at all levels to develop both local and global prevention strategies.

A Financial Burden

Societal costs of infectious diseases are staggering. In the United States, treatment of non-AIDS STDs alone costs $5 billion annually. The yearly price tags of other infectious diseases are $30 billion for intestinal infections, $17 billion for influenza, $1 billion for salmonella, and $720 million for Hepatitis B. Altogether, the cost of treatment and lost productivity associated with illness from infectious agents tops $120 billion each year.

Emerging and Reemerging Diseases

Although some infectious diseases, such as polio, have been nearly wiped out, the vast majority of these diseases will not be eliminated in our lifetime. Indeed, the World Health Organization reports that at least 30 new diseases have been scientifically recognized around the world in the last 20 years. These emerging diseases include Sin Nombre hantavirus, first identified in the US in 1993; cryptosporidiosis (a water-borne cause of diarrhea that recently affected more than 400,000 people in a single outbreak in the U.S.); the Ebola virus from Africa; and HIV.

Infectious diseases once thought under control are also reemerging. Diseases like tuberculosis, cholera, and even diphtheria are making a comeback.

How Do Microbes Make Us Sick?

Microbes are tiny organisms—too tiny to see without a microscope, yet they are abundant on Earth. They live everywhere—in air, soil, rock, and water. Some microbes cause disease in humans, plants, and animals. Others are essential for a healthy life, and we could not exist without them. Indeed, the relationship between microbes and humans is very delicate and complex.

Most microbes belong to one of four major groups: bacteria, viruses, fungi, or protozoa. A familiar, often-used word for microbes that cause disease is "germs." Some people refer to disease-causing microbes as "bugs." "I've got the flu bug," for example, is a phrase you may hear during the wintertime to describe an influenza virus infection.

Ways Microbes Can Infect Us

Through the Air: Microbes can be transmitted from person to person through the air, as in coughing or sneezing. These are common ways to get viruses that cause colds or flu or the bacterium that causes tuberculosis (TB). Interestingly, international airplane travel can expose passengers to germs not common in their own countries.

Table 1.1. Common Diseases and Infections with Their Microbial Causes

Bacteria	Fungus	Protozoa	Virus
Diarrheal disease	Athlete's foot	Diarrheal disease	Chickenpox
Meningitis	Pneumonia	Malaria	Common cold
Pneumonia	Sinusitis	Skin diseases	Diarrheal disease
Sinusitis	Skin diseases		Flu
Skin diseases	Vaginal infections		Genital herpes
Strep throat			Meningitis
Tuberculosis			Pneumonia
Urinary tract infection			Skin diseases
Vaginal infections			Viral hepatitis

From Person to Person: Scientists have identified more than 500 types of bacteria that live in the human mouth. Some keep the oral environment healthy, while others cause gum disease. One way to transmit oral bacteria from person to person is by kissing. Microbes such as HIV, herpes simplex virus 1, and gonorrhea bacteria are examples of germs that can be transmitted directly during sexual intercourse.

By Touching Infectious Material: A common way for some microbes to enter the body, especially when caring for young children, is to unintentionally pass feces on your hand to your mouth or the mouths of young children. Infant diarrhea is often spread in this way. Day care workers, for example, can pass diarrhea-causing rotavirus or *Giardia lamblia* (protozoa) from one baby to the next between diaper changes and other childcare practices. It also is possible to pick up cold viruses from shaking someone's hand or from touching surfaces such as a handrail or telephone.

A Healthy Person Can Be a Germ Carrier: The story of "Typhoid Mary" is a famous example from medical history about how a person can pass germs on to others, yet not be affected by them. The germs in this case were *Salmonella typhi* bacteria, which cause typhoid fever and are usually spread through food or water. Mary Mallon, an Irish immigrant who lived at the turn of the 20th century, worked as a cook for several New York City families. More than half of the first family she worked for came down with typhoid fever. Through a clever deduction, a researcher determined that the disease was caused by the family cook. He concluded that although Mary had no symptoms of the disease, she probably had had a mild typhoid infection sometime in the past. Though not sick, she still carried the bacteria and was able to spread them to others through the food she prepared.

Animals Can Carry Germs: You can catch a variety of germs from animals, especially household pets. The rabies virus, which can infect cats and dogs, is one of the most serious and deadly of these microbes. Fortunately, the rabies vaccine prevents animals from getting rabies. Vaccines also protect people from accidentally getting the virus from an animal and prevent people who have been exposed to the virus, such as through an animal bite, from getting sick.

Dog and cat saliva can contain any of more than 100 different germs that can make you sick. *Pasteurella* bacteria, the most common, can be transmitted through bites that break the skin causing serious, and sometimes fatal, diseases such as blood infections and meningitis.

Warm-blooded animals are not the only ones that can cause you harm. Pet reptiles such as turtles, snakes, and iguanas can transmit *Salmonella* bacteria to their unsuspecting owners.

Insects Can Carry Germs: Mosquitoes may be the most common insect carriers (vectors) of pathogens. *Anopheles* mosquitoes can pick up *Plasmodium*, which causes malaria, from the blood of an infected person and transmit the protozoan to an uninfected person. Fleas that pick up *Yersinia pestis* bacteria from rodents can then transmit plague to humans. Ticks, which are more closely related to crabs than to insects, are another common vector. The tiny deer tick can infect humans with *Borrelia burgdorferi*, the bacterium that causes Lyme disease, which it picks up from deer.

The Food You Eat or the Water You Drink Could Make You Sick: Every year, millions of people worldwide become ill from eating contaminated foods. Although many cases of foodborne illness or "food poisoning" are not reported, the U.S. Centers for Disease Control and Prevention (CDC) estimates there are 76 million illnesses, 325,000 hospitalizations, and 5,200 deaths in the United States each year that are caused by foodborne bacteria. Bacteria, viruses, and protozoa can cause these illnesses, some of which can be fatal if not treated properly.

Poor manufacturing processes or poor food preparation can allow microbes to grow in food and subsequently infect you. *Escherichia coli* (*E. coli*) bacteria sometimes persist in food products such as undercooked hamburger meat and unpasteurized fruit juice. These bacteria can have deadly consequences in vulnerable people, especially children and the elderly.

Cryptosporidia are bacteria found in fecal matter and can get into lake, river, and ocean water from sewage spills, animal waste, and water runoff. They can be released in the millions from infectious fecal matter. People who drink, swim, or play in infected water can get sick. People, including babies, with diarrhea caused by *Cryptosporidia* or other diarrhea-causing microbes, such as *Giardia* and *Salmonella*, can infect others while using swimming pools, waterparks, hot tubs, and spas.

Transplanted Animal Organs May Harbor Germs: As researchers investigate the possibility of transplanting animal organs, such as pig hearts, into people, they must guard against the risk that organs also may transmit microbes that were harmless to the animal into humans, where they indeed may cause disease.

7

Microbes Cause Different Kinds of Infections

Some disease-causing microbes can make you very sick very quickly and then not bother you again. Some can last for a long time and continue to damage tissues. Others can last forever, but you won't feel sick any more, or you will only feel sick once in a while. Most infections caused by microbes fall into three major groups: acute infections; chronic infections; and latent infections.

Acute Infections: Acute infections usually last a short time, but they can make you feel very uncomfortable, with signs and symptoms such as tiredness, achiness, coughing, and sneezing. The common cold is such an infection. The signs and symptoms of a cold can last for 2 to 24 days (but usually a week), though it may seem like a lot longer. Once your body's immune system has successfully fought off one of the many different types of rhinoviruses that caused your cold, the cold doesn't come back. If you get another cold, it's probably because you have been infected with someone else's rhinoviruses.

Chronic Infections: Chronic infections usually develop from acute infections and can last for days to months to a lifetime. Sometimes, people are totally unaware they are infected but still may be able to transmit the germ to others. For example, hepatitis C, which affects the liver, is a chronic viral infection. In fact, most people who have been infected with the hepatitis C virus don't know it until they have a blood test that shows antibodies to the virus. Recovery from this infection is rare—about 85 percent of infected persons become chronic carriers of the virus. In addition, serious signs of liver damage, like cirrhosis or cancer, may not appear until as long as 20 years after the infection began.

Latent Infections: Latent infections are "hidden" or "silent" and may or may not cause symptoms again after the initial acute episode. Some infectious microbes, usually viruses, can "wake up" and become active again, sometimes off and on for months or years, and cause symptoms. When active, these microbes can be transmitted to other people. Herpes simplex viruses, which cause genital herpes and common cold sores, can remain latent in nerve cells for short or long periods of time, or forever.

Chickenpox is another example of a latent infection. Before the chickenpox vaccine became available in the 1990s, most children in the United States got chickenpox. After the first acute episode, usually when children are very young, the *Varicella zoster* virus goes into hiding in the body. In many people, it emerges many years later when they are older adults and causes a painful disease of the nerves called herpes zoster, or shingles.

The Difference between Infection and Disease

A disease occurs when cells or molecules in a person's body stop working properly, causing symptoms of illness. Many things can cause a disease, including altered genes, chemicals, aging, and infections. An infection occurs when another organism—such as a virus, bacterium, or parasite—enters a person's body and begins to reproduce. The invading microbe can directly damage cells, or the immune system can cause disease symptoms, such as fever, as it tries to rid the body of the invader. Some infections do not cause disease because the microbe is quickly killed or it hides out where it cannot be detected.

Generally, you should consult a doctor or other health care professional if you have or think you may have contracted an infectious disease. These trained professionals can determine whether you have been infected, determine the seriousness of your infection, and give you the best advice for treating or preventing disease. Sometimes, however, a visit to the doctor may not be necessary.

Some infectious diseases, such as the common cold, usually do not require a visit to the doctor. They often last a short time and are not life-threatening, or there is no specific treatment. We've all heard the advice to rest and drink plenty of liquids to treat colds. Unless there are complications, most victims of colds find their immune systems successfully ward off the viral culprits. In fact, the coughing, sneezing, and fever that make you feel miserable are part of your immune system's way of fighting them off.

If, however, you have other conditions in which your immune system doesn't function properly, you should be in contact with your doctor whenever you suspect you have any infectious disease, even the common cold. Such conditions can include asthma and immunodeficiency diseases like HIV infection and AIDS. In addition, some common, usually mild infectious diseases, such as chickenpox or flu, can cause serious harm in very young children or the elderly.

Infectious Diseases Are Diagnosed in Many Ways

Sometimes a doctor or other health care professional can diagnose an infectious disease by listening to your medical history and doing a physical exam. For example, listening to a patient describe what happened and any symptoms they have noticed plays an important part in helping a doctor find out what's wrong.

Blood and urine tests are other ways to diagnose an infection. A laboratory expert can sometimes see the offending microbe in a sample of blood or urine viewed under a microscope. One or both of these tests may be the only way to determine what caused the infection, or they may be used to confirm a diagnosis that was made based on taking a history and doing a physical exam.

In another type of test, a doctor will take a sample of blood or other body fluid, such as vaginal secretion, and then put it into a special container called a Petri dish to see if any microbe "grows." This test is called a culture. Certain bacteria, such as chlamydia and strep, and viruses, such as herpes simplex, usually can be identified using this method.

X-rays, scans, and biopsies (taking a tiny sample of tissue from the infected area and inspecting it under a microscope) are among other tools the doctor can use to make an accurate diagnosis.

All of the above procedures are relatively safe, and some can be done in a doctor's office or a clinic. Others pose a higher risk to patients because they involve procedures that go inside the body. One such invasive procedure is taking a biopsy from an internal organ. For example, one way a doctor can diagnose *Pneumocystis carinii* pneumonia, a lung disease caused by a fungus, is by doing a biopsy on lung tissue and then examining the sample under a microscope.

Infectious Diseases Are Treated in Many Ways

How an infectious disease is treated depends on the microbe that caused it and sometimes on the age and medical condition of the person affected. Certain diseases are not treated at all, but are allowed to run their course, with the immune system doing its job alone. Some diseases, such as the common cold, are treated only to relieve the symptoms. Others, such as strep throat, are treated to destroy the offending microbe as well as to relieve symptoms.

Your Immune System

Your immune system has an arsenal of ways to fight off invading microbes. Most begin with B and T cells and antibodies whose sole purpose it is to keep your body healthy. Some of these cells sacrifice their lives to rid you of disease and restore your body to a healthy state. Some microbes normally present in your body also help destroy microbial invaders. For example, normal bacteria in your digestive system help destroy disease-causing microbes, such as *Listeria* in that hot dog you had at lunch. Other important ways your body reacts to an infection include fever and coughing and sneezing.

Fever: Fever is one of your body's special ways of fighting an infection. Many microbes are very sensitive to temperature changes and cannot survive in temperatures higher than normal body heat, which is usually around 98.6 degrees Fahrenheit. Your body uses fever to destroy flu viruses, for example.

Coughing and Sneezing: Another piece in your immune system's reaction to invading infection-causing microbes is mucus production. Coughing and sneezing help mucus move those germs out of your body efficiently and quickly.

Other Methods: Your body may also to fight off an infection by using these methods: inflammation; vomiting; diarrhea; fatigue; and cramping.

Your Doctor

Bacterial Illnesses: The last century saw an explosion in our knowledge about how microbes work and in our methods of treating infectious diseases. For example, the discovery of antibiotics to treat and cure many bacterial diseases was a major breakthrough in medical history. Doctors, however, sometimes prescribe antibiotics unnecessarily for a variety of reasons, including pressure from patients with viral infections. Patients may insist on being prescribed an antibiotic without knowing that it won't work on viruses. Colds and flu are two notable viral infections for which some doctors send their patients to the drugstore with a prescription for an antibiotic.

Because antibiotics have been overprescribed or inappropriately prescribed over the years, some bacteria have become resistant to the killing effects of these drugs. This resistance, called antimicrobial or drug resistance, has become a very serious problem, especially in hospital settings. Bacteria that are not killed by the antibiotic become strong enough to resist the same medicine the next time it's given.

Viral Illnesses: Viral diseases can be very difficult to treat because viruses live inside the body's cells where they are protected from medicines in the blood stream. Researchers developed the first antiviral drug in the late 20th century. The drug, acyclovir, was first approved by the U.S. Food and Drug Administration to treat herpes simplex virus infections. Only a few other antiviral medicines are available to prevent and treat viral infections and diseases.

Health care professionals treat HIV infection with a group of powerful medicines which can keep the virus in check. Known as highly active antiretroviral therapy, or HAART, the new treatment has improved the lives of many suffering from this deadly infection.

Viral diseases should never be treated with antibiotics. Sometimes a person with a viral disease will develop a bacterial disease as a complication of the initial viral disease. For example, children with chickenpox often scratch the skin sores caused by the viral infection. Bacteria such as staph can enter those lesions and cause a bacterial infection. The doctor may then prescribe an antibiotic to destroy the bacteria. The antibiotic, however, will not work on the chickenpox virus. It will work only against staph.

Unfortunately, safe and effective treatments and cures for most viral diseases have eluded researchers, but there are safe vaccines to protect you from viral infections and diseases.

Fungal Infections: Medicines applied directly to the infected area are available by prescription and over the counter for treating skin and nail fungal infections. Unfortunately, many people have had limited success with them. During the 1990s, oral prescription medicines became available for treating fungal infections of the skin and nails.

For many years, very powerful oral antifungal medicines were used only to treat systemic (within the body) fungal infections, such as histoplasmosis. Doctors usually prescribe oral antifungal medications cautiously because all of them, even the milder ones for skin and nail fungi, can have very serious side effects.

Protozoan Diseases: Diseases caused by protozoan parasites are among the leading causes of death and disease in tropical and subtropical regions of the world. Developing countries within these areas contain three-quarters of the world's population, and their populations suffer the most from these diseases. Controlling parasitic diseases is a problem because there are no vaccines for any of them.

In many cases, controlling the insects that transmit these diseases is difficult because of pesticide resistance, concerns regarding environmental damage, and lack of adequate public health systems to apply existing insect-control methods. Thus, control of these diseases relies heavily on the availability of medicines. Doctors usually use antiparasitic medicines to treat protozoal infections. Unfortunately, there are very few medicines that fight protozoal infections, and some of those are either harmful to humans or are becoming ineffective.

The fight against the protozoan *Plasmodium falciparum*, the cause of the most deadly form of malaria, is a good example. This protozoan has become resistant to most of the medicines currently available to destroy it. A major focus of malaria research is on developing a vaccine to prevent people from getting the disease. In the meantime, many worldwide programs hope to eventually control malaria by keeping people from contact with infected mosquitoes or from getting infected if contact can't be avoided.

New Microbes Emerge on the Scene and Old Ones Reappear

Emerging Microbes

From time to time, strange new disease-causing microbes seem to come out of nowhere. Scientists usually define newly emerging infectious diseases as those that have only recently appeared in a population or have existed but are rapidly increasing in incidence or geographic range. Recent examples include West Nile fever, *E. coli* infection, chronic hepatitis C, flu, hantavirus infection, and Lyme disease.

In addition, pathogens previously not seen in the United States, like West Nile virus, may become more common here because of the increased speed of international travel and because more people are traveling.

In the early summer of 1999, cases of encephalitis (inflammation of the brain) and death began to appear in New York City. Researchers later identified West Nile virus as the cause. Prior to that time, health care experts had never seen cases of illness caused by this virus in the United States. The virus is common in Africa, West Asia, and the Middle East. Mosquitoes become infected when they feed on infected birds, which may circulate the virus in their blood for a few days. Infected mosquitoes can then transmit West Nile virus to humans and animals while biting to take blood. Every summer since it first appeared, West Nile virus has been found in a continuously increasing number of states.

Identified in 1989, the hepatitis C virus causes approximately 20 percent of all cases of acute viral liver disease each year in the United States. CDC estimates that nearly 4 million Americans are infected with hepatitis C, many of whom are not aware of their infection. Chronic liver disease due to hepatitis C causes between 8,000 and 10,000 deaths and leads to about 1,000 liver transplants each year in the United States. Over the next two decades, the number of annual deaths from hepatitis C is expected to triple if there continues to be no effective treatment.

Within the past few years, many outbreaks of intestinal disease with bloody diarrhea have been reported in the United States and abroad. These outbreaks are often due to the newly pathogenic O157:H7 strain of *E. coli*, which was first recognized in 1982. Other strains of *E. coli* are common in other countries but less frequent in the United States. Approximately 10 to 15 percent of people infected with these organisms develop hemolytic uremic syndrome (HUS), a serious complication that can lead to kidney failure and death. Children and the elderly are particularly at risk for developing HUS.

Environmental changes can cause a microbe to become a health threat to humans. Lyme disease and hantavirus pulmonary syndrome are two examples.

Lyme disease emerged in 1975 in the northeastern United States as people expanded their communities into wooded areas occupied by infected deer ticks. It is the most common tickborne infection in this country, affecting people in almost every state. Although not deadly, Lyme disease can cause serious illness. In 1982, scientists at the National Institute of Allergy and Infectious Diseases identified *B. burgdorferi* bacteria as the cause of Lyme disease. From then until 1999, health care workers reported more than 128,000 cases of the disease to CDC.

In 1993, an outbreak of a mysterious, often fatal lung disease occurred in the southwestern United States. That outbreak occurred in part from weather changes like those brought about by El Niño, which fosters increases in the rodent populations that carry diseases. Scientists quickly determined the illness was caused by a previously unknown strain of hantavirus, a family of disease-causing viruses that occurs naturally in mice and other rodents. By April 2001, health care workers had reported that 283 people had developed the condition known as hantavirus pulmonary syndrome. More than a third have died from the disease.

Re-Emerging Microbes

The reappearance of microbes that had been successfully conquered or controlled by medicines is distressing to the scientific and medical communities as well as to the public. A major cause of this re-emergence is that microbes, which cause these diseases, are becoming resistant to the drugs used to treat them.

According to the World Health Organization (WHO), nearly 2 billion people—one-third of the world's population—have TB. This includes between 10 and 15 million people in the United States. TB is the world's leading cause of death from a single infectious organism, killing 2 million people each year. The TB crisis has intensified because multidrug-resistant (MDR) microbes have emerged. An incurable form of the disease may develop from infections caused by these organisms. WHO estimates more than 50 million people worldwide may be infected with MDR strains of TB.

Malaria, the most deadly of all tropical parasitic diseases, has been resurging dramatically. Increasing resistance of *Plasmodium protozoa* to inexpensive and effective medicines presents problems for treating active infections. WHO estimates between 300 million and 500 million new cases of malaria occur worldwide each year. At least 2.7 million people die annually. In the United States, approximately 1,000 cases are reported annually, which researchers estimate represent only 25 to 50 percent of actual cases. Although most of these cases occurred in people who had been infected while traveling abroad, others occurred in people bitten by infected mosquitoes in states such as New York.

In the United States, approximately 25 percent of the population has flu-associated illness annually, leading to an average of 20,000 to 40,000 deaths per year. Influenza viruses change from year to year and powerful strains have re-emerged throughout history to cause worldwide, catastrophic pandemics. Many scientists believe the next pandemic is long overdue. In addition, in the 1990s, people in Hong Kong became infected with avian influenza—the first known case of an influenza virus jumping directly from birds to people.

Chapter 2

What Is a Microbe?

"Microbe" is a term for tiny creatures that individually are too small to be seen with the unaided eye. Microbes include bacteria (back-tear-ee-uh), archaea (are-key-uh), fungi (fun-jeye), and protists (pro-tists). You've probably heard of bacteria and fungi before. Archaea are bacteria-like creatures that have some traits not found in any true bacteria. Protists include primitive algae (al-gee), amoebas (ah-me-buhs), slime molds, and protozoa (pro-toe-zoh-uh). We can also include viruses (vye-rus-is) as a major type of microbe, though there is a debate as to whether viruses can be considered living creatures or not.

Figures 2.1–2.4 show what microbes look like through a high-power microscope. As you can see, microbes come in many varieties. They may live as individuals or cluster together in communities.

So how small are microbes? Well, let's say we could enlarge an average virus, the smallest of all microbes, to the size of a baseball. An average bacterium would then be the size of the pitcher's mound. And just one of the millions of cells that make up your body would be the size of the ballpark.

Text in this chapter is from "Case #1: What Is a Microbe," and "Case #6: Virus or Bacterium?" © 1999 American Society for Microbiology (ASM). All rights reserved. For additional information about microbiology, visit the ASM educational website www.microbeworld.org. Reprinted with permission. Despite the date of this material, the explanations given still provide accurate information about understanding the nature and variety of microbes.

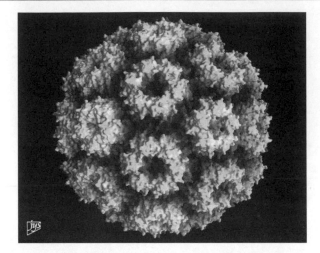

Figure 2.1. Virus. (© Jean-Yves Sgro, University of Wisconsin. PDP Entry: CWP 1. Image created with GRASP.)

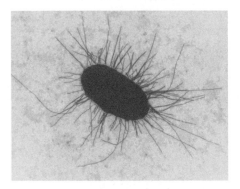

Figure 2.2. Bacterium. (Copyright Dennis Kunkel Microscopy, Inc.)

Figure 2.3. Alga. (Image Courtesy of Bowling Green State University Center for Algal Microscopy and Image Digitization)

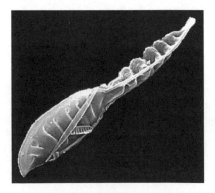

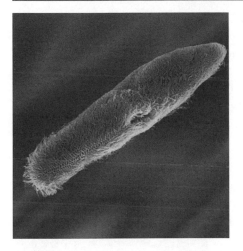

Figure 2.4. Protozoan. (Copyright Dennis Kunkel Microscopy, Inc.)

Bacteria

Bacteria consist of only a single cell, but don't let their small size and seeming simplicity fool you. They're an amazingly complex and fascinating group of creatures. Bacteria have been found that can live in temperatures above the boiling point and in cold that would freeze your blood. They "eat" everything from sugar and starch to sunlight, sulfur, and iron. There's even a species of bacteria—*Deinococcus radiodurans*—that can withstand blasts of radiation 1,000 times greater than would kill a human being.

Bacteria fall into a category of life called the Prokaryotes (pro-carry-oats). Prokaryotes' genetic material, or DNA, is not enclosed in a cellular compartment called the nucleus. Bacteria and archaea are the only prokaryotes. All other life forms are Eukaryotes (you-carry-oats), creatures whose cells have nuclei. (Viruses are not considered true cells, so they don't fit into either of these categories.)

Bacteria are among the earliest forms of life that appeared on earth billions of years ago. Scientists think that they helped shape and change the young planet's environment, eventually creating atmospheric oxygen that enabled other, more complex life forms to develop. Many believe that more complex cells developed as once free-living bacteria took up residence in other cells, eventually becoming the organelles in modern complex cells. The mitochondria (mite-oh-con-dree-uh) that make energy for your body cells is one example of such an organelle.

There are thousands of species of bacteria, but all of them are basically one of three different shapes. Some are rod- or stick-shaped and called bacilli (buh-sill-eye). Others are shaped like little balls and called cocci (cox-eye). Others still are helical or spiral in shape. Some bacterial cells exist as individuals while others cluster together to form pairs, chains, squares or other groupings.

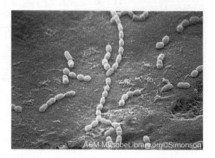

Figure 2.5. *Ball-shaped Streptococci.* (Streptococcus sobrinus *by Dr. Lloyd G. Simonson, Naval Institute for Dental and Biomedical Research.* © *Lloyd G. Simonson.)*

Bacteria live on or in just about every material and environment on earth from soil to water to air, and from your house to arctic ice to volcanic vents. Each square centimeter of your skin averages about 100,000 bacteria. A single teaspoon of topsoil contains more than a billion (1,000,000,000) bacteria.

Some bacteria move about their environment by means of long, whip-like structures called flagella. They rotate their flagella like tiny outboard motors to propel themselves through liquid environments. They may also reverse the direction in which their flagella rotate so that they tumble about in one place. Other bacteria secrete a slime layer and ooze over surfaces like slugs. Others are fairly stationary.

Some bacteria are photosynthetic (foe-toe-sin-theh-tick)—they can make their own food from sunlight, just like plants. Also like plants, they give off oxygen. Other bacteria absorb food from the material they live on or in. Some of these bacteria can live off unusual "foods" such as iron or sulfur. The microbes that live in your gut absorb nutrients from the digested food you've eaten.

Archaea

The archaea very much resemble bacteria, so much so that they were once thought to be a weird group of bacteria. However, by studying

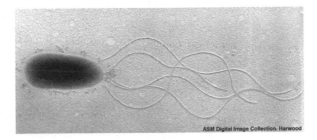

ASM Digital Image Collection. Harwood

Figure 2.6. *Bacterium with flagella. ("Flagella of* Pseudomonas putida*" by Caroline Harwood, Ph.D., University of Iowa. This micrograph was published in the* Journal of Bacteriology, *171:4063-4099, in July 1989 by C. S. Harwood, K. Fosnaugh, and M. Dispensa. Reprinted with permission of the author and the American Society of Microbiology.)*

archaeal cells on a molecular level, scientists have now come to think that these "weird bacteria" actually are a separate category of life altogether. While archaea resemble bacteria and have some genes that are similar to bacterial genes, they also contain other genes that are more like what you'd find in eukaryotes. Furthermore, they have some genes that aren't like any found in anything else.

Archaea are among the earliest forms of life that appeared on earth billions of years ago. It's now generally believed that the archaea and bacteria developed separately from a common ancestor nearly 4 billion years ago. Millions of years later, the ancestors of today's eukaryotes split off from the archaea. So historically, archaea are more closely related to us than they are to bacteria.

Many archaea thrive in conditions that would kill other creatures: boiling water, super-salty pools, sulfur-spewing volcanic vents, acidic water, and deep in Antarctic ice. These types of archaea are often labeled "extremophiles," meaning creatures that love extreme conditions. Archaea have been found that can live in temperatures above 212°F (100°C). In contrast, no known eukaryotes can survive over 140°F (60°C). Other archaea have been found in an Antarctic lake with a surface that is permanently frozen.

How do these extremophiles do it? They make a variety of protective molecules and enzymes (en-zimes). For example, some archaea live in highly acidic environments. If the acid got into the archaeal cells, it would destroy their DNA, so they have to keep it out. But the defensive molecules on their cellular surfaces do come into contact

21

with the acid and are uniquely designed not to break apart in it. Archaea that live in very salty water are able to keep all the fluid from dissolving out of their cells by producing or pulling in from the outside solutes such as potassium chloride that balance the inside of the cells with the salty water outside. Other enzymes allow other archaea to tolerate extreme hot or cold.

Not all the archaea are extremophiles. Many live in more ordinary temperatures and conditions. For example, scientists can find archaea alongside bacteria and algae floating about in the open ocean. Some archaea even live in your guts.

Archaea eat a variety of substances for energy, including hydrogen gas, carbon dioxide and sulfur. One type of salt-loving archaea uses sunlight to make energy, but not the way plants do it. This archaea has a light-harvesting pigment in the membrane surrounding its cell. This pigment, called bacteriorhodopsin (back-tear-ee-oh-row-dop-sin), reacts with light and enables the cell to make ATP, an energy molecule.

There are three main types of archaea: the crenarchaeota (kren-are-key-oh-ta), which are characterized by their ability to tolerate extremes in temperature and acidity; the euryarchaeota (you-ree-are-key-oh-ta), which include methane-producers and salt-lovers; and the korarchaeota (core-are-key-oh-ta), a catch-all group for archaea about which very little is known. Among these three main types of archaea are some subtypes, which include:

- Methanogens (meth-an-oh-jins): Archaea that produce methane gas as a waste product of their "digestion," or process of making energy.

- Halophiles (hal-oh-files): Those archaea that live in salty environments.

- Thermophiles (ther-mo-files): The archaea that live at extremely hot temperatures.

- Psychrophiles (sigh-crow-files): Those that live at unusually cold temperatures.

Fungi

When you hear the word fungus, you probably think of mushrooms. Did you know bread mold is a kind of fungus, too? And that the itchy burning of athlete's foot is caused by another fungus? And that when you take penicillin, you're taking a medicine made by a fungus?

Fungi come in a variety of shapes and sizes and different types. They can range from individual cells to enormous chains of cells that can stretch for miles. Fungi are eukaryotic organisms—their DNA is enclosed in a nucleus. Many of them may look plant-like, but fungi do not make their own food from sunlight like plants do.

Fungi include single-celled creatures that exist individually—the yeasts—and multicellular bunches, such as molds or mushrooms. Yeast cells look like little round or oval blobs under a microscope. They're too tiny to see as individuals, but you can see large clusters of them as a white powdery coating on fruits and leaves.

Molds are described as filament-like, or filamentous, because they form long filament-like, or thread-like, strands of cells called hyphae (high-fee). These hyphae are what give mold colonies their fuzzy appearance. They also form the fleshy body, or mushroom, that some species grow. It may seem odd to think of something as big as a mushroom as a microbe. But the cells of the hyphae making up that mushroom are connected in a closer way than the cells of other multicellular creatures are. The cell walls separating the cells in hyphae usually have openings that allow the protoplasm, or fluid that fills cells, to flow between them. Essentially, a fungal hypha is like a tube. Your cells, on the other hand, are completely walled off from each other and the cell fluid, or cytoplasm, inside doesn't mingle between cells.

Fungi usually grow best in environments that are slightly acidic (a pH measurement of 5 or so; a pH of 7 is neutral). They can grow on substances with very low moisture. Fungi live in the soil and on your body, in your house and on plants and animals, in freshwater and seawater. A single teaspoon of topsoil contains about 120,000 fungi.

Fungi are basically static. But they can spread either by forming reproductive spores that are carried on wind and rain or by growing and extending their hyphae. Remember that hyphae are chains of fungal cells. Hyphae grow as new cells form at the tips, creating ever longer and branching chains of cells. It takes a lot to stop them, too. Hyphae are tough enough to punch through plant cell walls and the hard exoskeletons of insects.

Fungi absorb nutrients from living or dead organic matter (plant or animal stuff) that they grow on. They absorb simple, easily dissolved nutrients, such as sugars, through their cell walls. They give off special digestive enzymes to break down complex nutrients into simpler forms that they can absorb.

Some fungi are quite useful to us. We've tapped several kinds to make antibiotics to fight bacterial infections. These antibiotics are based on natural compounds the fungi produce to compete against bacteria for nutrients and space. We use *Saccharomyces cerevisiae* (sack-air-oh-my-seas sair-uh-vis-ee-ay), more familiarly known as baker's yeast, to make bread rise and to brew beer. Fungi break down dead plants and animals and keep the world tidier. We're exploring ways to use natural fungal enemies of insect pests to get rid of these bugs.

There are some nasty fungi that cause diseases in plants, animals, and people. One of the most famous is *Phytophthora infestans* (fie-tof-thor-uh in-fes-tuhns), which caused the Great Potato Famine in Ireland in the mid-1800s that resulted in a million deaths. Fungi ruin about a quarter to half of harvested fruits and vegetables annually.

Protists

The category of Protists includes many widely ranging microbes, including slime molds, protozoa and primitive algae. They are all eukaryotic creatures, meaning their DNA is enclosed in a nucleus inside the cell (unlike bacteria, which are prokaryotic and have no nucleus to enclose their DNA).

Algae

When you think of algae, you probably think of seaweed or the green, slimy stuff that forms on the walls of untreated, dirty swimming pools. Here we'll focus on the microscopic algae. Algae are found in bodies of fresh and salt water across the globe. They can also grow on rocks and trees and in soil when enough moisture is available. (They also grow on the hair of the South American sloth, giving the animal a greenish color.)

Most algae are able to make energy from sunlight, like plants do. They produce a large amount of the oxygen we breathe. However, at some stages of their lives, some algae get their nutrients from other living things. You may have heard of large fish kills along the east coast of the U.S. caused by *Pfiesteria* (fis-teer-ee-uh). *Pfiesteria* belongs to a type of algae called the dinoflagellates (die-no-flah-geh-lets). Some dinoflagellates make their own energy from sunlight, like plants. But others like *Pfiesteria* produce toxic substances that stun passing fish and cause bleeding sores. The *Pfiesteria* then feed on the fish blood and fluids. This microbe has at least 24 different forms it cycles through during its life.

Diatoms (die-uh-toms) are another kind of algae. They have hard shells made out of silica, or glass. When they die, these shells sink to the bottom of their watery environments. We mine deposits of these silica shells that formed hundreds of thousands of years ago to make abrasives, shiny road paint, and grit in toothpaste. Diatoms come in all sorts of shapes—some are round and others are oval. Some look like leaves and others like fat commas.

Because photosynthetic algae make so much oxygen, these microbes are very helpful. But sometimes certain kinds of algae can also grow in such large numbers—called blooms or red tides—that when they suddenly die off en masse, the breaking down of their cells by bacteria depletes the amount of dissolved oxygen in the water, hurting the animals and plants that live there.

Protozoa

The word protozoa means "little animal." They are so named because many species behave like tiny animals—specifically, they hunt and gather other microbes as food. Protozoa mainly feed on bacteria, but they also eat other protozoa, bits of stuff that has come off of other living things—what's generally called organic matter—and sometimes fungi. Some protozoa absorb food through their cell membranes. Others, like the amoebas (ah-me-buhs), surround food and engulf it. Others have openings called mouth pores into which they sweep food. All protozoa digest their food in stomach-like compartments called vacuoles (vac-you-ohls). As they eat, they make and give off nitrogen, which is an element that plants and other higher creatures can use.

Protozoa range in size from 1/5,000 to 1/50 of an inch (5 to 500 μm) in diameter. They can be classified into three general groups based on their shape. One group is the ciliates (silly-ates), which are generally the largest protozoa. They have hair-like projections called cilia (silly-uh) and they eat the other two types of protozoa as well as bacteria. The second group is the amoebae (ah-me-bee), which can be subdivided into the testate amoebae, which have a shell-like covering, and the naked amoebae, which don't have this covering. Finally, the third group is the flagellates, which are generally the smallest of the protozoa and have one or several long, whip-like projections called flagella poking out of their cells.

To hunt, protozoa have to be able to move about. Amoebas ooze about by extending parts of their cells as pseudopods (sue-doh-pods) or "false feet." Amoebae have fluid cell membranes or coverings that they can stretch out, bend, and curve. As the membrane moves outward, the fluid and other parts inside the cell follow, flowing into the new bulge created by the moving membrane. Many ciliates swim along by beating their cilia in a rhythmic pattern, like so many tiny oars. Flagellates swim by waving their flagella, using them much like a fish uses its tail push itself through water.

Some protozoa prefer to latch themselves in one place. For example, a ciliate called *Vorticella* (vor-tih-sell-uh) attaches to a spot on a long, springy stalk. It creates a mini whirlpool around its mouth pore by beating the cilia ringing its bulbous top end so that food particles get sucked in. Whenever anything too big to be eaten hits a *Vorticella*, it springs back out of the way by rapidly coiling up its stalk.

The vast majority of protozoa do us no harm, but there are a few that cause disease. One type of amoeba can live in human intestines. It feeds on red blood cells and causes a disease known as dysentery (dis-in-tear-ee). The parasitic protozoan *Cryptosporidium parvum* (cryp-toe-spore-id-ee-um par-vum) sickened around 400,000 people in Milwaukee in 1993 when it got into the tap water. Perhaps the best-known protozoal menace is *Plasmodium* (plaz-mo-dee-um), the parasite that causes malaria.

Slime Molds

Slime molds have traits like both fungi and animals. They have very complex life cycles involving multiple forms and stages. During good times, they live as independent, amoeba-like cells, dining on fungi and bacteria. But if conditions become uncomfortable—not enough food available, the temperature isn't right, etc.—individual cells begin gathering together to form a single structure. This happens when the cells give off a chemical signal that tells all of them to gather together. The new communal structure produces a slimy covering and is called a slug because it so closely resembles the animal you sometimes see gliding across sidewalks. The slug oozes toward light. When the communal cells sense that they've come across more food or better conditions, the slug stops. It then slowly does a kind of headstand. Cells in the slug now begin to do different things. Some of the cells form an anchor for the upended slug. Others in the middle of the slug begin making a stalk and some at the tip turn into what's called a spore cap and others become spores in that cap. When a drop of rain or strong wind knocks the spore cap hard enough, the spores go flying out. These spores are like plant seeds. Each of them becomes a new amoeba-like cell when they land and each goes off on its merry way.

Viruses

Viruses are strange things that straddle the fence between living and non-living. On the one hand, if they're floating around in the air

Figure 2.7. *Slime mold stalk and spore cap (Copyright Dennis Kunkel Microscopy, Inc.).*

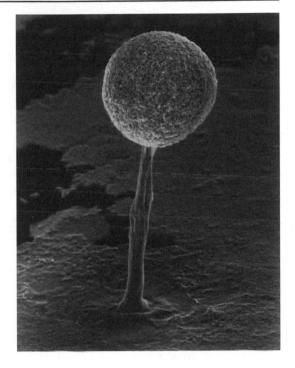

or sitting on a doorknob, they're inert. They're about as alive as a rock. But if they come into contact with a suitable plant, animal or bacterial cell, they spring into action. They infect and take over the cell like pirates hijacking a ship.

A virus is basically a tiny bundle of genetic material—either DNA or RNA—carried in a shell called the viral coat, or capsid, which is made up of bits of protein called capsomeres. Some viruses have an additional layer around this coat called an envelope. That's basically all there is to viruses.

There are thousands of different viruses that come in a variety of shapes. Many are polyhedral (polly-hee-drul), or multi-sided. If you've ever looked closely at a cut gem, like the diamond in an engagement ring, you've seen an example of a polyhedral shape. (Unlike the diamond in a ring, however, a virus does not taper to a point, but is shaped similarly all around.) Other viruses are shaped like spiky ovals or bricks with rounded corners. Some are like skinny sticks while others look like bits of looped string. Some are more complex and shaped like little lunar landing pods.

Viruses are found on or in just about every material and environment on earth from soil to water to air. They're basically found anywhere there are cells to infect. Viruses have evolved to infect every form of life, from animal to plant and from fungi to bacteria. Individual types of viruses tend to be somewhat picky about what type of cells they infect, however. Plant viruses are not equipped to infect animal cells, for example, though a certain plant virus could infect a number of related plants. Sometimes, a virus may infect one creature and do no harm, but cause havoc when it gets into a different but closely enough related creature. For example, the *Hantavirus* is carried by deer mice without much noticeable effect on the rodents. But if *Hantavirus* gets into a person, it causes a dramatic and frequently deadly disease marked by excessive bleeding.

Viruses exist for one purpose only: to reproduce. To do that, they have to take over the reproductive machinery of suitable host cells. Upon landing on an appropriate host cell, a virus gets its genetic material inside the cell either by tricking the host cell to pull it inside, like it would a nutrient molecule, or by fusing its viral coat with the host cell wall or membrane and releasing its genes inside. Some viruses inject their genes into the host cell, leaving their empty viral coats sitting outside.

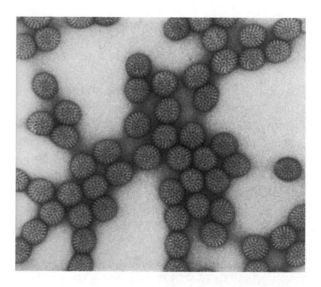

Figure 2.8. *Rotavirus ("Transmission electron micrograph of rotavirus," by Dr. Erskine Palmer, Centers for Disease Control and Prevention).*

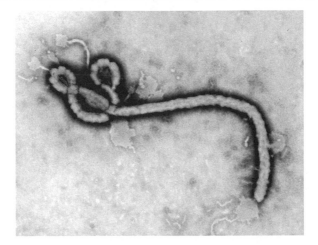

Figure 2.9. *Ebola virus ("Transmission electron micrograph of Ebola virus," by C. Goldsmith, Centers for Disease Control and Prevention).*

If a virus is a DNA virus, its genetic material then inserts itself into the host cell's DNA. If the virus is an RNA virus, it must first turn its RNA into DNA using the host cell's machinery before inserting into the host DNA. The viral genes are then copied many, many times, using the machinery the host cell would normally use to reproduce its own DNA. The virus uses the host cell's enzymes to build new viral capsids and other viral proteins. The new viral genes and proteins then come together and assemble into whole new viruses. The new viruses are either released from the host cell without destroying the cell or eventually build up to a large enough number that they burst the host cell like an overfilled water balloon.

Viruses may be referred to often as the smallest infectious things. But there are some smaller contenders. Some of the agents of plant disease lack even a viral coat and are merely small strings of plain, or "naked," RNA. These particles are called viroids. They are believed to be a more primitive version of ordinary viruses. But maybe viroids aren't the smallest infectious agents all.

Prions

Do you recall hearing about Mad Cow Disease? This is an ailment that affects the animals' brains and is also called bovine spongiform encephalopathy (boh-vine sponge-ee-form en-sef-uh-la-puth-ee) because it makes the brain appear full of holes, like a sponge. There is a human form of this disease called Creutzfeldt-Jakob (kroits-feld ya-cob) disease. Some scientists now believe these brain illnesses are among a few diseases caused by an infectious agents called prions (pree-ons). Prions are not even DNA or RNA, but simply proteins. They are thought to be misshapen or abnormal versions of proteins normally found in animals or people. Very little is known about prions. Scientists suggest that they spread when a prion comes into contact with the normal version of the protein and causes the normal protein to change shape and become a prion, too.

Virus or Bacterium?

Because bacteria and viruses cause many of the diseases we're familiar with, people often confuse these two microbes. But viruses are as different from bacteria as goldfish are from giraffes. For one thing, they differ greatly in size. The biggest viruses are only as large as the tiniest bacteria. Another difference is their structure. Bacteria are complex compared to viruses.

A typical bacterium has a rigid cell wall and a thin, rubbery cell membrane surrounding the fluid, or cytoplasm, inside the cell. A bacterium contains all of the genetic information needed to make copies of itself—its DNA—in a structure called a chromosome. In addition, it may have extra loose bits of DNA called plasmids floating in the cytoplasm. Bacteria also have ribosomes, tools necessary for copying DNA so bacteria can reproduce. Some have threadlike structures called flagella that they use to move. A virus may or may not have an outermost spiky layer called the envelope. All viruses have a protein coat and a core of genetic material, either DNA or RNA. And that's it. Period.

The main difference between viruses and bacteria, however, is the way they reproduce. Bacteria contain the genetic blueprint (DNA) and all the tools (ribosomes, proteins, etc.) they need to reproduce themselves. Viruses are moochers. They contain only a limited genetic blueprint and they don't have the necessary building tools. They have to invade other cells and hijack their cellular machinery to reproduce. Viruses invade by attaching to a cell and injecting their genes or by being swallowed up by the cell.

Chapter 3

Avoiding Infectious Diseases

Ten Tips for Preventing the Spread of Infection

Some diseases have become immune to the antibiotics we use. As a result, controlling diseases and preventing infections from spreading are more crucial than ever, and doing so begins with measures every individual can take. Here are ten tips to remember:

1. Wash your hands frequently—especially before preparing food, before eating, and after using the restroom. Insist that your health care providers wash their hands and use gloves, especially before any invasive treatment or procedure.

2. Don't insist that your physician give you antibiotics if you don't need them. Antibiotics have no effect on illnesses caused by viruses.

3. Take prescribed antibiotics exactly as instructed; do not stop taking them without checking with your physician, even if the medicine makes you feel better—or worse.

This chapter begins with "10 Tips for Preventing the Spread of Infection," which is reprinted with permission from the Association for Professionals in Infection Control and Epidemiology, Inc. (APIC), www.apic.org. © 2002 APIC. All rights reserved. Other sections are excerpted from "Fight The Bite!" Division of Vector-Borne Infectious Diseases, Centers for Disease Control and Prevention (CDC), July 2003; "Protection against Mosquitoes and Other Arthropods," National Center for Infectious Diseases (NCID), CDC, July 2003, "Risks from Food and Drink," NCID, CDC, July 2003, and "Healthy Swimming 2003," Division of Parasitic Diseases, CDC, May 2003.

4. Keep your immunizations—and those of your children—up to date.

5. Don't send your child to a day care center or to a school with symptoms of an infection—such as vomiting, diarrhea, and/or fever.

6. Follow safe sexual practices.

7. Do not use intravenous (I.V.) drugs; if you do, do not share needles.

8. Don't share personal items—such as razor blades, tooth brushes, combs, and hairbrushes—and don't eat or drink from others' plates or glasses.

9. Keep kitchen surfaces clean, especially when preparing meat, chicken, and fish; disinfect kitchen surfaces.

10. Keep hot foods hot and cold foods cold, especially when they will be left out for a long time.

Fight The Bite! Avoid Mosquito Bites to Avoid Infection

Fighting mosquito bites reduces your risk of getting diseases that mosquitoes can carry. Take the commonsense steps below to reduce your risk:

- **Apply insect repellent containing DEET** (N,N-diethyl-meta-toluamide) to exposed skin when you go outdoors. Even a short time being outdoors can be long enough to get a mosquito bite. In general, the more DEET a repellent contains, the longer time it can protect against mosquito bites. However, there appears to be no added benefit of concentrations greater than 50%. A microencapsulated, sustained-release formulation can have a longer period of activity than liquid formulations at the same concentrations. Length of protection also varies with ambient temperature, amount of perspiration, any water exposure, abrasive removal, and other factors.

  No definitive studies have been published about what concentration of DEET is safe for children. No serious illness has arisen from use of DEET according the manufacturer's recommendations. DEET formulations as high as 50% are recommended for both adults and children older than 2 months of age. Lower concentrations are not as long lasting, offering short-term protection only and necessitating more frequent reapplication. Repellent products that do not contain DEET are not likely to offer the same degree of protection from mosquito bites as products containing DEET. Non-DEET repellents have not necessarily been as thoroughly studied as DEET and may not be safer for use on children. Parents should choose the type and concentration of repellent to be used by taking into account the amount of time that a child will be outdoors, exposure to mosquitoes, and the risk of mosquito-transmitted disease in the area. The recommendations for DEET use in pregnant women do not differ from those for non-pregnant adults.

DEET is toxic when ingested and may cause skin irritation in sensitive persons. High concentrations applied to skin can cause blistering.

- **Clothing can help reduce mosquito bites.** When possible, wear long-sleeves, long pants and socks when outdoors. Mosquitoes may bite through thin clothing, so spraying clothes with repellent containing permethrin or DEET will give extra protection. Don't apply repellents containing permethrin directly to skin. Do not spray repellent containing DEET on the skin under your clothing.

- **Be aware of peak mosquito hours.** The hours from dusk to dawn are peak mosquito biting times for many species of mosquitoes. Take extra care to use repellent and protective clothing during evening and early morning—or consider avoiding outdoor activities during these times.

- **Drain standing water from around your home.** Mosquitoes lay their eggs in standing water. Limit the number of places around your home for mosquitoes to breed by getting rid of items that hold water.

- **Install or repair screens.** Some mosquitoes like to come indoors. Keep them outside by having well-fitting screens on both windows and doors. Offer to help neighbors whose screens might be in bad shape.

- **Report dead birds to local authorities.** Dead birds may be a sign that West Nile virus is circulating between birds and the mosquitoes in an area. Over 130 species of birds are known to have been infected with West Nile virus, though not all infected birds will die. It's important to remember that birds die from many other causes besides West Nile virus.

- **Clean up.** Mosquito breeding sites can be everywhere. Neighborhood clean up days can be organized by civic or youth organizations to pick up containers from vacant lots and parks, and to encourage people to keep their yards free of standing water. Mosquitoes don't care about fences, so it's important to control breeding sites anywhere in the neighborhood.

Protection against Ticks and Other Biting Insects

When exposure to ticks or biting insects is a possibility, people should be advised to tuck their pants into their socks and to wear boots, not sandals. Permethrin-based repellents applied as directed will enhance protection. People should be advised to inspect themselves and their clothing for ticks, both during outdoor activity and at the end of the day. Ticks are detected more easily on light-colored or white clothing. Prompt removal of attached ticks can prevent some infections.

While traveling, when accommodations are not adequately screened or air conditioned, bed nets are essential to provide protection and comfort. Bed nets should be tucked under mattresses and can be sprayed with a repellent, such as permethrin. The permethrin will be effective for several months if the bed net is not washed.

Travelers should be advised that permethrin-containing repellents (for example, Permanone or deltamethrin) are recommended for use on clothing, shoes, bed nets, and camping gear. Permethrin is highly effective as an insecticide and as a repellent. Permethrin-treated clothing repels and kills ticks, mosquitoes, and other arthropods and retains this effect after repeated laundering. There appears to be little potential for toxicity from permethrin-treated clothing. The insecticide should be reapplied after every five washings.

Most authorities also recommend repellents containing N,N-diethyl-meta-toluamide (DEET). DEET repels mosquitoes, ticks, and other arthropods when applied to the skin or clothing.

Risks from Food and Drink

Contaminated food and drink are common sources for the introduction of infection into the body. Among the more common infections that people can acquire from contaminated food and drink are *Escherichia coli* infections, shigellosis or bacillary dysentery, giardiasis, cryptosporidiosis, Norwalk-like viruses, and hepatitis A. Other less common infectious disease risks include typhoid fever and other salmonelloses, cholera, rotavirus infections, and a variety of protozoan and helminthic parasites (other than those that cause giardiasis and cryptosporidiosis). Many of the infectious diseases transmitted in food and water can also be acquired directly through the fecal-oral route.

Food

All raw food is subject to contamination. Particularly in areas where hygiene and sanitation are inadequate, travelers should be advised to avoid salads, uncooked vegetables, and unpasteurized milk and milk products such as cheese, and to eat only food that has been cooked and is still hot or fruit that has been peeled by the traveler personally. Undercooked and raw meat, fish, and shellfish can carry various intestinal pathogens. Cooked food that has been allowed to stand for several hours at ambient temperature can provide a fertile medium for bacterial growth and should be thoroughly reheated before serving. Consumption of food and beverages obtained from street food vendors has been associated with an increased risk of illness.

Some species of fish and shellfish can contain poisonous biotoxins, even when well cooked. The most common type of biotoxin in fish is ciguatoxin. The flesh of the barracuda is the most toxic laden and should always be avoided. Red snapper, grouper, amberjack, sea bass, and a wide range of tropical reef fish contain the toxin at unpredictable times. The potential for ciguatera poisoning exists in all subtropical and tropical insular areas of the Caribbean and the Pacific and Indian Oceans where the implicated fish species are eaten. Symptoms of ciguatera poisoning include gastroenteritis followed by neurologic problems such as dysesthesias (sensation impairments), temperature reversal, weakness, and, rarely, hypotension (low blood pressure). Scombroid is another common fish poisoning that occurs worldwide in tropical as well as temperate regions. Fish of the *Scombridae* family (for example, bluefin, yellowfin tuna, mackerel, and bonito), as well as some nonscombroid fish (such as mahi mahi, herring, amberjack, and bluefish) may contain high levels of histidine in their flesh. With improper refrigeration or preservation, histidine is converted to histamine, which can cause flushing, headache, nausea, vomiting, diarrhea, and urticaria.

Cholera cases have occurred in people who ate crab brought back from Latin America by travelers. Travelers should be advised not to bring perishable seafood with them when they return to the United States from high-risk areas. Also, the incorrect assumption is often made that food and water aboard commercial aircraft are safe. Food and water may be obtained in the country of departure where items may be contaminated as well.

Water

Water that has been adequately chlorinated, by using minimum recommended water treatment standards used in the United States, will afford substantial protection against viral and bacterial water-borne diseases. However, chlorine treatment alone, as used in the routine disinfection of water, might not kill some enteric viruses and the parasitic organisms that cause giardiasis, amebiasis, and cryptosporidiosis. In areas where chlorinated tap water is not available or where hygiene and sanitation are poor, people should be advised that only the following might be safe to drink:

- Beverages, such as tea and coffee, made with boiled water.
- Canned or bottled carbonated beverages, including carbonated bottled water and soft drinks.
- Beer and wine.

When traveling to places where water might be contaminated, travelers should be advised that ice should also be considered contaminated and should not be used in beverages. If ice has been in contact with containers used for drinking, travelers should be advised to thoroughly clean the containers, preferably with soap and hot water, after the ice has been discarded.

It is safer to drink a beverage directly from the can or bottle than from a questionable container. However, water on the outside of beverage cans or bottles might also be contaminated. Therefore, travelers should be advised to dry wet cans or bottles before they are opened and to wipe clean surfaces with which the mouth will have direct contact. Where water might be contaminated, travelers should be advised to avoid brushing their teeth with tap water.

Travelers should be advised of the following methods for treating water to make it safe for drinking and other purposes.

- **Boiling.** Boiling is by far the most reliable method to make water of uncertain purity safe for drinking. Water should be brought to a vigorous rolling boil for 1 minute and allowed to cool to room temperature; ice should not be added. This procedure will kill bacterial and parasitic causes of diarrhea at all altitudes and viruses at low altitudes. To kill viruses at altitudes of more than 2,000 m (6,562 feet), water should be boiled for 3 minutes or chemical disinfection should be used after the water has boiled for 1 minute. Adding a pinch of salt to each quart or pouring the water several times from one clean container to another will improve the taste.

- **Chemical disinfection.** Chemical disinfection with iodine is an alternative method of water treatment when it is not feasible to boil water. However, this method cannot be relied on to kill *Cryptosporidium* unless the water is allowed to sit for 15 hours before it is drunk. Two well-tested methods for disinfection with iodine are the use of tincture of iodine and tetraglycine hydroperiodide tablets (such as Globaline, Potable-Aqua, or Coghlan's). These tablets are available from pharmacies and sporting goods stores. The manufacturers' instructions should be followed. Chlorine, in various forms, can also be used for chemical disinfection. However, its germicidal activity varies greatly with the pH, temperature, and organic content of the water to be purified; therefore, it can produce less consistent levels of disinfection in many types of water. Chemically treated water is intended for short-term use only. If iodine-disinfected water is the only water available, it should be used for only a few weeks.

Water Filters

Portable filters currently on the market will provide various degrees of protection against microbes. Reverse-osmosis filters provide protection against viruses, bacteria, and protozoa, but they are expensive, are larger than most filters used by backpackers, and the small pores on this type of filter are rapidly plugged by muddy or cloudy water. In addition, the membranes in some filters can be damaged by chlorine in water. Microstrainer filters with pore sizes in the 0.1- to 0.3-µm range can remove bacteria and protozoa from drinking water, but they do not remove viruses. To kill viruses, travelers using microstrainer filters should be advised to disinfect the water with iodine or chlorine after filtration, as described previously. Filters with iodine-impregnated resins are most effective against bacteria, and the iodine will kill some viruses; however, the contact time with the iodine in the filter is too short to kill the protozoa *Cryptosporidium* and, in cold water, *Giardia*.

Avoiding Recreational Water Illnesses

Swimming, one of the most popular activities in the country, is a fun, active, and healthy way to spend leisure time. Every year, millions of people visit "recreational water" sites, such as swimming pools, water parks, hot tubs, lakes, rivers, or the ocean. Over the past century, the use of modern disinfection systems in pools and environmental improvements in our lakes, rivers, and oceans has improved the quality of recreational water. Despite this, there has been an increase over the past decade in the number of outbreaks of illness associated with swimming.

What are recreational water illnesses (RWIs)?

RWIs are illnesses that are spread by swallowing, breathing, or having contact with contaminated water from swimming pools, spas, lakes, rivers, or oceans. Recreational water illnesses can cause a wide variety of symptoms, including skin, ear, respiratory, eye, and wound infections. The most commonly reported RWI is diarrhea. Diarrheal illnesses can be caused by germs such as crypto, short for *Cryptosporidium*, or *Giardia*, *Shigella*, and *E. coli* O157:H7.

How are RWIs spread?

Keep in mind that you share the water with everyone else in the pool, lake, or ocean. If swimmers are ill with diarrhea, the germs that they carry can contaminate the water if they have an "accident" in the pool. On average people have about 0.14 grams of feces on their bottoms which, when rinsed off, can contaminate recreational water. When people are ill with diarrhea, their stool can contain millions of germs. Therefore, swimming when ill with diarrhea can easily contaminate large pools or waterparks. In addition, lakes, rivers, and the ocean can be contaminated by sewage spills, animal waste and water runoff following rainfall. Some common germs can also live for long periods of time in salt water. If someone swallows water that has been contaminated with feces, he/she may become sick. Many of these diarrhea-causing germs do not have to be swallowed in large amounts to cause illness.

Many other RWIs (eye, skin, ear, and respiratory infections) are caused by germs that live naturally in the environment (water, soil). In the pool or hot tub, if disinfectant is not maintained at the appropriate levels, these germs can increase to the point where they can cause illness when swimmers breathe or have contact with water containing these germs.

Why doesn't chlorine kill these RWI germs?

Chlorine in swimming pools does kill the germs that may make people sick, but it takes time. Chlorine in properly disinfected pools kills most germs that can cause RWIs in less than an hour. Chlorine takes longer to kill some germs such as crypto, which can survive for days in even a properly disinfected pool. This means that without your help, illness can spread even in well-maintained pools. Healthy swimming behaviors are needed to protect you and your family from RWIs and will help stop germs from getting in the pool.

Where are RWIs found?

In addition to swimming pools, swimming in contaminated hot tubs, oceans, lakes, rivers, and playing in decorative water fountains can also spread RWIs.

Hot tubs. Skin infections like "hot tub rash" are the most common RWIs spread through hot tubs and spas. Chlorine and other disinfectant levels evaporate more quickly because of the higher temperature of the water in the tubs. It is important to check disinfectant levels even more regularly than in swimming pools. "Hot tub rash" can also occur in pools and at the lake or beach.

Decorative water fountains: Not all decorative or interactive fountains are chlorinated or filtered. Therefore, when people, especially diaper-aged children, play in the water, they can contaminate the water with fecal matter. Swallowing this contaminated water can then cause diarrheal illness.

Lakes, rivers, and oceans: Lakes, rivers, and oceans can become contaminated with germs from sewage, animal waste, water runoff following rainfall, fecal accidents, and germs rinsed off the bottoms of swimmers. It is important to avoid swallowing the water because natural recreational water is not disinfected. Avoid swimming after rainfalls or in areas identified as unsafe by health departments.

Who is most likely to get ill from an RWI?

Children, pregnant women, and people with compromised immune systems (such as those living with AIDS, those who have received an organ transplant, or those receiving certain types of chemotherapy) can suffer from more severe illness if infected. People with compromised immune systems should be aware that recreational water might be contaminated with human or animal waste that contains *Cryptosporidium* (or crypto), which can be life threatening in persons with weakened immune systems. People with a compromised immune system

39

should consult their health care provider before participating in behaviors that place them at risk for illness.

Chapter 4

What Is an Infectious Diseases Specialist?

An infectious diseases (ID) specialist is a physician with advanced training in the diagnosis and treatment of illnesses caused by micro-organisms or germs. Because their training and experience cover a unique cross-section of medicine, ID specialists often are asked to evaluate and oversee challenging cases. ID specialists practice both in hospitals and in office settings.

What kind of training do ID specialists have?

Your ID physician has undergone nine to ten years of education and training. After four years of medical school, he or she spent three more years being trained as a doctor of internal medicine or pediat-rics. This was followed by two to three years of specialized training in infectious diseases. Most ID specialists who treat patients also are board certified, which means they have passed a difficult examina-tion and are certified by the American Board of Internal Medicine in both internal medicine and infectious diseases or by the American Board of Pediatrics in both pediatrics and infectious diseases.

What kinds of patients and cases do ID specialists treat?

ID specialists diagnose and treat conditions resulting from all types of infections, including those caused by germs such as bacteria, viruses, fungi and parasites. These microscopic organisms penetrate the body's natural barriers and multiply, creating symptoms ranging from sore throat and fever (as in the case of strep throat) to more serious and even deadly problems (such as AIDS or meningitis).

ID specialists also see patients to determine whether the symptoms are due to an infection or not. Most commonly, the patient has a fever.

Some ID specialists serve as primary care physicians, treating most illnesses and coordinating their patients' overall care.

When should I see an ID specialist?

Not all infectious diseases require you to see an ID specialist. Many common infections can be treated by your personal physician. Your doctor might refer you to an ID specialist in cases where an infection is difficult to diagnose, is accompanied by a high fever or does not respond to treatment. The specialized training and diagnostic tools of the ID specialist can help determine the cause of your infection and the best approach to treatment.

ID specialists also see healthy people who plan to travel to foreign countries or locations where infection risk is higher. In these cases, ID specialists can help determine whether special immunizations or other preventive measures are necessary to protect travelers from disease.

What kinds of tests, procedures and treatments are typical?

Infectious diseases specialists are like medical detectives. They examine difficult cases, looking for clues to identify the culprit and solve the problem. If you are in the hospital or ICU with a severe illness, you may not be aware of your ID specialist's visits, constant attention and care. Much of their work is done behind the scenes. Examining germs carefully under the microscope, ID specialists make a diagnosis and coordinate a plan to treat your disease. They will review your medical data, including X-rays and laboratory reports such as blood work and culture data. They also may perform a physical exam to help determine the cause of the problem.

ID specialists often order laboratory tests to examine samples of blood or other body fluids or cultures from wounds. A blood serum analysis can help the ID specialist detect antibodies that indicate what type of infection you have. Often these advanced studies can further explain the results of earlier tests, helping to pinpoint the problem.

Treatments consist of medicines—usually antibiotics—to help battle the infection and prevent it from returning. These medicines may be given to you orally (in the form of pills or liquids) or administered directly into your veins, via an IV tube. Many ID specialists have IV antibiotic therapy available in their offices, which decreases the likelihood that the patient will need to be hospitalized. ID specialists do not perform surgical procedures.

How does my ID specialist work with other medical professionals?

The ID specialist works with your personal physician to determine which diagnostic tests are appropriate. If treatment is necessary, your doctor and the ID specialist will work together to develop a treatment plan best suited to your needs. Often you will be asked to return to the ID specialist for a follow-up visit. This allows the specialist to check on your progress, confirm that the infection is gone, and help prevent it from coming back.

If you acquire an infection while in the hospital, the ID specialist will work with other hospital physicians to help direct your care. The specialist also might provide follow-up care after you go home.

If your ID specialist is also your personal physician, he or she will coordinate your care, referring you to other specialists when necessary.

What information should I give my ID specialist?

Be sure to give your ID specialist all medical records related to your condition, including X-rays, laboratory reports and immunization records. Often your personal physician will forward this information to the specialist before your scheduled appointment. You should also provide the ID specialist with a complete list of all medications you are taking and any allergies you have. This list should include over-the-counter (nonprescription) medications as well. Also, be sure to tell the ID specialist if you are taking birth control pills; some antibiotics may interfere with the effectiveness of oral contraceptives.

What can I do to help reduce the risk of getting an infectious disease?

One of the best strategies for preventing infectious diseases is immunization. Make sure you and your children receive all recommended vaccinations. Ask your doctor for advice about other things you and your family can do to prevent infectious diseases.

Where can I get more information about prevention and treatment of infectious diseases?

Your doctor is your best source of information. In addition, the Infectious Diseases Society of America (IDSA), a professional organization of more than 5,000 ID physicians, scientists and other infectious diseases experts, can help point you in the direction of resources and additional information.

Infectious Diseases Society of America
66 Canal Center Plaza, Suite 600
Alexandria, VA 22314
Phone: (703) 299-0200
Fax: (703) 299-0204
E-mail: info@idsociety.org

Chapter 5

The Immune System: The Body's First Line of Defense

The immune system is a complex of organs—highly specialized cells and even a circulatory system separate from blood vessels—all of which work together to clear infection from the body. The organs of the immune system, which are positioned throughout the body, are called lymphoid organs. The word "lymph" in Greek means a pure, clear stream—an appropriate description considering its appearance and purpose.

Lymphatic vessels and lymph nodes are the parts of the special circulatory system that carries lymph, a transparent fluid containing white blood cells (chiefly lymphocytes). Lymph bathes the tissues of the body, and the lymphatic vessels collect and move it eventually back into the blood circulation. Lymph nodes dot the network of lymphatic vessels and provide meeting grounds for the immune system cells that defend against invaders. The spleen, at the upper left of the abdomen, is also a staging ground and a place where immune system cells confront foreign microbes.

Pockets of lymphoid tissue are in many other locations throughout the body, such as the bone marrow and thymus. Tonsils, adenoids, Peyer's patches, and the appendix are also lymphoid tissues. Once in the bloodstream, lymphocytes are transported to tissues throughout the body, where they act as sentries on the lookout for foreign antigens.

From "The Immune System," National Institute of Allergy and Infectious Diseases (NIAID), Last updated July 7, 1999. The explanation of immune system functioning is still valid despite the older date of this document.

How the Immune System Works

Cells of the lymphatic system that will grow into the many types of more specialized cells that circulate throughout the immune system are produced in the bone marrow. This nutrient-rich, spongy tissue is found in the center shafts of certain long, flat bones of the body, such as the bones of the pelvis. The cells most relevant for understanding immune function are the lymphocytes. There are two major classes of lymphocytes: B cells and T cells.

B cells grow to maturity in the bone marrow. They produce antibodies that circulate in the blood and lymph streams. These antibodies attach to foreign antigens to mark them for destruction by other immune cells. B cells are part of what is known as "antibody-mediated" or "humoral" immunity, so called because the antibodies circulate in blood and lymph, which the ancient Greeks called, the body's "humors."

T cells mature in the thymus, which is high in the chest behind the breastbone. T cells also patrol the body and lymph for foreign invaders, but certain T cells can do more than just mark the antigens: they attack and destroy cells they recognize as foreign. T lymphocytes are responsible for "cell-mediated" immunity (or "cellular immunity"). T cells also orchestrate, regulate, and coordinate the overall immune response. T cells depend on unique cell surface molecules, called the major histocompatibility complex (MHC), to help them recognize antigen fragments.

Antibodies

The antibodies produced by B cells are basic templates with a special region that is highly specific to target a given antigen. Much like a car coming off a production line, the antibody's frame remains constant, but through chemical and cellular messages, the immune system selects a green sedan, a red convertible, or a white truck to combat a particular invader. In contrast to cars, however, the variety of antibodies is very large.

Different antibodies are destined for different purposes.

- Some coat the foreign invaders to make them attractive to the circulating scavenger cells (called "phagocytes") that will engulf an unwelcome microbe.

- Some antibodies combine with antigens. When this happens they activate a cascade of nine proteins that have been circulating

46

in inactive form in the blood (the complex that comprises the nine components is known as "complement"). Once antibodies have reacted with an antigen, a partnership with complement forms to help destroy foreign invaders and remove them from the body.

Still other types of antibodies block viruses from entering cells.

T Cells

T cells have two major roles in immune defense: regulating the body's immune response and attacking invading cells. Regulatory T cells are essential for orchestrating the response of an elaborate system of different types of immune cells. Helper T cells, for example, also known as CD4 positive T cells (CD4+ T cells), alert B cells to start making antibodies. They also can activate other T cells and immune system scavenger cells (called macrophages; macrophages are one class of phagocytes) and influence which type of antibody is produced.

Certain other T cells, called CD8 positive T cells (CD8+ T cells), can become killer cells that attack and destroy infected cells. The killer T cells are also called cytotoxic T cells (or CTLs [cytotoxic lymphocytes]).

Immune System Process

The immune system process functions in different ways depending on the type of response:

- **Activation of cytotoxic T cells:** After a macrophage engulfs and processes an antigen, the macrophage displays the antigen fragments combined with a Class I MHC protein on the macrophage cell surface. A receptor on a circulating, resting cytotoxic T cell recognizes the antigen-protein complex and binds to it. The binding process and a helper T cell activate the cytotoxic T cell so that it can attack and destroy the diseased cell.

- **Activation of helper T cells:** After a macrophage engulfs and processes an antigen, it displays the antigen fragments combined with a Class II MHC protein on the macrophage cell surface. The antigen-protein combination attracts a helper T cell, and promotes its activation.

- **Activation of B cells to make antibody:** A B cell uses one of its receptors to bind to its matching antigen, which the B cell engulfs and processes. The B cell then displays a piece of the antigen, bound to a Class II MHC protein, on the cell surface. This whole complex then binds to an activated helper T cell. This binding process stimulates the transformation of the B cell into an antibody-secreting plasma cell.

Part Two

Diseases Acquired from Food and Drinking Water

Chapter 6

Botulism

What is botulism?

Botulism is a rare but serious paralytic illness caused by a nerve toxin that is produced by the bacterium *Clostridium botulinum.* There are three main kinds of botulism. Foodborne botulism is caused by eating foods that contain the botulism toxin. Wound botulism is caused by toxin produced from a wound infected with *Clostridium botulinum.* Infant botulism is caused by consuming the spores of the botulinum bacteria, which then grow in the intestines and release toxin. All forms of botulism can be fatal and are considered medical emergencies. Foodborne botulism can be especially dangerous because many people can be poisoned by eating a contaminated food.

What kind of germ is Clostridium botulinum*?*

Clostridium botulinum is the name of a group of bacteria commonly found in soil. These rod-shaped organisms grow best in low oxygen conditions. The bacteria form spores which allow them to survive in a dormant state until exposed to conditions that can support their growth. There are seven types of botulism toxin designated by the letters A through G; only types A, B, E and F cause illness in humans.

"Botulism," Division of Bacterial and Mycotic Diseases, Centers for Disease Control and Prevention (CDC), reviewed October 18, 2001.

How common is botulism?

In the United States an average of 110 cases of botulism are reported each year. Of these, approximately 25% are foodborne, 72% are infant botulism, and the rest are wound botulism. Outbreaks of foodborne botulism involving two or more persons occur most years and usually caused by eating contaminated home-canned foods. The number of cases of foodborne and infant botulism has changed little in recent years, but wound botulism has increased because of the use of black-tar heroin, especially in California.

What are the symptoms of botulism?

The classic symptoms of botulism include double vision, blurred vision, drooping eyelids, slurred speech, difficulty swallowing, dry mouth, and muscle weakness. Infants with botulism appear lethargic, feed poorly, are constipated, and have a weak cry and poor muscle tone. These are all symptoms of the muscle paralysis caused by the bacterial toxin. If untreated, these symptoms may progress to cause paralysis of the arms, legs, trunk, and respiratory muscles. In foodborne botulism, symptoms generally begin 18 to 36 hours after eating a contaminated food, but they can occur as early as 6 hours or as late as 10 days.

How is botulism diagnosed?

Physicians may consider the diagnosis if the patient's history and physical examination suggest botulism. However, these clues are usually not enough to allow a diagnosis of botulism. Other diseases such as Guillain-Barré syndrome, stroke, and myasthenia gravis can appear similar to botulism, and special tests may be needed to exclude these other conditions. These tests may include a brain scan, spinal fluid examination, nerve conduction test (electromyography, or EMG), and a Tensilon test for myasthenia gravis. The most direct way to confirm the diagnosis is to demonstrate the botulinum toxin in the patient's serum or stool by injecting serum or stool into mice and looking for signs of botulism. The bacteria can also be isolated from the stool of persons with foodborne and infant botulism. These tests can be performed at some state health department laboratories and at CDC.

How can botulism be treated?

The respiratory failure and paralysis that occur with severe botulism may require a patient to be on a breathing machine (ventilator) for weeks, plus intensive medical and nursing care. After several weeks, the paralysis slowly improves. If diagnosed early, foodborne and wound botulism can be treated with an antitoxin which blocks the action of toxin circulating in the blood. This can prevent patients from worsening, but recovery still takes many weeks. Physicians may try to remove contaminated food still in the gut by inducing vomiting or by using enemas. Wounds should be treated, usually surgically, to remove the source of the toxin-producing bacteria. Good supportive care in a hospital is the mainstay of therapy for all forms of botulism. Currently, antitoxin is not routinely given for treatment of infant botulism.

Are there complications from botulism?

Botulism can result in death due to respiratory failure. However, in the past 50 years the proportion of patients with botulism who die has fallen from about 50% to 8%. A patient with severe botulism may require a breathing machine as well as intensive medical and nursing care for several months. Patients who survive an episode of botulism poisoning may have fatigue and shortness of breath for years and long-term therapy may be needed to aid recovery.

How can botulism be prevented?

Botulism can be prevented. Foodborne botulism has often been from home-canned foods with low acid content, such as asparagus, green beans, beets, and corn. However, outbreaks of botulism from more unusual sources such as chopped garlic in oil, chile peppers, tomatoes, improperly handled baked potatoes wrapped in aluminum foil, and home-canned or fermented fish. Persons who do home canning should follow strict hygienic procedures to reduce contamination of foods. Oils infused with garlic or herbs should be refrigerated. Potatoes which have been baked while wrapped in aluminum foil should be kept hot until served or refrigerated. Because the botulism toxin is destroyed by high temperatures, persons who eat home-canned foods should consider boiling the food for 10 minutes before eating it to ensure safety. Instructions on safe home canning can be obtained from county extension services or from the US Department of Agriculture. Because honey can contain spores of *Clostridium botulinum* and this has been a source of infection for infants, children less than 12 months old should not be fed honey. Honey is safe for persons 1 year of age and older. Wound botulism can be prevented by promptly seeking medical care for infected wounds and by not using injectable street drugs.

What are public health agencies doing to prevent or control botulism?

Public education about botulism prevention is an ongoing activity. Information about safe canning is widely available for consumers. State health departments and CDC have persons knowledgeable about botulism available to consult with physicians 24 hours a day. If antitoxin is needed to treat a patient, it can be quickly delivered to a physician anywhere in the country. Suspected outbreaks of botulism are quickly investigated, and if they involve a commercial product, the appropriate control measures are coordinated among public health and regulatory agencies. Physicians should report suspected cases of botulism to a state health department.

Chapter 7

Brucellosis

What is brucellosis?

Brucellosis is an infectious disease caused by the bacteria of the genus *Brucella*. These bacteria are primarily passed among animals, and they cause disease in many different vertebrates. Various *Brucella* species affect sheep, goats, cattle, deer, elk, pigs, dogs, and several other animals. Humans become infected by coming in contact with animals or animal products that are contaminated with these bacteria. In humans brucellosis can cause a range of symptoms that are similar to the flu and may include fever, sweats, headaches, back pains, and physical weakness. Sever infections of the central nervous systems or lining of the heart may occur. Brucellosis cab also cause long-lasting or chronic symptoms that include recurrent fevers, joint pain, and fatigue.

How common is brucellosis?

Brucellosis is not very common in the United States, where 100 to 200 cases occur each year. But brucellosis can be very common in countries where animal disease control programs have not reduced the amount of disease among animals.

Where is brucellosis usually found?

Although brucellosis can be found worldwide, it is more common in countries that do not have good standardized and effective public

"Brucellosis," Division of Bacterial and Mycotic Diseases, Centers for Disease Control and Prevention (CDC), reviewed June 20, 2001.

health and domestic animal health programs. Areas currently listed as high risk are the Mediterranean Basin (Portugal, Spain, Southern France, Italy, Greece, Turkey, North Africa), South and Central America, Eastern Europe, Asia, Africa, the Caribbean, and the Middle East. Unpasteurized cheeses, sometimes called "village cheeses," from these areas may represent a particular risk for tourists.

How is brucellosis transmitted to humans, and who is likely to become infected?

Humans are generally infected in one of three ways: eating or drinking something that is contaminated with *Brucella*, breathing in the organism (inhalation), or having the bacteria enter the body through skin wounds. The most common way to be infected is by eating or drinking contaminated milk products. When sheep, goats, cows, or camels are infected, their milk is contaminated with the bacteria. If the milk is not pasteurized, these bacteria can be transmitted to persons who drink the milk or eat cheeses made from it. Inhalation of *Brucella* organisms is not a common route of infection, but it can be a significant hazard for people in certain occupations, such as those working in laboratories where the organism is cultured. Inhalation is often responsible for a significant percentage of cases in abattoir employees. Contamination of skin wounds may be a problem for persons working in slaughterhouses or meat packing plants or for veterinarians. Hunters may be infected through skin wounds or by accidentally ingesting the bacteria after cleaning deer, elk, moose, or wild pigs that they have killed.

Can brucellosis be spread from person to person?

Direct person-to-person spread of brucellosis is extremely rare. Mothers who are breast-feeding may transmit the infection to their infants. Sexual transmission has also been reported. For both sexual and breast-feeding transmission, if the infant or person at risk is treated for brucellosis, their risk of becoming infected will probably be eliminated within 3 days. Although uncommon, transmission may also occur via contaminated tissue transplantation.

Is there a way to prevent infection?

Yes. Do not consume unpasteurized milk, cheese, or ice cream while traveling. If you are not sure that the dairy product is pasteurized, don't eat it. Hunters and animal herdsman should use rubber gloves when handling viscera of animals. There is no vaccine available for humans.

My dog has been diagnosed with brucellosis. Is that a risk for me?

B. canis is the species of *Brucella* species that can infect dogs. This species has occasionally been transmitted to humans, but the vast majority of dog infections do not result in human illness. Although veterinarians exposed to blood of infected animals are at risk, pet owners are not considered to be at risk for infection. This is partly because it is unlikely that they will come in contact with blood, semen, or placenta of the dog. The bacteria may be cleared from the animal within a few days of treatment; however re-infection is common and some animal body fluids may be infectious for weeks. Immunocompromised persons (cancer patients, HIV-infected individuals, or transplantation patients) should not handle dogs known to be infected with *B. canis*.

How is brucellosis diagnosed?

Brucellosis is diagnosed in a laboratory by finding *Brucella* organisms in samples of blood or bone marrow. Also, blood tests can be done to detect antibodies against the bacteria. If this method is used, two blood samples should be collected 2 weeks apart.

Is there a treatment for brucellosis?

Yes, but treatment can be difficult. Doctors can prescribe effective antibiotics. Usually, doxycycline and rifampin are used in combination for 6 weeks to prevent reoccurring infection. Depending on the timing of treatment and severity of illness, recovery may take a few weeks to several months. Mortality is low (<2%), and is usually associated with endocarditis.

I am a veterinarian, and I recently accidentally jabbed myself with the animal vaccine (RB-51 or B-19, or REV-1) while I was vaccinating cows (or sheep, goats). What do I need to do?

These are live vaccines, and B-19 is known to cause disease in humans. Although we know less about the other vaccines, the recommendations are the same. You should see a health care provider. A baseline blood sample should be collected for testing for antibodies. We recommend that you take antibiotics (doxycycline and rifampin for B-19 and REV-1, or doxycycline alone for RB-51) for 3 weeks. At the end of that time you should be rechecked and a second blood sample should be collected. (The sample can also be collected at 2 weeks.) The same recommendations hold true for spraying vaccine in the eyes (6 weeks of treatment in this case) or spraying onto open wounds on the skin.

Chapter 8

Campylobacter *Infections*

What is campylobacteriosis?

Campylobacteriosis is an infectious disease caused by bacteria of the genus *Campylobacter*. Most people who become ill with campylobacteriosis get diarrhea, cramping, abdominal pain, and fever within 2 to 5 days after exposure to the organism. The diarrhea may be bloody and can be accompanied by nausea and vomiting. The illness typically lasts 1 week. Some persons who are infected with *Campylobacter* don't have any symptoms at all. In persons with compromised immune systems, *Campylobacter* occasionally spreads to the bloodstream and causes a serious life-threatening infection.

How common is Campylobacter?

Campylobacter is one of the most common bacterial causes of diarrheal illness in the United States. Virtually all cases occur as isolated, sporadic events, not as a part of large outbreaks. Active surveillance through FoodNet indicates about 15 cases are diagnosed each year for each 100,000 persons in the population. Many more cases go undiagnosed or unreported, and campylobacteriosis is estimated to affect over 1 million persons every year, or 0.5% of the general population. Campylobacteriosis occurs much more frequently in the summer months than in the winter. The organism is isolated from infants

---

"*Campylobacter* Infection," Division of Bacterial and Mycotic Diseases, Centers for Disease Control and Prevention (CDC), reviewed July 21, 2003.

and young adults more frequently than from other age groups and from males more frequently than females. Although *Campylobacter* doesn't commonly cause death, it has been estimated that approximately 100 persons with *Campylobacter* infections may die each year.

What sort of germ is Campylobacter?

The *Campylobacter* organism is actually a group of spiral-shaped bacteria that can cause disease in humans and animals. Most human illness is caused by one species, called *Campylobacter jejuni*, but 1% of human *Campylobacter* cases are caused by other species. *Campylobacter jejuni* grows best at the body temperature of a bird, and seems to be well adapted to birds, who carry it without becoming ill. The bacterium is fragile. It cannot tolerate drying and can be killed by oxygen. It grows only if there is less than the atmospheric amount of oxygen present. Freezing reduces the number of *Campylobacter* bacteria present on raw meat.

How is the infection diagnosed?

Many different kinds of infections can cause diarrhea and bloody diarrhea. Doctors can look for bacterial causes of diarrhea by asking a laboratory to culture a sample of stool from an ill person. Diagnosis of *Campylobacter* requires special laboratory culture procedures, which doctors may need to specifically request.

How can campylobacteriosis be treated?

Virtually all persons infected with *Campylobacter* will recover without any specific treatment. Patients should drink plenty of fluids as long as the diarrhea lasts. In more severe cases, antibiotics such as erythromycin or a fluoroquinolone can be used, and can shorten the duration of symptoms if they are given early in the illness. Your doctor will make the decision about whether antibiotics are necessary.

Are there long-term consequences?

Most people who get campylobacteriosis recover completely within 2 to 5 days, although sometimes recovery can take up to 10 days. Rarely, some long-term consequences can result from a *Campylobacter* infection. Some people may have arthritis following campylobacteriosis; others may develop a rare disease that affects the nerves of the body beginning several weeks after the diarrheal illness. This disease, called Guillain-Barré syndrome, occurs when a person's immune system is "triggered" to attack the body's own nerves, and can lead to paralysis that lasts several weeks and usually requires intensive care. It is estimated that approximately one in every 1000 reported campylobacteriosis cases leads to Guillain-Barré syndrome. As many as 40% of Guillain-Barré syndrome cases in this country may be triggered by campylobacteriosis.

How do people get infected with this germ?

Campylobacteriosis usually occurs in single, sporadic cases, but it can also occur in outbreaks, when a number of people become ill at one time. Most cases of campylobacteriosis are associated with handling raw poultry or eating raw or undercooked poultry meat. A very small number of *Campylobacter* organisms (fewer than 500) can cause illness in humans. Even one drop of juice from raw chicken meat can infect a person. One way to become infected is to cut poultry meat on a cutting board, and then use the unwashed cutting board or utensil to prepare vegetables or other raw or lightly cooked foods. The *Campylobacter* organisms from the raw meat can then spread to the other foods. The organism is not usually spread from person to person, but this can happen if the infected person is a small child or is producing a large volume of diarrhea. Larger outbreaks due to *Campylobacter* are not usually associated with raw poultry but are usually related to drinking unpasteurized milk or contaminated water. Animals can also be infected, and some people have acquired their infection from contact with the infected stool of an ill dog or cat.

How does food or water get contaminated with Campylobacter?

Many chicken flocks are silently infected with *Campylobacter*; that is, the chickens are infected with the organism but show no signs of illness. *Campylobacter* can be easily spread from bird to bird through a common water source or through contact with infected feces. When an infected bird is slaughtered, *Campylobacter* can be transferred from the intestines to the meat. More than half of the raw chicken in the United States market has *Campylobacter* on it. *Campylobacter* is also present in the giblets, especially the liver.

Unpasteurized milk can become contaminated if the cow has an infection with *Campylobacter* in her udder or the milk is contaminated

61

with manure. Surface water and mountain streams can become contaminated from infected feces from cows or wild birds. This infection is common in the developing world, and travelers to foreign countries are also at risk for becoming infected with *Campylobacter*.

What can be done to prevent the infection?

There are some simple food handling practices for preventing *Campylobacter* infections. Physicians who diagnose campylobacteriosis and clinical laboratories that identify this organism should report their findings to the local health department. If many cases occur at the same time, it may mean that many people were exposed to a common contaminated food item or water source which might still be available to infect more people. When outbreaks occur, community education efforts can be directed at proper food handling techniques, especially thorough cooking of all poultry and other foods of animal origin, and common sense kitchen hygiene practices. Some data suggest that *Campylobacter* can spread through a chicken flock in their drinking water. Providing clean, chlorinated water sources for the chickens might prevent *Campylobacter* infections in poultry flocks and thereby decrease the amount of contaminated meat reaching the market place.

Some Tips for Preventing Campylobacteriosis

- Cook all poultry products thoroughly. Make sure that the meat is cooked throughout (no longer pink), any juices run clear, and the inside is cooked to 170°F (77°C) for breast meat, and 180°F (82°C) for thigh meat.

- If you are served undercooked poultry in a restaurant, send it back for further cooking.

- Wash hands with soap before handling raw foods of animal origin. Wash hands with soap after handling raw foods of animal origin and before touching anything else.

- Make sure that persons with diarrhea, especially children, wash their hands carefully and frequently with soap to reduce the risk of spreading the infection.

- Wash hands with soap after having contact with pet feces.

- Avoid consuming unpasteurized milk and untreated surface water.

Prevent cross-contamination in the kitchen:

- Use separate cutting boards for foods of animal origin and other foods.

- Carefully clean all cutting boards, countertops and utensils with soap and hot water after preparing raw food of animal origin.

What are public health agencies doing to prevent or control campylobacteriosis?

To learn more about how *Campylobacter* causes disease and is spread, CDC began a national surveillance program in 1982. A more detailed active surveillance system was instituted in 1996; this will provide more information on how often this disease occurs and what the risk factors are for getting it. CDC is also making an effort to inform the public about campylobacteriosis and ways to avoid getting this disease. The U.S. Department of Agriculture conducts research on how to prevent the infection in chickens. The Food and Drug Administration has produced the Model Food Code, which could decrease the risk of contaminated chicken being served in commercial food establishments.

Chapter 9

Cryptosporidiosis

What is **Cryptosporidium***?*

Cryptosporidiosis (krip-toc-spo-rid-e-o-sis), is a diarrheal disease caused by a microscopic parasite, *Cryptosporidium parvum*. It can live in the intestine of humans and animals and is passed in the stool of an infected person or animal. Both the disease and the parasite are also known as "crypto." The parasite is protected by an outer shell that allows it to survive outside the body for long periods of time and makes it very resistant to chlorine disinfection. During the past two decades, crypto has become recognized as one of the most common causes of waterborne disease (drinking and recreational) in humans in the United States. The parasite is found in every region of the United States and throughout the world.

What are the symptoms of crypto?

Symptoms include diarrhea, loose or watery stool, stomach cramps, upset stomach, and a slight fever. Some people have no symptoms.

How long after infection do symptoms appear?

Symptoms generally begin 2–10 days after being infected.

"Cryptosporidiosis," Division of Parasitic Diseases, Centers for Disease Control and Prevention (CDC), reviewed May 2001.

How long will symptoms last?

In persons with average immune systems, symptoms usually last about 2 weeks; the symptoms may go in cycles in which you may seem to get better for a few days, then feel worse, before the illness ends.

How is crypto spread?

Crypto lives in the intestine of infected humans or animals. Millions of crypto can be released in a bowel movement from an infected human or animal. You can become infected after accidentally swallowing the parasite. Crypto may be found in soil, food, water, or surfaces that have been contaminated with the feces from infected humans or animals. Crypto is not spread by contact with blood. Crypto can be spread:

- By putting something in your mouth or accidentally swallowing something that has come in contact with the stool of a person or animal infected with crypto.

- By swallowing recreational water contaminated with crypto. Recreational water is water in swimming pools, hot tubs, Jacuzzis, fountains, lakes, rivers, springs, ponds, or streams that can be contaminated with sewage or feces from humans or animals. Note: Crypto is chlorine resistant and can live for days in pools.

- By eating uncooked food contaminated with crypto. Thoroughly wash with uncontaminated water all vegetables and fruits you plan to eat raw. See below for information on making water safe.

- By accidentally swallowing crypto picked up from surfaces (such as toys, bathroom fixtures, changing tables, diaper pails) contaminated with stool from an infected person.

I have been diagnosed with crypto. Should I worry about spreading infection to others?

Yes, crypto can be very contagious. Follow these guidelines to avoid spreading crypto to others.

- Wash your hands with soap and water after using the toilet, changing diapers, and before eating or preparing food.

- Avoid swimming in recreational water (pools, hot tubs, lakes or rivers, the ocean, etc.) if you have crypto and for at least 2 weeks after diarrhea stops. You can pass crypto in your stool and contaminate water for several weeks after your symptoms have ended. This has resulted in many outbreaks of crypto among recreational water users. Note: you are not protected in a chlorinated pool because crypto is chlorine resistant and can live for days in pools.

- Avoid fecal exposure during sex.

Am I at risk for severe disease?

Although crypto can infect all people, some groups are more likely to develop more serious illness. Young children and pregnant women may be more susceptible to the dehydration resulting from diarrhea and should drink plenty of fluids while ill.

If you have a severely weakened immune system, you are at risk for more serious disease. Your symptoms may be more severe and could lead to serious or life-threatening illness. Examples of persons with weakened immune systems include those with HIV/AIDS; cancer and transplant patients who are taking certain immunosuppressive drugs; and those with inherited diseases that affect the immune system. If you have a severely weakened immune system, consult with your health care provider for additional guidance. You can also call the CDC AIDS HOTLINE toll-free at 1-800-342-2437 and ask for more information on cryptosporidiosis.

What should I do if I think I have crypto?

See your health care provider.

How is a crypto infection diagnosed?

Your health care provider will ask you to submit stool samples to see if you are infected. Because testing for crypto can be difficult, you may be asked to submit several stool specimens over several days. Because tests for crypto are not routinely done in most laboratories, your health care provider should specifically request testing for the parasite.

What is the treatment for crypto?

There is no effective treatment. Most people with a healthy immune system will recover on their own. If you have diarrhea, drink plenty of fluids to prevent dehydration. Rapid loss of fluids because of diarrhea can be life-threatening in babies; parents should consult their health care provider about fluid replacement therapy options for babies. Antidiarrheal medicine may help slow down diarrhea, but consult with your health care provider before taking it.

People who are in poor health or who have a weakened immune system are at higher risk for more severe and more prolonged illness. For persons with AIDS, anti-retroviral therapy that improves immune status will also decrease or eliminate symptoms of crypto. However, crypto is usually not cured and may come back if the immune status worsens. See your health care provider to discuss anti-retroviral therapy used to improve immune status.

How can I prevent crypto?

Practice good hygiene

- Wash hands thoroughly with soap and water.
    - Wash hands after using the toilet and before handling or eating food (especially for persons with diarrhea).
    - Wash hands after every diaper change, especially if you work with diaper-aged children, even if you are wearing gloves.
- Protect others by not swimming if experiencing diarrhea (essential for children in diapers).

Avoid water that might be contaminated

- Avoid swallowing recreational water. Click here for information on recreational water illnesses.
- Avoid drinking untreated water from shallow wells, lakes, rivers, springs, ponds, and streams.
- Avoid drinking untreated water during community-wide outbreaks of disease caused by contaminated drinking water. In the United States, nationally distributed brands of bottled or canned carbonated soft drinks are safe to drink. Commercially packaged noncarbonated soft drinks and fruit juices that do not require refrigeration until after they are opened (for example, those that can be stored unrefrigerated on grocery shelves) also are safe. Click here to find out how to choose bottled water that is also safe to drink.

- Avoid using ice or drinking untreated water when traveling in countries where the water supply might be unsafe.

- If you are unable to avoid drinking or using water that might be contaminated, then treat the water yourself by:

  - Heating the water to a rolling boil for at least 1 minute.

  - Using a filter that has an absolute pore size of at least 1 micron or one that has been NSF-rated for "cyst removal."

Do not rely on chemical disinfection of crypto because it is highly resistant to inactivation by chlorine or iodine.

Avoid food that might be contaminated

- Wash and/or peel all raw vegetables and fruits before eating.

- Use uncontaminated water to wash all food that is to be eaten raw.

- Avoid eating uncooked foods when traveling in countries with minimal water treatment and sanitation systems.

Avoid fecal exposure during sex

Chapter 10

Cysticercosis

What is cysticercosis?

Cysticercosis (SIS-tuh-sir-KO-sis) is an infection caused by the pork tapeworm, *Taenia solium*. Infection occurs when the tapeworm larvae enter the body and form cysticerci (SIS-tuh-sir-KEY) (cysts). When cysticerci are found in the brain, the condition is called neurocysticercosis (NEW-row SIS-tuh-sir-KO-sis).

Where is cysticercosis found?

The tapeworm that causes cysticercosis is found worldwide. Infection is found most often in rural, developing countries with poor hygiene where pigs are allowed to roam freely and eat human feces. This allows the tapeworm infection to be completed and the cycle to continue. However, there are over 1,000 cases reported in the United States every year, mostly in the Southwest.

How can I get cysticercosis?

By accidentally swallowing pork tapeworm eggs. This happens as a result of drinking water containing eggs, or eating food with eggs

Division of Parasitic Diseases, National Center for Infectious Diseases, Centers for Disease Control and Prevention (CDC). This page last reviewed August 31, 1999. This text reviewed and revised by David A. Cooke, M.D. on January 26, 2004.

on them. Although pigs are part of the pork tapeworm lifecycle, the eggs are not in the meat, so even vegetarians, Muslims, or Jews who do not eat pork can develop cysticercosis.

Infected people pass tapeworm eggs into their bowel movements. In areas with poor sanitation, their feces may get mixed into the drinking water. Insufficient hand washing after a bowel movement may also leave eggs on the hands of an infected person.

Fruits and vegetables may be grown in fields with unclean water, be handled by infected people with eggs on their hands, or may be washed with unsanitary water. When a person eats or drinks contaminated food or water contaminated, the eggs pass into the body. Once inside the stomach, the tapeworm eggs hatch, penetrate the intestine, travel through the bloodstream and may develop into cysticerci in the muscles, brain, or eyes.

What are the signs and symptoms of cysticercosis?

Signs and symptoms will depend on the location and number of cysticerci in your body.

Cysticerci in the muscles: Cysticerci in the muscles generally do not cause symptoms. However, you may be able to feel lumps under your skin.

Cysticerci in the eyes: Although rare, cysticerci may float in the eye and cause blurry or disturbed vision. Infection in the eyes may cause swelling or detachment of the retina.

Neurocysticercosis (cysticerci in the brain, spinal cord): Symptoms of neurocysticercosis depend upon where and how many cysticerci (often called lesions) are found in the brain. Seizures, and headaches are the most common symptoms. However, confusion, lack of attention to people and surroundings, difficulty with balance, swelling of the brain (called hydrocephalus) may also occur. Death can occur suddenly with heavy infections.

How long will I be infected before symptoms begin?

Symptoms can occur months to years after infection, usually when the cysts are in the process of dying. When this happens, the brain can swell. The pressure caused by swelling is what causes most of the symptoms of neurocysticercosis. Most people with cysticerci in muscles won't have symptoms of infection.

How is cysticercosis diagnosed?

Diagnosis can be difficult and may require several testing methods. Your health care provider will ask you about where you have traveled and your eating habits. Diagnosis of neurocysticercosis is usually made by MRI or CT brain scans. Blood tests are available to help diagnose an infection, but may not always be accurate. If surgery is necessary, confirmation of the diagnosis can be made by the laboratory.

What should I do if I think I have cysticercosis?

See your health care provider.

Is there treatment for cysticercosis?

Yes. Infections are generally treated with anti-parasitic drugs in combination with anti-inflammatory drugs. Surgery is sometimes necessary to treat cases in the eyes, cases that are not responsive to drug treatment, or to reduce brain edema (swelling). Not all cases of cysticercosis are treated.

I have been diagnosed with neurocysticercosis. My health care provider has decided not to treat me. How was this decision made?

Often, the decision of whether or not to treat neurocysticercosis is based upon the number of lesions found in the brain and the symptoms you have. When only one lesion is found, often treatment is not given. If you have more than one lesion, specific anti-parasitic treatment is generally recommended.

If the brain lesion is considered calcified (this means that a hard shell has formed around the tapeworm larvae), the cysticerci is considered dead and specific anti-parasitic treatment is not beneficial.

As the cysticerci die, the lesion will shrink. The swelling will go down, and often symptoms (such as seizures) will go away.

Can infection be spread from person to person?

No. Cysticercosis is not spread from person to person. However, a person infected with the intestinal tapeworm stage of the infection (*T. solium*) will shed tapeworm eggs in their bowel movements. Tapeworm eggs that are accidentally swallowed by another person can cause infection.

Should I be tested for an intestinal tapeworm infection?

Yes. Family members may also be tested. Because the tapeworm infection can be difficult to diagnose, your health care provider may ask you to submit several stool specimens over several days or to examine your stools for evidence of a tapeworm.

How can I prevent cysticercosis and other disease causing germs?

- Avoid eating raw or undercooked pork and other meats.

- Don't eat meat of pigs that are likely to be infected with the tapeworm.

- Wash hands with soap and water after using the toilet and before handling food, especially when traveling in developing countries.

- Wash and peel all raw vegetables and fruits before eating. Avoid food that may be contaminated with feces.

- Drink only bottled or boiled (1 minute) water or carbonated (bubbly) drinks in cans or bottles. Do not drink fountain drinks or any drinks with ice cubes. Another way to make water safe is by filtering it through an "absolute 1 micron or less" filter *and* dissolving iodine tablets in the filtered water. "Absolute 1 micron" filters can be found in camping/outdoor supply stores.

For More Information

McCormick GF. Cysticercosis: review of 230 patients. *Bulletin of Clinical Neurosciences* 1985; 50:76-101.

Padma MV, Behari M, Misra NK, Ahuja GK. Albendazole in single CT ring lesions in epilepsy. *Neurology* 1994;44:1344-6.

Schantz PM, Moore AC, Munoz JL, Hartman BJ, Schaefer JA, Aron AM, et al. Neurocysticercosis in an orthodox Jewish community in New York City. *N Engl J Med* 1992;327:692-5.

Vazquez V, Sotelo J. The course of seizures after treatment for cerebral cysticercosis. *N Engl J Med* 1992;327:696-702.

Chapter 11

Escherichia Coli (E. Coli)

Escherichia coli O157:H7 is an emerging cause of foodborne illness. An estimated 73,000 cases of infection and 61 deaths occur in the United States each year. Infection often leads to bloody diarrhea, and occasionally to kidney failure. Most illness has been associated with eating undercooked, contaminated ground beef. Person-to-person contact in families and child care centers is also an important mode of transmission. Infection can also occur after drinking raw milk and after swimming in or drinking sewage-contaminated water.

Consumers can prevent *E. coli* O157:H7 infection by thoroughly cooking ground beef, avoiding unpasteurized milk, and washing hands carefully.

Because the organism lives in the intestines of healthy cattle, preventive measures on cattle farms and during meat processing are being investigated.

What is Escherichia coli *O157:H7?*

E. coli O157:H7 is one of hundreds of strains of the bacterium *Escherichia coli*. Although most strains are harmless and live in the intestines of healthy humans and animals, this strain produces a powerful toxin and can cause severe illness.

E. coli O157:H7 was first recognized as a cause of illness in 1982 during an outbreak of severe bloody diarrhea; the outbreak was traced

Division of Bacterial and Mycotic Diseases, National Center for Infectious Diseases, Centers for Disease Control and Prevention (CDC). Last reviewed July 3, 2003.

to contaminated hamburgers. Since then, most infections have come from eating undercooked ground beef.

The combination of letters and numbers in the name of the bacterium refers to the specific markers found on its surface and distinguishes it from other types of *E. coli*.

How is E. coli *O157:H7 spread?*

The organism can be found on a small number of cattle farms and can live in the intestines of healthy cattle. Meat can become contaminated during slaughter, and organisms can be thoroughly mixed into beef when it is ground. Bacteria present on the cow's udders or on equipment may get into raw milk.

Eating meat, especially ground beef, that has not been cooked sufficiently to kill *E. coli* O157:H7 can cause infection. Contaminated meat looks and smells normal. Although the number of organisms required to cause disease is not known, it is suspected to be very small.

Among other known sources of infection are consumption of sprouts, lettuce, salami, unpasteurized milk and juice, and swimming in or drinking sewage-contaminated water.

Bacteria in diarrheal stools of infected persons can be passed from one person to another if hygiene or handwashing habits are inadequate.

This is particularly likely among toddlers who are not toilet trained. Family members and playmates of these children are at high risk of becoming infected.

Young children typically shed the organism in their feces for a week or two after their illness resolves. Older children rarely carry the organism without symptoms.

What illness does E. coli *O157:H7 cause?*

E. coli O157:H7 infection often causes severe bloody diarrhea and abdominal cramps; sometimes the infection causes nonbloody diarrhea or no symptoms. Usually little or no fever is present, and the illness resolves in 5 to 10 days.

In some persons, particularly children under 5 years of age and the elderly, the infection can also cause a complication called hemolytic uremic syndrome, in which the red blood cells are destroyed and the kidneys fail. About 2%–7% of infections lead to this complication. In the United States, hemolytic uremic syndrome is the principal cause of acute kidney failure in children, and most cases of hemolytic uremic syndrome are caused by *E. coli* O157:H7.

How is E. coli *O157:H7 infection diagnosed?*

Infection with *E. coli* O157:H7 is diagnosed by detecting the bacterium in the stool. Most laboratories that culture stool do not test for *E. coli* O157:H7, so it is important to request that the stool specimen be tested on sorbitol-MacConkey (SMAC) agar for this organism. All persons who suddenly have diarrhea with blood should get their stool tested for *E. coli* O157:H7.

How is the illness treated?

Most persons recover without antibiotics or other specific treatment in 5–10 days. There is no evidence that antibiotics improve the course of disease, and it is thought that treatment with some antibiotics may precipitate kidney complications. Antidiarrheal agents, such as loperamide (Imodium), should also be avoided.

Hemolytic uremic syndrome is a life-threatening condition usually treated in an intensive care unit. Blood transfusions and kidney dialysis are often required. With intensive care, the death rate for hemolytic uremic syndrome is 3%–5%.

What are the long-term consequences of infection?

Persons who only have diarrhea usually recover completely.

About one-third of persons with hemolytic uremic syndrome have abnormal kidney function many years later, and a few require long-term dialysis. Another 8% of persons with hemolytic uremic syndrome have other lifelong complications, such as high blood pressure, seizures, blindness, paralysis, and the effects of having part of their bowel removed.

What can be done to prevent the infection?

E. coli O157:H7 will continue to be an important public health concern as long as it contaminates meat. Preventive measures may reduce the number of cattle that carry it and the contamination of meat during slaughter and grinding. Research into such prevention measures is just beginning.

What can you do to prevent E. coli *O157:H7 infection?*

- Cook all ground beef and hamburger thoroughly. Because ground beef can turn brown before disease-causing bacteria are killed, use a digital instant-read meat thermometer to ensure thorough cooking. Ground beef should be cooked until a thermometer inserted into several parts of the patty, including the thickest part, reads at least 160° F. Persons who cook ground beef without using a thermometer can decrease their risk of illness by not eating ground beef patties that are still pink in the middle.

- If you are served an undercooked hamburger or other ground beef product in a restaurant, send it back for further cooking. You may want to ask for a new bun and a clean plate, too.

- Avoid spreading harmful bacteria in your kitchen. Keep raw meat separate from ready-to-eat foods. Wash hands, counters, and utensils with hot soapy water after they touch raw meat. Never place cooked hamburgers or ground beef on the unwashed plate that held raw patties. Wash meat thermometers in between tests of patties that require further cooking.

- Drink only pasteurized milk, juice, or cider. Commercial juice with an extended shelf-life that is sold at room temperature (e.g. juice in cardboard boxes, vacuum sealed juice in glass containers) has been pasteurized, although this is generally not indicated on the label. Juice concentrates are also heated sufficiently to kill pathogens.

- Wash fruits and vegetables thoroughly, especially those that will not be cooked. Children under 5 years of age, immunocompromised persons, and the elderly should avoid eating alfalfa sprouts until their safety can be assured. Methods to decontaminate alfalfa seeds and sprouts are being investigated.

- Drink municipal water that has been treated with chlorine or other effective disinfectants.

- Avoid swallowing lake or pool water while swimming.

- Make sure that persons with diarrhea, especially children, wash their hands carefully with soap after bowel movements to reduce the risk of spreading infection, and that persons wash hands after changing soiled diapers. Anyone with a diarrheal illness should avoid swimming in public pools or lakes, sharing baths with others, and preparing food for others.

For more information about reducing your risk of foodborne illness, visit the U.S. Department of Agriculture's Food Safety and Inspection Service website at: http://www.fsis.usda.gov/. For more advice on cooking ground beef, visit the U.S. Department of Agriculture web site at: http://www.fsis.usda.gov/OA/topics/gb.htm

Chapter 12

Gastroenteritis

Viral Gastroenteritis

What is viral gastroenteritis?

Gastroenteritis means inflammation of the stomach and small and large intestines. Viral gastroenteritis is an infection caused by a variety of viruses that results in vomiting or diarrhea. It is often called the "stomach flu," although it is not caused by the influenza viruses.

What causes viral gastroenteritis?

Many different viruses can cause gastroenteritis, including rotaviruses, adenoviruses, caliciviruses, astroviruses, Norwalk virus, and a group of Noroviruses. Viral gastroenteritis is not caused by bacteria (such as *Salmonella* or *Escherichia coli*) or parasites (such as *Giardia*), or

"Viral Gastroenteritis," reviewed August 20, 2001, "Rotavirus," reviewed August 20, 2001, and "Norovirus: Q&A," reviewed January 21, 2003, Respiratory and Enteric Viruses Branch, Division of Viral and Rickettsial Diseases, National Center for Infectious Diseases, Centers for Disease Control and Prevention (CDC). The section titled "Norwalk Virus Infection" is reprinted with permission from *Model Emergency Response Communications Planning for Infectious Disease Outbreaks and Bioterrorist Events, Second Edition*, October 2001, p. 216–217. © 2001 Association of State and Territorial Directors of Health Promotion and Public Health Education. All rights reserved. Developed with funding from the Centers for Disease Control and Prevention (CDC) through cooperative agreement #U50/CCU012359 to the Directors of Health Promotion and Education.

by medications or other medical conditions, although the symptoms may be similar. Your doctor can determine if the diarrhea is caused by a virus or by something else.

What are the symptoms of viral gastroenteritis?

The main symptoms of viral gastroenteritis are watery diarrhea and vomiting. The affected person may also have headache, fever, and abdominal cramps ("stomach ache"). In general, the symptoms begin 1 to 2 days following infection with a virus that causes gastroenteritis and may last for 1 to 10 days, depending on which virus causes the illness.

Is viral gastroenteritis a serious illness?

For most people, it is not. People who get viral gastroenteritis almost always recover completely without any long-term problems. Gastroenteritis is a serious illness, however, for persons who are unable to drink enough fluids to replace what they lose through vomiting or diarrhea. Infants, young children, and persons who are unable to care for themselves, such as the disabled or elderly, are at risk for dehydration from loss of fluids. Immune compromised persons are at risk for dehydration because they may get a more serious illness, with greater vomiting or diarrhea. They may need to be hospitalized for treatment to correct or prevent dehydration.

Is the illness contagious? How are these viruses spread?

Yes, viral gastroenteritis is contagious. The viruses that cause gastroenteritis are spread through close contact with infected persons (for example, by sharing food, water, or eating utensils). Individuals may also become infected by eating or drinking contaminated foods or beverages.

How does food get contaminated by gastroenteritis viruses?

Food may be contaminated by food preparers or handlers who have viral gastroenteritis, especially if they do not wash their hands regularly after using the bathroom. Shellfish may be contaminated by sewage, and persons who eat raw or undercooked shellfish harvested from contaminated waters may get diarrhea. Drinking water can also be contaminated by sewage and be a source of spread of these viruses.

Where and when does viral gastroenteritis occur?

Viral gastroenteritis affects people in all parts of the world. Each virus has its own seasonal activity. For example, in the United States, rotavirus and astrovirus infections occur during the cooler months of the year (October to April), whereas adenovirus infections occur throughout the year. Viral gastroenteritis outbreaks can occur in institutional settings, such as schools, child care facilities, and nursing homes, and can occur in other group settings, such as banquet halls, cruise ships, dormitories, and campgrounds.

Who gets viral gastroenteritis?

Anyone can get it. Viral gastroenteritis occurs in people of all ages and backgrounds. However, some viruses tend to cause diarrheal disease primarily among people in specific age groups. Rotavirus infection is the most common cause of diarrhea in infants and young children under 5 years old. Adenoviruses and astroviruses cause diarrhea mostly in young children, but older children and adults can also be affected. Norwalk and Noroviruses are more likely to cause diarrhea in older children and adults.

How is viral gastroenteritis diagnosed?

Generally, viral gastroenteritis is diagnosed by a physician on the basis of the symptoms and medical examination of the patient. Rotavirus infection can be diagnosed by laboratory testing of a stool specimen. Tests to detect other viruses that cause gastroenteritis are not in routine use.

How is viral gastroenteritis treated?

The most important of treating viral gastroenteritis in children and adults is to prevent severe loss of fluids (dehydration). This treatment should begin at home. Your physician may give you specific instructions about what kinds of fluid to give. Centers for Disease Control and Prevention, (CDC) recommends that families with infants and young children keep a supply of oral rehydration solution (ORS) at home at all times and use the solution when diarrhea first occurs in the child. ORS is available at pharmacies without a prescription. Follow the written directions on the ORS package, and use clean or boiled water. Medications, including antibiotics (which have no effect on viruses) and other treatments, should be avoided unless specifically recommended by a physician.

Can viral gastroenteritis be prevented?

Yes. Persons can reduce their chance of getting infected by frequent handwashing, prompt disinfection of contaminated surfaces with household chlorine bleach-based cleaners, and prompt washing of soiled articles of clothing. If food or water is thought to be contaminated, it should be avoided.

Is there a vaccine for viral gastroenteritis?

There is no vaccine or medicine currently available that prevents viral gastroenteritis. A vaccine is being developed, however, that protects against severe diarrhea from rotavirus infection in infants and young children.

Rotavirus

What is rotavirus?

Rotavirus is the most common cause of severe diarrhea among children, resulting in the hospitalization of approximately 55,000 children each year in the United States and the death of over 600,000 children annually worldwide. The incubation period for rotavirus disease is approximately 2 days. The disease is characterized by vomiting and watery diarrhea for 3–8 days, and fever and abdominal pain occur frequently. Immunity after infection is incomplete, but repeat infections tend to be less severe than the original infection.

What does rotavirus look like?

A rotavirus has a characteristic wheel-like appearance when viewed by electron microscopy (the name rotavirus is derived from the Latin *rota*, meaning "wheel"). Rotaviruses are nonenveloped, double-shelled viruses. The genome is composed of 11 segments of double-stranded RNA, which code for six structural and five nonstructural proteins. The virus is stable in the environment.

How is rotavirus spread?

The primary mode of transmission is fecal-oral, although some have reported low titers of virus in respiratory tract secretions and other body fluids. Because the virus is stable in the environment, transmission can occur through ingestion of contaminated water or food and contact with contaminated surfaces. In the United States and other countries with a temperate climate, the disease has a winter seasonal pattern, with annual epidemics occurring from November to April. The highest rates of illness occur among infants and young children, and most children in the United States are infected by 2 years of age. Adults can also be infected, though disease tends to be mild.

How is rotavirus diagnosed?

Diagnosis may be made by rapid antigen detection of rotavirus in stool specimens. Strains may be further characterized by enzyme immunoassay or reverse transcriptase polymerase chain reaction, but such testing is not commonly done.

How is rotavirus treated?

For persons with healthy immune systems, rotavirus gastroenteritis is a self-limited illness, lasting for only a few days. Treatment is nonspecific and consists of oral rehydration therapy to prevent dehydration. About one in 40 children with rotavirus gastroenteritis will require hospitalization for intravenous fluids.

Can rotavirus be prevented?

In 1998, the U.S. Food and Drug Administration approved a live virus vaccine (Rotashield) for use in children. However, the Advisory Committee on Immunization Practices (ACIP) recommended that Rotashield no longer be recommended for infants in the United States because of data that indicated a strong association between Rotashield and intussusception (bowel obstruction) among some infants during the first 1–2 weeks following vaccination.

Norwalk Virus Infection

What is Norwalk virus infection?

Norwalk virus infection is an intestinal illness that often occurs in outbreaks.

What is the infectious agent that causes Norwalk virus infection?

Norwalk virus infection is caused by the Norwalk virus. The virus was first identified in 1972 after an outbreak of gastrointestinal illness in Norwalk, Ohio. Later, other viruses with similar features were described and called Norwalk-like viruses. These have since been classified as members of the calicivirus family.

Where is Norwalk virus found?

Norwalk and Norwalk-like viruses are found worldwide. Humans are the only known hosts. The viruses are passed in the stool of infected persons.

How do people get Norwalk virus infection?

People get Norwalk virus infection by swallowing food or water that has been contaminated with stool from an infected person. Outbreaks in the United States are often linked to eating raw shellfish, especially oysters and clams. Shellfish become contaminated via stool from sick food handlers or from raw sewage dumped overboard by recreational and/or commercial boaters. Contaminated water, ice, eggs, salad ingredients, and ready-to-eat foods are other sources of infection.

Who is at risk for Norwalk virus infection?

Anyone can get Norwalk virus infection, but it may be more common in adults and older children.

What are the signs and symptoms of Norwalk virus infection?

- Nausea
- Vomiting
- Diarrhea
- Stomach cramps

Symptoms usually appear in 1 to 2 days after swallowing contaminated food or water. Infected persons usually recover in 2 to 3 days without serious or long-term health effects. Severe illness or hospitalization is uncommon.

How is Norwalk virus infection diagnosed and treated?

Laboratory diagnosis is difficult. Diagnosis is often based on the combination of symptoms and the short time of illness.

No specific treatment is available. Persons who are severely dehydrated might need rehydration therapy.

How common is Norwalk virus infection?

Norwalk and Norwalk-like viruses are increasingly being recognized as leading causes of foodborne disease in the United States. However, since no routine diagnostic test is available, the true prevalence is not known. Norwalk and Norwalk-like viruses have been linked to outbreaks of intestinal illness on cruise ships and in communities, camps, schools, institutions, and families.

Many oyster-related outbreaks of intestinal illness linked to Norwalk-like viruses have been reported in Louisiana, Florida, Maryland, and other states where oyster harvesting is common. In 1993, 73 people in Louisiana and about 130 others in the United States who ate oysters from Louisiana became ill. A malfunctioning sewage system was the cause of an outbreak in 1996. An outbreak in 1997 was linked to sewage from oyster-harvesting boats.

How can Norwalk virus be prevented?

- Wash hands with soap and warm water after toilet visits and before preparing or eating food.

- Cook all shellfish thoroughly before eating.

- Wash raw vegetables before eating.

- Dispose of sewage in a sanitary manner.

- Food handlers with symptoms of Norwalk-like illness should not prepare or touch food.

Norovirus: Questions and Answers

What are noroviruses?

Noroviruses are a group of viruses that cause the "stomach flu," or gastroenteritis, in people. The term norovirus was recently approved as the official name for this group of viruses. Several other names have been used for noroviruses, including:

- Norwalk-like viruses (NLVs)

- caliciviruses (because they belong to the virus family *Caliciviridae*)

- small round structured viruses

Viruses are very different from bacteria and parasites, some of which can cause illnesses similar to nororvirus infection. Viruses are much smaller, are not affected by treatment with antibiotics, and cannot grow outside of a person's body.

What are the symptoms of illness caused by noroviruses?

The symptoms of norovirus illness usually include nausea, vomiting, diarrhea, and some stomach cramping. Sometimes people additionally have a low-grade fever, chills, headache, muscle aches, and a general sense of tiredness. The illness often begins suddenly, and the infected person may feel very sick. The illness is usually brief, with symptoms lasting only about 1 or 2 days. In general, children experience more vomiting than adults.

What is the name of the illness caused by noroviruses?

Illness caused by norovirus infection has several names, including:

- stomach flu—this "stomach flu" is not related to the flu (or influenza), which is a respiratory illness caused by influenza virus.
- viral gastroenteritis—the most common name for illness caused by norovirus. Gastroenteritis refers to an inflammation of the stomach and intestines.
- acute gastroenteritis
- non-bacterial gastroenteritis
- food poisoning (although there are other causes of food poisoning)
- calicivirus infection

How serious is norovirus disease?

Norovirus disease is usually not serious, although people may feel very sick and vomit many times a day. Most people get better within 1 or 2 days, and they have no long-term health effects related to their illness. However, sometimes people are unable to drink enough liquids to replace the liquids they lost because of vomiting and diarrhea. These persons can become dehydrated and may need special medical attention. This problem with dehydration is usually only seen among the very young, the elderly, and persons with weakened immune systems. There is no evidence to suggest that an infected person can become a long-term carrier of norovirus.

How do people become infected with noroviruses?

Noroviruses are found in the stool or vomit of infected people. People can become infected with the virus in several ways, including:

- eating food or drinking liquids that are contaminated with norovirus;

- touching surfaces or objects contaminated with norovirus, and then placing their hand in their mouth;

- having direct contact with another person who is infected and showing symptoms (for example, when caring for someone with illness, or sharing foods or eating utensils with someone who is ill).

Persons working in day-care centers or nursing homes should pay special attention to children or residents who have norovirus illness. This virus is very contagious and can spread rapidly throughout such environments.

When do symptoms appear?

Symptoms of norovirus illness usually begin about 24 to 48 hours after ingestion of the virus, but they can appear as early as 12 hours after exposure.

Are noroviruses contagious?

Noroviruses are very contagious and can spread easily from person to person. Both stool and vomit are infectious. Particular care should be taken with young children in diapers who may have diarrhea.

How long are people contagious?

People infected with norovirus are contagious from the moment they begin feeling ill to at least 3 days after recovery. Some people may be contagious for as long as 2 weeks after recovery. Therefore, it is particularly important for people to use good handwashing and other hygienic practices after they have recently recovered from norovirus illness.

Who gets norovirus infection?

Anyone can become infected with these viruses. There are many different strains of norovirus, which makes it difficult for a person's body to develop long-lasting immunity. Therefore, norovirus illness can recur throughout a person's lifetime. In addition, because of differences in genetic factors, some people are more likely to become infected and develop more severe illness than others.

What treatment is available for people with norovirus infection?

Currently, there is no antiviral medication that works against norovirus and there is no vaccine to prevent infection. Norovirus infection cannot be treated with antibiotics. This is because antibiotics work to fight bacteria and not viruses.

Norovirus illness is usually brief in healthy individuals. When people are ill with vomiting and diarrhea, they should drink plenty of fluids to prevent dehydration. Dehydration among young children, the elderly, the sick, can be common, and it is the most serious health effect that can result from norovirus infection. By drinking oral rehydration fluids (ORF), juice, or water, people can reduce their chance of becoming dehydrated. Sports drinks do not replace the nutrients and minerals lost during this illness.

Can norovirus infections be prevented?

Yes. You can decrease your chance of coming in contact with noroviruses by following these preventive steps:

- Frequently wash your hands, especially after toilet visits and changing diapers and before eating or preparing food.

- Carefully wash fruits and vegetables, and steam oysters before eating them.

- Thoroughly clean and disinfect contaminated surfaces immediately after an episode of illness by using a bleach-based household cleaner.

- Immediately remove and wash clothing or linens that may be contaminated with virus after an episode of illness (use hot water and soap).

- Flush or discard any vomitus and/or stool in the toilet and make sure that the surrounding area is kept clean.

Persons who are infected with norovirus should not prepare food while they have symptoms and for 3 days after they recover from their illness. Food that may have been contaminated by an ill person should be disposed of properly.

Chapter 13

Giardiasis

What is giardiasis?

Giardiasis (GEE-are-DYE-uh-sis) is a diarrheal illness caused by *Giardia intestinalis* (also known as *Giardia lamblia*), a one-celled, microscopic parasite that lives in the intestine of people and animals. The parasite is passed in the stool of an infected person or animal. The parasite is protected by an outer shell that allows it to survive outside the body and in the environment for long periods of time. During the past 2 decades, *Giardia* has become recognized as one of the most common causes of waterborne disease (drinking and recreational) in humans in the United States. The parasite is found in every region of the United States and throughout the world.

What are the symptoms of giardiasis?

Symptoms include diarrhea, loose or watery stool, stomach cramps, and upset stomach. These symptoms may lead to weight loss and dehydration. Some people have no symptoms.

How long after infection do symptoms appear?

Symptoms generally begin 1–2 weeks after being infected.

"Giardiasis," Division of Parasitic Diseases, Centers for Disease Control and Prevention (CDC), reviewed May 2001.

How long will symptoms last?

In otherwise healthy persons, symptoms may last 2–6 weeks. Occasionally, symptoms last longer.

How is giardiasis spread?

Giardia lives in the intestine of infected humans or animals. Millions of germs can be released in a bowel movement from an infected human or animal. You can become infected after accidentally swallowing the parasite. *Giardia* may be found in soil, food, water, or surfaces that have been contaminated with the feces from infected humans or animals. *Giardia* is not spread by contact with blood. *Giardia* can be spread:

- By putting something in your mouth or accidentally swallowing something that has come in contact with the stool of a person or animal infected with *Giardia*.

- By swallowing recreational water contaminated with *Giardia*. Recreational water is water in swimming pools, hot tubs, Jacuzzis, fountains, lakes, rivers, springs, ponds, or streams that can be contaminated with sewage or feces from humans or animals.

- By eating uncooked food contaminated with *Giardia*. Thoroughly wash with uncontaminated water all vegetables and fruits you plan to eat raw. See below for information on making water safe.

- By accidentally swallowing *Giardia* picked up from surfaces (such as toys, bathroom fixtures, changing tables, diaper pails) contaminated with stool from an infected person.

Who is at risk?

Everyone. Persons at increased risk for giardiasis include child care workers; children who attend day care centers, including diaper-aged children; international travelers; hikers; campers; swimmers; and others who drink or accidentally swallow water from contaminated sources that is untreated (no heat inactivation, filtration, or chemical disinfection). Several community-wide outbreaks of giardiasis have been linked to drinking municipal water or recreational water contaminated with *Giardia*.

I have been diagnosed with a Giardia infection. Should I worry about spreading infection to others?

Yes, *Giardia* can be very contagious. Follow these guidelines to avoid spreading *Giardia* to others.

- Wash your hands with soap and water after using the toilet, changing diapers, and before eating or preparing food.

- Avoid swimming in recreational water (pools, hot tubs, lakes or rivers, the ocean, etc.) if you have *Giardia* and for at least 2 weeks after diarrhea stops. You can pass *Giardia* in your stool and contaminate water for several weeks after your symptoms have ended. This has resulted in outbreaks of *Giardia* among recreational water users.

- Avoid fecal exposure during sex.

What should I do if I think I have giardiasis?

See your health care provider.

How is a Giardia infection diagnosed?

Your health care provider will likely ask you to submit stool samples to see if you have the parasite. Because *Giardia* can be difficult to diagnose, he or she may ask you to submit several stool specimens over several days.

What is the treatment for giardiasis?

Several prescription drugs are available to treat *Giardia*. Consult with your health care provider. Although *Giardia* can infect all people, young children and pregnant women may be more susceptible to the dehydration resulting from diarrhea and should drink plenty of fluids while ill.

How can I prevent Giardia infection?

Practice good hygiene.

- Wash hands thoroughly with soap and water.
  - Wash hands after using the toilet and before handling or eating food (especially for persons with diarrhea).

91

- Wash hands after every diaper change, especially if you work with diaper-aged children, even if you are wearing gloves.

- Protect others by not swimming if experiencing diarrhea (essential for children in diapers).

Avoid water that might be contaminated

- Avoid swallowing recreational water.

- Avoid drinking untreated water from shallow wells, lakes, rivers, springs, ponds, and streams.

- Avoid drinking untreated water during community-wide outbreaks of disease caused by contaminated drinking water. In the United States, nationally distributed brands of bottled or canned carbonated soft drinks are safe to drink. Commercially packaged noncarbonated soft drinks and fruit juices that do not require refrigeration until after they are opened (those that are stored unrefrigerated on grocery shelves) also are safe.

- Avoid using ice or drinking untreated water when traveling in countries where the water supply might be unsafe.

- If you are unable to avoid drinking or using water that might be contaminated, then treat the water yourself by:
  - Heating the water to a rolling boil for at least 1 minute.
  - Using a filter that has an absolute pore size of at least 1 micron or one that has been NSF rated for "cyst removal."

    If the methods above cannot be used, then try chemical inactivation of *Giardia* by chlorination or iodination. Chemical disinfection may be less effective than other methods because it is highly dependent on the temperature, pH, and cloudiness of the water.

Avoid food that might be contaminated

- Wash and/or peel all raw vegetables and fruits before eating.
- Use uncontaminated water to wash all food that is to be eaten raw.
- Avoid eating uncooked foods when traveling in countries with minimal water treatment and sanitation systems.

Avoid fecal exposure during sex

My water comes from a well; should I have my well water tested?

If you answer yes to the following questions, consider having your well water tested.

- Are other members of your family or users of your well water ill?

If yes, your well may be the source of infection.

- Is your well located at the bottom of a hill or is it considered shallow?

If so, runoff from rain or flood water may be draining directly into your well causing contamination.

- Is your well in a rural area where animals graze?

Well water can become fecally contaminated if animal waste seepage contaminates the ground water. This can occur if your well has cracked casings, is poorly constructed, or is too shallow.

Tests specifically for *Giardia* are expensive, difficult, and usually require hundreds of gallons of water to be pumped through a filter. If you answered yes to the above questions, consider testing your well for fecal coliforms or *E. coli* instead of *Giardia*. Although fecal coliforms or *E. coli* tests do not specifically test for *Giardia*, testing will show if your well has fecal contamination.

These tests are only useful if your well is not routinely disinfected with chlorine since chlorine kills fecal coliforms and *E. coli*. If the tests are positive, the water may also be contaminated with *Giardia*, as well as other harmful bacteria and viruses. Look in your local telephone directory for a laboratory or cooperative extension that offers water testing. If the fecal coliform test comes back positive, indicating that your well is fecally contaminated, contact your local water authority for instructions on how to disinfect your well.

My child was recently diagnosed as having giardiasis, but does not have any diarrhea. My health care provider says treatment is not necessary. Is this true?

In general, the answer by the American Academy of Pediatrics is that treatment is not necessary. However, there are a few exceptions.

If your child does not have diarrhea, but is having nausea, or is fatigued, losing weight, or has a poor appetite, you and your health care provider may wish to consider treatment. If your child attends a day care center where an outbreak is continuing to occur despite efforts to control it, screening and treatment of children without obvious symptoms may be a good idea. The same is true if several family members are ill, or if a family member is pregnant and therefore not able to take the most effective anti-*Giardia* medications.

For More Information

1. Giardiasis Surveillance, United States, 1992–1997. *MMWR* 2000; 49, SS-7: 1-13.

2. Addiss DG, Juranek DD, Spencer HC. Treatment of children with asymptomatic and nondiarrheal *Giardia* infection. *Pediatr Infect Dis J* 1991;10:843-6.

3. Addiss DG, Davis JP, Roberts JM, Mast EE. Epidemiology of giardiasis in Wisconsin. Increasing incidence of reported cases and unexplained seasonal trends. *Am J Trop Med Hyg* 1992;47:13-9.

4. Bartlett AV, Englander SJ, Jarvis BA, Ludwig L, Carlson JF, Topping JP. Controlled trial of *Giardia lamblia*: Control strategies in day care centers. *Am J Public Health* 1991;81:1001-6.

5. Kreuter AK, Del Bene VE, Amstey MS. Giardiasis in pregnancy. *Am J Obstet Gynecol* 1981;40:895-901.

6. Lengerich EJ, Addiss DG, Juranek DD. Severe giardiasis in the United States. *Clin Infect Dis* 1994; 18:760-3.

Chapter 14

Helicobacter pylori
and Peptic Ulcers

What is a peptic ulcer?

A peptic ulcer is a sore on the lining of the stomach or duodenum, which is the beginning of the small intestine. Peptic ulcers are common: One in 10 Americans develops an ulcer at some time in his or her life. One cause of peptic ulcer is bacterial infection, but some ulcers are caused by long-term use of nonsteroidal anti-inflammatory agents (NSAIDs), like aspirin and ibuprofen. In a few cases, cancerous tumors in the stomach or pancreas can cause ulcers. Peptic ulcers are not caused by stress or eating spicy food.

What is **H. pylori?**

Helicobacter pylori (*H. pylori*) is a type of bacteria. Researchers believe that *H. pylori* is responsible for the majority of peptic ulcers.

H. pylori infection is common in the United States: About 20 percent of people under 40 years old and half of those over 60 years have it. Most infected people, however, do not develop ulcers. Why *H. pylori* does not cause ulcers in every infected person is not known. Most likely, infection depends on characteristics of the infected person, the type of *H. pylori*, and other factors yet to be discovered.

"*H. pylori* and Peptic Ulcer," National Digestive Diseases Information Clearinghouse (NDDIC), National Institute of Diabetes and Digestive and Kidney Diseases (NIDDK), National Institutes of Health (NIH), U.S. Department of Health and Human Services. NIH Pub. No. 03-4225, December 2002.

Researchers are not certain how people contract *H. pylori*, but they think it may be through food or water.

Researchers have found *H. pylori* in the saliva of some infected people, so the bacteria may also spread through mouth-to-mouth contact such as kissing.

How does H. pylori *cause a peptic ulcer?*

H. pylori weakens the protective mucous coating of the stomach and duodenum, which allows acid to get through to the sensitive lining beneath. Both the acid and the bacteria irritate the lining and cause a sore, or ulcer.

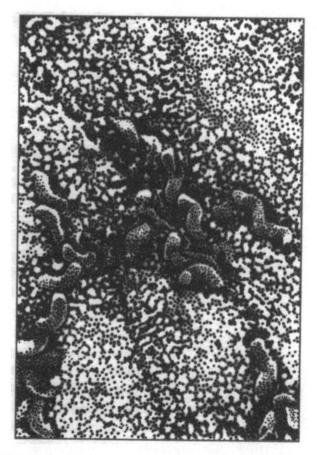

Figure 14.1. Helicobacter pylori (H. pylori) *bacteria.*

H. pylori is able to survive in stomach acid because it secretes enzymes that neutralize the acid. This mechanism allows *H. pylori* to make its way to the "safe" area—the protective mucous lining. Once there, the bacterium's spiral shape helps it burrow through the lining.

What are the symptoms of an ulcer?

Abdominal discomfort is the most common symptom. This discomfort usually

- is a dull, gnawing ache
- comes and goes for several days or weeks
- occurs 2 to 3 hours after a meal
- occurs in the middle of the night (when the stomach is empty)
- is relieved by eating
- is relieved by antacid medications

Other symptoms include

- weight loss
- poor appetite
- bloating
- burping
- nausea
- vomiting

Some people experience only very mild symptoms, or none at all.

Emergency Symptoms. If you have any of these symptoms, call your doctor right away:

- sharp, sudden, persistent stomach pain
- bloody or black stools
- bloody vomit or vomit that looks like coffee grounds

They could be signs of a serious problem, such as

- perforation—when the ulcer burrows through the stomach or duodenal wall

- bleeding—when acid or the ulcer breaks a blood vessel

- obstruction—when the ulcer blocks the path of food trying to leave the stomach

How is an H. pylori-*related ulcer diagnosed?*

Diagnosing an ulcer. To see whether symptoms are caused by an ulcer, the doctor may do an upper gastrointestinal (GI) series or an endoscopy. An upper GI series is an x-ray of the esophagus, stomach, and duodenum. The patient drinks a chalky liquid called barium to make these organs and any ulcers show up more clearly on the x-ray.

An endoscopy is an exam that uses an endoscope, a thin, lighted tube with a tiny camera on the end. The patient is lightly sedated, and the doctor carefully eases the endoscope into the mouth and down the throat to the stomach and duodenum. This allows the doctor to see the lining of the esophagus, stomach, and duodenum. The doctor can use the endoscope to take photos of ulcers or remove a tiny piece of tissue to view under a microscope.

Diagnosing *H. pylori.* If an ulcer is found, the doctor will test the patient for *H. pylori*. This test is important because treatment for an ulcer caused by *H. pylori* is different from that for an ulcer caused by NSAIDs.

H. pylori is diagnosed through blood, breath, stool, and tissue tests. Blood tests are most common. They detect antibodies to *H. pylori* bacteria. Blood is taken at the doctor's office through a finger stick.

Urea breath tests are an effective diagnostic method for *H. pylori*. They are also used after treatment to see whether it worked. In the doctor's office, the patient drinks a urea solution that contains a special carbon atom. If *H. pylori* is present, it breaks down the urea, releasing the carbon. The blood carries the carbon to the lungs, where the patient exhales it. The breath test is 96 percent to 98 percent accurate.

Stool tests may be used to detect *H. pylori* infection in the patient's fecal matter. Studies have shown that this test, called the *Helicobacter pylori* stool antigen (HpSA) test, is accurate for diagnosing *H. pylori*.

Tissue tests are usually done using the biopsy sample that is removed with the endoscope. There are three types:

- The rapid urease test detects the enzyme urease, which is produced by *H. pylori*.

- A histology test allows the doctor to find and examine the actual bacteria.

- A culture test involves allowing *H. pylori* to grow in the tissue sample.

In diagnosing *H. pylori*, blood, breath, and stool tests are often done before tissue tests because they are less invasive. However, blood tests are not used to detect *H. pylori* following treatment because a patient's blood can show positive results even after *H. pylori* has been eliminated.

How are H. pylori *peptic ulcers treated?*

H. pylori peptic ulcers are treated with drugs that kill the bacteria, reduce stomach acid, and protect the stomach lining. Antibiotics are used to kill the bacteria. Two types of acid-suppressing drugs might be used: H2 blockers and proton pump inhibitors.

H_2 blockers work by blocking histamine, which stimulates acid secretion. They help reduce ulcer pain after a few weeks. Proton pump inhibitors suppress acid production by halting the mechanism that pumps the acid into the stomach. H_2 blockers and proton pump inhibitors have been prescribed alone for years as treatments for ulcers. But used alone, these drugs do not eradicate *H. pylori* and therefore do not cure *H. pylori*-related ulcers. Bismuth subsalicylate, a component of Pepto-Bismol, is used to protect the stomach lining from acid. It also kills *H. pylori*.

Treatment usually involves a combination of antibiotics, acid suppressors, and stomach protectors. Antibiotic regimens recommended for patients may differ across regions of the world because different areas have begun to show resistance to particular antibiotics.

The use of only one medication to treat *H. pylori* is not recommended. At this time, the most proven effective treatment is a 2-week

Table 14.1. Drugs used to treat *H. pylori* peptic ulcers.

Antibiotics: metronidazole, tetracycline, clarithromycin, amoxicillin

H$_2$ blockers: cimetidine, ranitidine, famotidine, nizatidine

Proton pump inhibitors: omeprazole, lansoprazole, rabeprazole, esomeprazole, pantoprazole

Stomach-lining protector: bismuth subsalicylate

course of treatment called triple therapy. It involves taking two antibiotics to kill the bacteria and either an acid suppressor or stomach-lining shield. Two-week triple therapy reduces ulcer symptoms, kills the bacteria, and prevents ulcer recurrence in more than 90 percent of patients.

Unfortunately, patients may find triple therapy complicated because it involves taking as many as 20 pills a day. Also, the antibiotics used in triple therapy may cause mild side effects such as nausea, vomiting, diarrhea, dark stools, metallic taste in the mouth, dizziness, headache, and yeast infections in women. (Most side effects can be treated with medication withdrawal.) Nevertheless, recent studies show that 2 weeks of triple therapy is ideal.

Early results of studies in other countries suggest that 1 week of triple therapy may be as effective as the 2-week therapy, with fewer side effects.

Another option is 2 weeks of dual therapy. Dual therapy involves two drugs: an antibiotic and an acid suppressor. It is not as effective as triple therapy.

Two weeks of quadruple therapy, which uses two antibiotics, an acid suppressor, and a stomach-lining shield, looks promising in research studies. It is also called bismuth triple therapy.

Can H. pylori *infection be prevented?*

No one knows for sure how *H. pylori* spreads, so prevention is difficult. Researchers are trying to develop a vaccine to prevent infection.

Why don't all doctors automatically check for H. pylori?

Changing medical belief and practice takes time. For nearly 100 years, scientists and doctors thought that ulcers were caused by stress, spicy food, and alcohol. Treatment involved bed rest and a bland diet. Later, researchers added stomach acid to the list of causes and began treating ulcers with antacids.

Since *H. pylori* was discovered in 1982, studies conducted around the world have shown that using antibiotics to destroy *H. pylori* cures peptic ulcers. The prevalence of *H. pylori* ulcers is changing. The infection is becoming less common in people born in developed countries. The medical community, however, continues to debate *H. pylori*'s role in peptic ulcers. If you have a peptic ulcer and have not been tested for *H. pylori* infection, talk to your doctor.

Points to Remember

- A peptic ulcer is a sore in the lining of the stomach or duodenum.

- The majority of peptic ulcers are caused by the *H. pylori* bacterium. Many of the other cases are caused by NSAIDs. None are caused by spicy food or stress.

- *H. pylori* can be transmitted from person to person through close contact and exposure to vomit.

- Always wash your hands after using the bathroom and before eating.

- A combination of antibiotics and other drugs is the most effective treatment for *H. pylori* peptic ulcers.

Additional Readings

Graham DY, Rakel RE, Fendrick AM, et al. Recognizing peptic ulcer disease: keys to clinical and laboratory diagnosis. *Postgraduate Medicine*. 1999;105(3):113–133.

Lahaie RG, Gaudreau C. *Helicobacter pylori* antibiotic resistance: trends over time. *Canadian Journal of Gastroenterology*. 2000;14(10): 895–899.

Manes G, Balzano A, Iaquinto G, et al. Accuracy of the stool antigen test in the diagnosis of *Helicobacter pylori* infection before treatment and in patients on omeprazole therapy. *Alimentary Pharmacology and Therapeutics*. 2001;15(1):73–79.

McManus TJ. *Helicobacter pylori*: an emerging infectious disease. *Nurse Practitioner*. 2000;25(8):42–46.

National Institutes of Health, Office of the Director. *NIH Consensus Statement*: Helicobacter pylori *in Peptic Ulcer Disease*. Vol. 12, No. 1. Bethesda, MD: National Institutes of Health; 1994.

Saunders CS. *H. pylori* infection: simplifying management. *Patient Care*. 1999;(20):118–134.

Vaira D, Holton J, Menegatti M, et al. Review article: invasive and noninvasive tests for *Helicobacter pylori* infection. *Alimentary Pharmacology and Therapeutics*. 2000;14(suppl 3):13–22.

appearing in this document are used only because they are considered necessary in the context of the information provided. If a product is not mentioned, this does not mean or imply that the product is unsatisfactory.

Chapter 15

Listeriosis

Listeria: The Bacterium, The Disease

What is **Listeria monocytogenes?**

Listeria monocytogenes is a bacterium that can cause listeriosis, a serious bacterial infection in humans. *L. monocytogenes* is commonly found in soil and water and on plant material, particularly decaying plant material. These environments are regarded as the natural habitat of this organism. The bacterium often moves through the animal and human intestinal tract without causing illness, and has been found in many domestic and wild animals, including birds and fish. *L. monocytogenes* may enter a food processing environment through incoming food materials and on the shoes and clothing of personnel. Once *L. monocytogenes* is in a food processing environment, it may become established on food contact surfaces and non-food contact surfaces (for example, floors and floor drains).

What is listeriosis?

Listeriosis is a serious and potentially fatal infection caused by eating food contaminated with the bacterium *L. monocytogenes*. The disease affects primarily pregnant women, older adults and persons

From "*Listeria monocytogenes* Risk Assessment Questions and Answers," Center for Food Safety and Applied Nutrition, U.S. Food and Drug Administration, and Food Safety and Inspection Service, U.S. Department of Agriculture, October 21, 2003.

with weakened immune systems due to a disease (for example, diabetes, organ transplant, cancer, age) or due to medications (such as steroids). A person with listeriosis initially has fever, muscle aches, and sometimes gastrointestinal symptoms, such as nausea or diarrhea. If infection spreads to the nervous system, symptoms such as headache, stiff neck, confusion, loss of balance, or convulsions can occur. In some instances other organ systems within the body can become infected. Infected pregnant women may experience only a mild, flu-like illness; however, their unborn children are at risk. Infections during pregnancy can lead to premature delivery, infection of the newborn, or even stillbirth.

Listeriosis is a significant public health concern because it is life-threatening. Death occurs in about 20 percent of the cases. The Centers for Disease Control and Prevention estimates that approximately 2500 persons become seriously ill and 500 persons die each year from listeriosis.

What is the incubation period for Listeria infection?

There can be a substantial delay between the time of ingestion of contaminated food and the onset of serious symptoms. The average time from exposure to illness is approximately 30 days, but symptoms can appear as long as 90 days after exposure. It is important for consumers to know that the infection can occur as much as 90 days later, so that they can seek appropriate treatment if they have symptoms of *Listeria* infection.

What foods have been associated with cases of listeriosis?

Cases of listeriosis in the U.S. have been associated with frankfurters (hot dogs), deli/luncheon meats, pâté, salami, brie cheese, Mexican-style soft cheese, shrimp, butter, raw vegetables, and pasteurized milk. Additionally, outside the U.S., shellfish, raw fish, smoked seafood, pork tongue, cream, rice salad, coleslaw, soft cheeses, pâté, rillettes, unpasteurized milk, and butter were associated with outbreaks of listeriosis.

How does L. monocytogenes survive in ready-to-eat foods?

L. monocytogenes is a remarkably tough organism. It resists heat, salt, nitrite and acidity much better than many organisms. This bacterium survives on cold surfaces and also can multiply slowly at 0°C

(32°F), defeating one traditional food safety defense—refrigeration. Optimal refrigeration temperatures of 40°F (4.4°C) or below stops the multiplication of most other foodborne bacteria. Refrigeration does not kill most bacteria. The risk from *L. monocytogenes* in foods that support its growth is increased substantially when such foods are stored in refrigerators that are too warm (at temperatures above 40°F) or when foods are stored for extended periods.

Commercial freezer temperatures of 0°F (-18°C) stop *L. monocytogenes* from multiplying.

What advice do you give to consumers to reduce their risk of contracting listeriosis?

Because *Listeria monocytogenes* can grow at refrigerator temperatures the U.S. Food and Drug Administration (FDA) and the U.S. Department of Agriculture's Food Safety and Inspection Service (FSIS) advise all consumers to reduce the risk of illness by:

- Using a refrigerator thermometer to make sure that the refrigerator always stays at 40 degrees F or below.

- Using perishable items that are precooked or ready-to-eat as soon as possible.

The following additional advice is provided for pregnant women, older adults, and people with weakened immune systems who are at a higher risk for foodborne disease, including listeriosis:

- Do not eat hot dogs and luncheon meats, unless they are reheated until steaming hot.

- Do not eat soft cheese such as Feta, Brie, and Camembert cheeses, blue-veined cheeses, queso blanco, queso fresco, and Panela unless it is labeled as made with pasteurized milk.

- Do not eat refrigerated smoked seafood, unless it is contained in a cooked dish, such as a casserole. Refrigerated smoked seafood, such as salmon, trout, whitefish, cod, tuna, or mackerel, is most often labeled as "nova-style," "lox," "kippered," "smoked," or "jerky." The fish is found in the refrigerator section or sold at deli counters of grocery stores and delicatessens. Canned or shelf-stable smoked seafood may be eaten.

- Do not drink raw (unpasteurized) milk or eat foods that contain unpasteurized milk.

What has been the trend in the incidence of foodborne listeriosis over the past several years.

The Centers for Disease Control and Prevention has been evaluating the incidence of foodborne listeriosis since 1996 through its FoodNet active foodborne disease surveillance program. The program has shown a decline in the incidence of *Listeria monocytogenes* infections of approximately 40% during the period from 1996 to 2002, and further improvements are anticipated. The improvement in public health appears to be the direct result of changes instituted by the food industry and new regulatory initiatives developed by the FDA and the FSIS. With this progress, the regulatory agencies are on target for meeting the Administration's Healthy People 2010 goal of reducing the incidence of foodborne listeriosis by 50%.

Where can I purchase a refrigerator thermometer and are they expensive?

Refrigerator thermometers are available for purchase at grocery stores, department stores, kitchen stores, on the internet and a variety of other places. The cost generally ranges from $2 to $20 depending on the type of thermometer purchased.

The Listeria Risk Assessment

Why did FDA and FSIS conduct a risk assessment of L. monocytogenes?

FDA's risk assessment, conducted with FSIS and the Centers for Disease Control and Prevention, was designed to predict the potential relative risk of listeriosis from eating certain ready-to-eat foods among three age-based groups of people—perinatal (16 weeks after fertilization to 30 days after birth), elderly (60 years of age and older), and intermediate-age (general population, less than 60 years of age). This assessment evaluated foods within 23 categories considered to be principal potential sources of *Listeria*. The results of this assessment will assist both FDA and FSIS in the evaluation of the adequacy and focus of current programs, help in the development of new programs to ensure that these programs protect the public health and to evaluate the effectiveness of new strategies to minimize the public health impact of food-borne *Listeria*.

How were the food categories selected for the risk assessment?

Scientific and medical literature were reviewed to identify foods associated with *Listeria monocytogenes*. The published and unpublished literature included studies on outbreaks, sporadic cases, and food surveys. The identified foods were grouped into categories within five commodity groups including seafood, produce, dairy, meats, and combination foods (mainly salads that are composed of a mixture of ingredients, such as meat, poultry, seafood, egg and pasta).

What are the conclusions of the risk assessment?

The main findings from the risk assessment are:

- The risk assessment reinforces past conclusions that foodborne listeriosis is a moderately rare although severe disease.

- The risk assessment supports the findings of epidemiological investigations of both sporadic illness and outbreaks of listeriosis, for example, pâté, fresh soft cheeses, smoked seafood, frankfurters, and foods typically purchased from deli counters as potential vehicles of listeriosis for susceptible populations.

- New case control studies and other advanced epidemiological investigations are needed to reflect changes in food processing, distribution patterns, preparation, and consumption practices.

- From the exposure models and "what-if scenarios", it is apparent that five factors affect consumer exposure to *L. monocytogenes* at the time of food consumption: #1) Amount and frequency of consumption of a food; #2) Frequency and levels of L. monocytogenes in ready-to-eat food; #3) Potential to support growth of *L. monocytogenes* in food during refrigerated storage; #4) Refrigerated storage temperature; and #5) Duration of refrigerated storage before consumption.

Why has there been change in the advice to consumers relative to soft cheeses?

The risk assessment includes substantial new data from surveys of soft cheeses at retail and from outbreaks of listeriosis associated with these food categories. This new information indicates that the consumers' risk of listeriosis from soft cheeses, such as queso blanco, queso fresco, Panela, Camembert, Feta, Brie, and blue-veined cheeses, is primarily associated with cheeses made from unpasteurized milk. Thus, the consumer who wants to eat soft cheeses should make a healthy food choice by purchasing only those soft cheeses that are clearly labeled as being made from pasteurized milk.

Chapter 16

Shigellosis

What is shigellosis?

Shigellosis is an infectious disease caused by a group of bacteria called *Shigella*. Most who are infected with *Shigella* develop diarrhea, fever, and stomach cramps starting a day or two after they are exposed to the bacterium. The diarrhea is often bloody. Shigellosis usually resolves in 5 to 7 days. In some persons, especially young children and the elderly, the diarrhea can be so severe that the patient needs to be hospitalized. A severe infection with high fever may also be associated with seizures in children less than 2 years old. Some persons who are infected may have no symptoms at all, but may still pass the *Shigella* bacteria to others.

What sort of germ is Shigella?

The *Shigella* germ is actually a family of bacteria that can cause diarrhea in humans. They are microscopic living creatures that pass from person to person. *Shigella* were discovered over 100 years ago by a Japanese scientist named Shiga, for whom they are named. There are several different kinds of *Shigella* bacteria: *Shigella sonnei*, also known as "Group D" *Shigella*, accounts for over two-thirds of the shigellosis in the United States. A second type, *Shigella flexneri*, or "group B" *Shigella*, accounts for almost all of the rest. Other types of

"Shigellosis," Division of Bacterial and Mycotic Diseases, Centers for Disease Control and Prevention (CDC), reviewed March 7, 2003.

Shigella are rare in this country, though they continue to be important causes of disease in the developing world. One type found in the developing world, *Shigella dysenteriae* type 1, causes deadly epidemics there.

How can **Shigella** *infections be diagnosed?*

Many different kinds of diseases can cause diarrhea and bloody diarrhea, and the treatment depends on which germ is causing the diarrhea. Determining that *Shigella* is the cause of the illness depends on laboratory tests that identify *Shigella* in the stools of an infected person. These tests are sometimes not performed unless the laboratory is instructed specifically to look for the organism. The laboratory can also do special tests to tell which type of *Shigella* the person has and which antibiotics, if any, would be best to treat it.

How can **Shigella** *infections be treated?*

Shigellosis can usually be treated with antibiotics. The antibiotics commonly used for treatment are ampicillin, trimethoprim/sulfamethoxazole (also known as Bactrim* or Septra*), nalidixic acid, or ciprofloxacin. Appropriate treatment kills the *Shigella* bacteria that might be present in the patient's stools, and shortens the illness. Unfortunately, some *Shigella* bacteria have become resistant to antibiotics and using antibiotics to treat shigellosis can actually make the germs more resistant in the future. Persons with mild infections will usually recover quickly without antibiotic treatment. Therefore, when many persons in a community are affected by shigellosis, antibiotics are sometimes used selectively to treat only the more severe cases. Antidiarrheal agents such as loperamide (Imodium*) or diphenoxylate with atropine (Lomotil*) are likely to make the illness worse and should be avoided.

Are there long term consequences to a **Shigella** *infection?*

Persons with diarrhea usually recover completely, although it may be several months before their bowel habits are entirely normal. About 3% of persons who are infected with one type of *Shigella*, *Shigella flexneri*, will later develop pains in their joints, irritation of the eyes, and painful urination. This is called Reiter's syndrome. It can last for months or years, and can lead to chronic arthritis which is difficult to treat. Reiter's syndrome is caused by a reaction to *Shigella* infection that happens only in people who are genetically predisposed to it.

Once someone has had shigellosis, they are not likely to get infected with that specific type again for at least several years. However, they can still get infected with other types of *Shigella*.

How do people catch **Shigella?**

The *Shigella* bacteria pass from one infected person to the next. *Shigella* are present in the diarrheal stools of infected persons while they are sick and for a week or two afterwards. Most *Shigella* infections are the result of the bacterium passing from stools or soiled fingers of one person to the mouth of another person. This happens when basic hygiene and handwashing habits are inadequate. It is particularly likely to occur among toddlers who are not fully toilet-trained. Family members and playmates of such children are at high risk of becoming infected.

Shigella infections may be acquired from eating contaminated food. Contaminated food may look and smell normal. Food may become contaminated by infected food handlers who forget to wash their hands with soap after using the bathroom. Vegetables can become contaminated if they are harvested from a field with sewage in it. Flies can breed in infected feces and then contaminate food. *Shigella* infections can also be acquired by drinking or swimming in contaminated water. Water may become contaminated if sewage runs into it, or if someone with shigellosis swims in it.

What can a person do to prevent this illness?

There is no vaccine to prevent shigellosis. However, the spread of *Shigella* from an infected person to other persons can be stopped by frequent and careful handwashing with soap. Frequent and careful handwashing is important among all age groups. Frequent, supervised handwashing of all children should be followed in day care centers and in homes with children who are not completely toilet-trained (including children in diapers). When possible, young children with a *Shigella* infection who are still in diapers should not be in contact with uninfected children.

People who have shigellosis should not prepare food or pour water for others until they have been shown to no longer be carrying the *Shigella* bacterium.

If a child in diapers has shigellosis, everyone who changes the child's diapers should be sure the diapers are disposed of properly in a closed-lid garbage can, and should wash his or her hands carefully with soap and warm water immediately after changing the diapers.

After use, the diaper changing area should be wiped down with a disinfectant such as household bleach, Lysol* or bactericidal wipes.

Basic food safety precautions and regular drinking water treatment prevents shigellosis. At swimming beaches, having enough bathrooms near the swimming area helps keep the water from becoming contaminated.

Simple precautions taken while traveling to the developing world can prevent getting shigellosis. Drink only treated or boiled water, and eat only cooked hot foods or fruits you peel yourself. The same precautions prevent traveler's diarrhea in general.

How common is shigellosis?

Every year, about 18,000 cases of shigellosis are reported in the United States. Because many milder cases are not diagnosed or reported, the actual number of infections may be twenty times greater. Shigellosis is particularly common and causes recurrent problems in settings where hygiene is poor and can sometimes sweep through entire communities. Shigellosis is more common in summer than winter. Children, especially toddlers aged 2 to 4, are the most likely to get shigellosis. Many cases are related to the spread of illness in childcare settings, and many more are the result of the spread of the illness in families with small children.

In the developing world, shigellosis is far more common and is present in most communities most of the time.

What else can be done to prevent shigellosis?

It is important for the public health department to know about cases of shigellosis. It is important for clinical laboratories to send isolates of *Shigella* to the City, County, or State Public Health Laboratory so the specific type can be determined and compared to other *Shigella*. If many cases occur at the same time, it may mean that a restaurant, food, or water supply has a problem which needs correction by the public health department. If a number of cases occur in a day-care center, the public health department may need to coordinate efforts to improve handwashing among the staff, children, and their families. When a community-wide outbreak occurs, a community-wide approach to promote handwashing and basic hygiene among children can stop the outbreak. Improvements in hygiene for vegetables and fruit picking and packing may prevent shigellosis caused by contaminated produce.

Some prevention steps occur everyday, without you thinking about it. Making municipal water supplies safe and treating sewage are highly effective prevention measures that have been in place for many years.

What is the government doing about shigellosis?

The Centers for Disease Control and Prevention (CDC) monitors the frequency of *Shigella* infections in the country, and assists local and State health departments to investigate outbreaks, determine means of transmission, and devise control measures. CDC also conducts research to better understand how to identify and treat shigellosis. The Food and Drug Administration inspects imported foods and promotes better food preparation techniques in restaurants and food processing plants. The Environmental Protection Agency regulates and monitors the safety of our drinking water supplies. The government has also maintained active research into the development of a *Shigella* vaccine.

How can I learn more about this and other public health problems?

You can discuss any medical concerns you may have with your doctor or other heath care provider. Your local city or county health department can provide more information about this and other public health problems that are occurring in your area. General information about the public health of the nation is published every week in the *Morbidity and Mortality Weekly Report*, by the CDC in Atlanta, GA. Epidemiologists in your local and State Health Departments are tracking a number of important public health problems, investigating special problems that arise, and helping to prevent them form occurring in the first place, or from spreading if they do occur.

Some Tips for Preventing the Spread of Shigellosis

- wash hands with soap carefully and frequently, especially after going to the bathroom, after changing diapers, and before preparing foods or beverages
- dispose of soiled diapers properly
- disinfect diaper changing areas after using them
- keep children with diarrhea out of child care settings

- supervise handwashing of toddlers and small children after they use the toilet

- persons with diarrheal illness should not prepare food for others

- if you are traveling to the developing world, "boil it, cook it, peel it, or forget it"

- avoid drinking pool water

Chapter 17

Salmonellosis

What is salmonellosis?

Salmonellosis is an infection with a bacteria called *Salmonella*. Most persons infected with *Salmonella* develop diarrhea, fever, and abdominal cramps 12 to 72 hours after infection. The illness usually lasts 4 to 7 days, and most persons recover without treatment. However, in some persons the diarrhea may be so severe that the patient needs to be hospitalized. In these patients, the *Salmonella* infection may spread from the intestines to the blood stream, and then to other body sites and can cause death unless the person is treated promptly with antibiotics. The elderly, infants, and those with impaired immune systems are more likely to have a severe illness.

What sort of germ is Salmonella?

The *Salmonella* germ is actually a group of bacteria that can cause diarrheal illness in humans. They are microscopic living creatures that pass from the feces of people or animals, to other people or other animals. There are many different kinds of *Salmonella* bacteria. *Salmonella* serotype *Typhimurium* and *Salmonella* serotype *Enteritidis* are the most common in the United States. *Salmonella* has been known to cause illness for over 100 years. They were discovered by a American scientist named Salmon, for whom they are named.

"Salmonellosis," Division of Bacterial and Mycotic Diseases, Centers for Disease Control and Prevention (CDC), reviewed June 9, 2003.

How can Salmonella *infections be diagnosed?*

Many different kinds of illnesses can cause diarrhea, fever, or abdominal cramps. Determining that *Salmonella* is the cause of the illness depends on laboratory tests that identify *Salmonella* in the stools of an infected person. These tests are sometimes not performed unless the laboratory is instructed specifically to look for the organism. Once *Salmonella* has been identified, further testing can determine its specific type, and which antibiotics could be used to treat it.

How can Salmonella *infections be treated?*

Salmonella infections usually resolve in 5–7 days and often do not require treatment unless the patient becomes severely dehydrated or the infection spreads from the intestines. Persons with severe diarrhea may require rehydration, often with intravenous fluids. Antibiotics are not usually necessary unless the infection spreads from the intestines, then it can be treated with ampicillin, gentamicin, trimethoprim/sulfamethoxazole, or ciprofloxacin. Unfortunately, some *Salmonella* bacteria have become resistant to antibiotics, largely as a result of the use of antibiotics to promote the growth of feed animals.

Are there long term consequences to a Salmonella *infection?*

Persons with diarrhea usually recover completely, although it may be several months before their bowel habits are entirely normal. A small number of persons who are infected with *Salmonella*, will go on to develop pains in their joints, irritation of the eyes, and painful urination. This is called Reiter's syndrome. It can last for months or years, and can lead to chronic arthritis which is difficult to treat. Antibiotic treatment does not make a difference in whether or not the person later develops arthritis.

How do people catch Salmonella?

Salmonella live in the intestinal tracts of humans and other animals, including birds. Salmonella are usually transmitted to humans by eating foods contaminated with animal feces. Contaminated foods usually look and smell normal. Contaminated foods are often of animal origin, such as beef, poultry, milk, or eggs, but all foods, including vegetables may become contaminated. Many raw foods of animal origin are frequently contaminated, but fortunately, thorough cooking kills *Salmonella*. Food may also become contaminated by the unwashed hands of an infected food handler, who forgot to wash his or her hands with soap after using the bathroom.

Salmonella may also be found in the feces of some pets, especially those with diarrhea, and people can become infected if they do not wash their hands after contact with these feces. Reptiles are particularly likely to harbor *Salmonella* and people should always wash their hands immediately after handling a reptile, even if the reptile is healthy. Adults should also be careful that children wash their hands after handling a reptile.

What can a person do to prevent this illness?

There is no vaccine to prevent salmonellosis. Since foods of animal origin may be contaminated with *Salmonella*, people should not eat raw or undercooked eggs, poultry, or meat. Raw eggs may be unrecognized in some foods such as homemade hollandaise sauce, caesar and other salad dressings, tiramisu, homemade ice cream, homemade mayonnaise, cookie dough, and frostings. Poultry and meat, including hamburgers, should be well-cooked, not pink in the middle. Persons also should not consume raw or unpasteurized milk or other dairy products. Produce should be thoroughly washed before consuming.

Cross-contamination of foods should be avoided. Uncooked meats should be keep separate from produce, cooked foods, and ready-to-eat foods. Hands, cutting boards, counters, knives, and other utensils should be washed thoroughly after handling uncooked foods. Hands should be washed before handling any food, and between handling different food items.

People who have salmonellosis should not prepare food or pour water for others until they have been shown to no longer be carrying the *Salmonella* bacterium.

People should wash their hands after contact with animal feces. Since reptiles are particularly likely to have *Salmonella*, everyone should immediately wash their hands after handling reptiles. Reptiles (including turtles) are not appropriate pets for small children and should not be in the same house as an infant.

How common is salmonellosis?

Every year, approximately 40,000 cases of salmonellosis are reported in the United States. Because many milder cases are not diagnosed or reported, the actual number of infections may be thirty or more times greater. Salmonellosis is more common in the summer than winter.

Children are the most likely to get salmonellosis. Young children, the elderly, and the immunocompromised are the most likely to have severe infections. It is estimated that approximately 600 persons die each year with acute salmonellosis.

What else can be done to prevent salmonellosis?

It is important for the public health department to know about cases of salmonellosis. It is important for clinical laboratories to send isolates of *Salmonella* to the City, County, or State Public Health Laboratories so the specific type can be determined and compared with other *Salmonella* in the community. If many cases occur at the same time, it may mean that a restaurant, food, or water supply has a problem which needs correction by the public health department.

Some prevention steps occur everyday without you thinking about it. Pasteurization of milk and treating municipal water supplies are highly effective prevention measures that have been in place for many years. In the 1970s, small pet turtles were a common source of salmonellosis in the United States, and in 1975, the sale of small turtles was halted in this country. Improvements in farm animal hygiene, in slaughter plant practices, and in vegetable and fruit harvesting and packing operations may help prevent salmonellosis caused by contaminated foods. Better education of food industry workers in basic food safety and restaurant inspection procedures, may prevent cross-contamination and other food handling errors that can lead to outbreaks. Wider use of pasteurized egg in restaurants, hospitals, and nursing homes is an important prevention measure. In the future, irradiation or other treatments may greatly reduce contamination of raw meat.

What is the government doing about salmonellosis?

The Centers for Disease Control and Prevention (CDC) monitors the frequency of *Salmonella* infections in the country and assists the local and State Health Departments to investigate outbreaks and devise control measures. CDC also conducts research to better identify specific types of *Salmonella*. The Food and Drug Administration inspects imported foods, milk pasteurization plants, promotes better food preparation techniques in restaurants and food processing plants, and regulates the sale of turtles. The FDA also regulates the use of specific antibiotics as growth promotants in food animals. The U.S. Department of Agriculture monitors the health of food animals, inspects egg pasteurization plants, and is responsible for the quality of slaughtered and processed meat. The U.S. Environmental Protection Agency regulates and monitors the safety of our drinking water supplies.

How can I learn more about this and other public health problems?

You can discuss any medical concerns you may have with your doctor or other heath care provider. Your local City or County Health Department can provide more information about this and other public health problems that are occurring in your area. General information about the public health of the nation is published every week in the *Morbidity and Mortality Weekly Report*, by the CDC in Atlanta, GA. Epidemiologists in your local and State Health Departments are tracking a number of important public health problems, investigating special problems that arise, and helping to prevent them from occurring in the first place, or from spreading if they do occur.

What can I do to prevent salmonellosis?

- Cook poultry, ground beef, and eggs thoroughly before eating. Do not eat or drink foods containing raw eggs, or raw unpasteurized milk.

- If you are served undercooked meat, poultry or eggs in a restaurant, don't hesitate to send it back to the kitchen for further cooking.

- Wash hands, kitchen work surfaces, and utensils with soap and water immediately after they have been in contact with raw meat or poultry.

- Be particularly careful with foods prepared for infants, the elderly, and the immunocompromised.

- Wash hands with soap after handling reptiles or birds, or after contact with pet feces.

- Avoid direct or even indirect contact between reptiles (turtles, iguanas, other lizards, snakes) and infants or immunocompromised persons.

- Don't work with raw poultry or meat, and an infant (e.g., feed, change diaper) at the same time.

- Mother's milk is the safest food for young infants. Breast-feeding prevents salmonellosis and many other health problems.

Chapter 18

Travelers' Diarrhea

Who gets travelers' diarrhea?

Travelers' diarrhea (TD) is the most common illness affecting travelers. Each year between 20%–50% of international travelers, an estimated 10 million persons, develop diarrhea. The onset of TD usually occurs within the first week of travel but may occur at any time while traveling, and even after returning home. The most important determinant of risk is the traveler's destination. High-risk destinations are the developing countries of Latin America, Africa, the Middle East, and Asia. Persons at particular high-risk include young adults, immunosuppressed persons, persons with inflammatory-bowel disease, or diabetes, and persons taking H-2 blockers or antacids. Attack rates are similar for men and women. The primary source of infection is ingestion of fecally contaminated food or water.

What are common symptoms of travelers' diarrhea?

Most TD cases begin abruptly. The illness usually results in increased frequency, volume, and weight of stool. Altered stool consistency also is common. Typically, a traveler experiences four to five loose or watery bowel movements each day. Other commonly associated symptoms are nausea, vomiting, diarrhea, abdominal cramping, bloating, fever, urgency, and malaise. Most cases are benign and resolve in

"Travelers' Diarrhea," Division of Bacterial and Mycotic Diseases, Centers for Disease Control and Prevention (CDC), reviewed July 27, 2000.

1–2 days without treatment. TD is rarely life-threatening. The natural history of TD is that 90% of cases resolve within 1 week, and 98% resolve within 1 month.

What causes travelers' diarrhea?

Infectious agents are the primary cause of TD. Bacterial enteropathogens cause approximately 80% of TD cases. The most common causative agent isolated in countries surveyed has been enterotoxigenic *Escherichia coli* (ETEC). ETEC produce watery diarrhea with associated cramps and low-grade or no fever. Besides ETEC and other bacterial pathogens, a variety of viral and parasitic enteric pathogens also are potential causative agents.

What preventive measures are effective for travelers' diarrhea?

Travelers can minimize their risk for TD by practicing the following effective preventive measures:

- Avoid eating foods or drinking beverages purchased from street vendors or other establishments where unhygienic conditions are present.

- Avoid eating raw or undercooked meat and seafood.

- Avoid eating raw fruits (e.g., oranges, bananas, avocados) and vegetables unless the traveler peels them.

If handled properly, well-cooked and packaged foods usually are safe. Tap water, ice, unpasteurized milk, and dairy products are associated with increased risk for TD. Safe beverages include bottled carbonated beverages, hot tea or coffee, beer, wine, and water boiled or appropriately treated with iodine or chlorine.

Is prophylaxis of travelers' diarrhea recommended?

CDC does not recommend antimicrobial drugs to prevent TD. Studies show a decrease in the incidence of TD with use of bismuth subsalicylate and with use of antimicrobial chemoprophylaxis. Several studies show that bismuth subsalicylate taken as either 2 tablets 4 times daily or 2 fluid ounces 4 times daily reduces the incidence of travelers' diarrhea. The mechanism of action appears to be both antibacterial and antisecretory. Use of bismuth subsalicylate should be avoided by persons who are allergic to aspirin, during pregnancy, and by persons taking certain other medications (e.g., anticoagulants, probenecid, or methotrexate). In addition, persons should be informed about potential side effects, in particular about temporary blackening of the tongue and stool, and rarely, ringing in the ears. Because of potential adverse side effects, prophylactic bismuth subsalicylate should not be used for more than 3 weeks.

Some antibiotics administered in a once-a-day dose are 90% effective at preventing travelers' diarrhea; however, antibiotics are not recommended as prophylaxis. Routine antimicrobial prophylaxis increases the traveler's risk for adverse reactions and for infections with resistant organisms. Because antimicrobials can increase a traveler's susceptibility to resistant bacterial pathogens and provide no protection against either viral or parasitic pathogens, they can give travelers a false sense of security. As a result, strict adherence to preventive measures is encouraged, and bismuth subsalicylate should be used as an adjunct if prophylaxis is needed.

What treatment measures are effective for travelers' diarrhea?

TD usually is a self-limited disorder and often resolves without specific treatment; however, oral rehydration is often beneficial to replace lost fluids and electrolytes. Clear liquids are routinely recommended for adults. Travelers who develop three or more loose stools in an 8-hour period—especially if associated with nausea, vomiting, abdominal cramps, fever, or blood in stools—may benefit from antimicrobial therapy. Antibiotics usually are given for 3–5 days. Currently, fluoroquinolones are the drugs of choice. Commonly prescribed regimens are 500 mg of ciprofloxacin twice a day or 400 mg of norfloxacin twice a day for 3–5 days. Trimethoprim-sulfamethoxazole and doxycycline are no longer recommended because of the high level of resistance to these agents. Bismuth subsalicylate also may be used as treatment: 1 fluid ounce or two 262 mg tablets every 30 minutes for up to eight doses in a 24-hour period, which can be repeated on a second day. If diarrhea persists despite therapy, travelers should be evaluated by a doctor and treated for possible parasitic infection.

When should antimotility agents not be used to treat travelers' diarrhea?

Antimotility agents (loperamide, diphenoxylate, and paregoric) primarily reduce diarrhea by slowing transit time in the gut, and thus, allows more time for absorption. Some persons believe diarrhea is the body's defense mechanism to minimize contact time between gut pathogens and intestinal mucosa. In several studies, antimotility agents have been useful in treating travelers' diarrhea by decreasing the duration of diarrhea. However, these agents should never be used by persons with fever or bloody diarrhea, because they can increase the severity of disease by delaying clearance of causative organisms. Because antimotility agents are now available over the counter, their injudicious use is of concern. Adverse complications (toxic megacolon, sepsis, and disseminated intravascular coagulation) have been reported as a result of using these medications to treat diarrhea.

What is CDC doing to prevent travelers' diarrhea?

CDC, in collaboration with the World Health Organization and several Ministries of Health, is working to improve food and water safety around the world. CDC also investigates risk factors associated with acquisition of TD, to assist in identifying more effective preventive measures. CDC continues to monitor antimicrobial resistance in other countries and in the United States. In addition, CDC, in collaboration with international agencies, is working to improve sanitary conditions in foreign accommodations (e.g., tourist resorts) and frequently consults with travel medicine specialists and local and state health departments. CDC is responsible for evaluating sanitation on cruise ships docking in US ports.

Please visit CDC's Traveler's Health site for more information about the vessel sanitation program and for a summary of recent vessel inspections.

How can I learn more about travelers' diarrhea?

Potential travelers should consult with a doctor or a travel medicine specialist before departing on a trip abroad. Information about TD is available from your local or state health departments or the World Health Organization (WHO).

Other information that may be of interest to travelers can be found at the CDC Travelers' Health homepage at http://www.cdc.gov/travel.

Chapter 19

Trichinellosis

What is Trichinellosis?

Trichinellosis, also called trichinosis (TRICK-a-NO-sis), is caused by eating raw or undercooked pork and wild game products infected with the larvae of a species of worm called *Trichinella*. Infection occurs worldwide, but is most common in areas where raw or undercooked pork, such as ham or sausage, is eaten.

What are the symptoms of a trichinellosis infection?

Nausea, diarrhea, vomiting, fatigue, fever, and abdominal discomfort are the first symptoms of trichinellosis. Headaches, fevers, chills, cough, eye swelling, aching joints and muscle pains, itchy skin, diarrhea, or constipation follow the first symptoms. If the infection is heavy, patients may experience difficulty coordinating movements, and have heart and breathing problems. In severe cases, death can occur.

For mild to moderate infections, most symptoms subside within a few months. Fatigue, weakness, and diarrhea may last for months.

How soon after infection will symptoms appear?

Abdominal symptoms can occur 1–2 days after infection. Further symptoms usually start 2–8 weeks after eating contaminated meat.

"Trichinellosis," Division of Parasitic Diseases, Centers for Disease Control and Prevention (CDC), reviewed January 18, 2003.

Symptoms may range from very mild to severe and relate to the number of infectious worms consumed in meat. Often, mild cases of trichinellosis are never specifically diagnosed and are assumed to be the flu or other common illnesses.

How does infection occur in humans and animals?

When a human or animal eats meat that contains infective *Trichinella* cysts, the acid in the stomach dissolves the hard covering of the cyst and releases the worms. The worms pass into the small intestine and, in 1–2 days, become mature. After mating, adult females lay eggs. Eggs develop into immature worms, travel through the arteries, and are transported to muscles. Within the muscles, the worms curl into a ball and encyst (become enclosed in a capsule). Infection occurs when these encysted worms are consumed in meat.

Am I at risk for trichinellosis?

If you eat raw or undercooked meats, particularly pork, bear, wild feline (such as a cougar), fox, dog, wolf, horse, seal, or walrus, you are at risk for trichinellosis.

Can I spread trichinellosis to others?

No. Infection can only occur by eating raw or undercooked meat containing *Trichinella* worms.

What should I do if I think I have trichinellosis?

See your health care provider who can order tests and treat symptoms of trichinellosis infection. If you have eaten raw or undercooked meat, you should tell your health care provider.

How is trichinellosis infection diagnosed?

A blood test or muscle biopsy can show if you have trichinellosis.

How is trichinellosis infection treated?

Several safe and effective prescription drugs are available to treat trichinellosis. Treatment should begin as soon as possible and the decision to treat is based upon symptoms, exposure to raw or undercooked meat, and laboratory test results.

Is trichinellosis common in the United States?

Infection was once very common; however, infection is now relatively rare. From 1991–1996, an annual average of 38 cases per year were reported. The number of cases has decreased because of legislation prohibiting the feeding of raw meat garbage to hogs, commercial and home freezing of pork, and the public awareness of the danger of eating raw or undercooked pork products. Cases are less commonly associated with pork products and more often associated with eating raw or undercooked wild game meats.

How can I prevent trichinellosis?

- Cook meat products until the juices run clear or to an internal temperature of 170° F.

- Freeze pork less than 6 inches thick for 20 days at 5° F to kill any worms.

- Cook wild game meat thoroughly. Freezing wild game meats, unlike freezing pork products, even for long periods of time, may not effectively kill all worms.

- Cook all meat fed to pigs or other wild animals.

- Do not allow hogs to eat uncooked carcasses of other animals, including rats, which may be infected with trichinellosis.

- Clean meat grinders thoroughly if you prepare your own ground meats.

Curing (salting), drying, smoking, or microwaving meat does not consistently kill infective worms.

For More Information

1. Centers for Disease Control. Trichinosis Surveillance, United States, 1987-1990, *MMWR* 1991;40:(SS-3)35-42.

2. Moorhead A, Grunenwald PE, Dietz VJ, Schantz PM. Trichinellosis in the United States, 1991-1996: Declining but not gone. *Am J Trop Med Hyg* 1999; 60:66-69.

Chapter 20

Typhoid Fever

Typhoid fever is a life-threatening illness caused by the bacterium *Salmonella typhi*. In the United States about 400 cases occur each year, and 70% of these are acquired while traveling internationally. Typhoid fever is still common in the developing world, where it affects about 12.5 million persons each year.

Typhoid fever can be prevented and can usually be treated with antibiotics. If you are planning to travel outside the United States, you should know about typhoid fever and what steps you can take to protect yourself.

How is typhoid fever spread?

Salmonella typhi lives only in humans. Persons with typhoid fever carry the bacteria in their bloodstream and intestinal tract. In addition, a small number of persons, called carriers, recover from typhoid fever but continue to carry the bacteria. Both ill persons and carriers shed *S. typhi* in their feces (stool).

You can get typhoid fever if you eat food or drink beverages that have been handled by a person who is shedding *S. typhi* or if sewage contaminated with *S. typhi* bacteria gets into the water you use for drinking or washing food. Therefore, typhoid fever is more common

"Typhoid Fever," Division of Bacterial and Mycotic Diseases, Centers for Disease Control and Prevention (CDC), reviewed June 20, 2001. For the most current updates about typhoid fever, please visit CDC Travelers' Health at http://www.cdc.gov/travel/diseases/typhoid.htm

in areas of the world where handwashing is less frequent and water is likely to be contaminated with sewage.

Once *S. typhi* bacteria are eaten or drunk, they multiply and spread into the bloodstream. The body reacts with fever and other signs and symptoms.

Where in the world do you get typhoid fever?

Typhoid fever is common in most parts of the world except in industrialized regions such as the United States, Canada, western Europe, Australia, and Japan. Therefore, if you are traveling to the developing world, you should consider taking precautions. Over the past 10 years, travelers from the United States to Asia, Africa, and Latin America have been especially at risk.

How can you avoid typhoid fever?

Two basic actions can protect you from typhoid fever:

1. Avoid risky foods and drinks.

2. Get vaccinated against typhoid fever.

It may surprise you, but watching what you eat and drink when you travel is as important as being vaccinated. This is because the vaccines are not completely effective. Avoiding risky foods will also help protect you from other illnesses, including travelers' diarrhea, cholera, dysentery, and hepatitis A.

"Boil It, Cook It, Peel It, or Forget It"

- If you drink water, buy it bottled or bring it to a rolling boil for one minute before you drink it. Bottled carbonated water is safer than uncarbonated water.

- Ask for drinks without ice unless the ice is made from bottled or boiled water. Avoid popsicles and flavored ices that may have been made with contaminated water.

- Eat foods that have been thoroughly cooked and that are still hot and steaming.

- Avoid raw vegetables and fruits that cannot be peeled. Vegetables like lettuce are easily contaminated and are very hard to wash well.

- When you eat raw fruit or vegetables that can be peeled, peel them yourself. (Wash your hands with soap first.) Do not eat the peelings.

- Avoid foods and beverages from street vendors. It is difficult for food to be kept clean on the street, and many travelers get sick from food bought from street vendors.

Getting Vaccinated

If you are traveling to a country where typhoid is common, you should consider being vaccinated against typhoid. Visit a doctor or travel clinic to discuss your vaccination options.

Remember that you will need to complete your vaccination at least 1 week before you travel so that the vaccine has time to take effect. Typhoid vaccines lose effectiveness after several years; if you were vaccinated in the past, check with your doctor to see if it is time for a booster vaccination. Taking antibiotics will not prevent typhoid fever; they only help treat it.

Table 20.1 provides basic information on typhoid vaccines that are available in the United States.

The parenteral heat-phenol-inactivated vaccine (manufactured by Wyeth-Ayerst) has been discontinued.

Table 20.1. Typhoid vaccines available in the United States.

Vaccine Name: Ty21a (Vivotif Berna, Swiss Serum and Vaccine Institute)
  How given: 1 capsule by mouth
  Number of doses necessary: 4
  Time between doses: 2 days
  Total time needed to set aside for vaccination: 2 weeks
  Minimum age for vaccination: 6 years
  Booster needed every: 5 years

Vaccine Name: ViCPS (Typhim Vi, Pasteur Merieux)
  How given: Injection
  Number of doses necessary: 1
  Time between doses: N/A
  Total time needed to set aside for vaccination: 1 week
  Minimum age for vaccination: 2 years
  Booster needed every: 2 years

What are the signs and symptoms of typhoid fever?

Persons with typhoid fever usually have a sustained fever as high as 103° to 104° F (39° to 40° C). They may also feel weak, or have stomach pains, headache, or loss of appetite. In some cases, patients have a rash of flat, rose-colored spots. The only way to know for sure if an illness is typhoid fever is to have samples of stool or blood tested for the presence of *S. typhi*.

What do you do if you think you have typhoid fever?

If you suspect you have typhoid fever, see a doctor immediately. If you are traveling in a foreign country, you can usually call the U.S. consulate for a list of recommended doctors.

You will probably be given an antibiotic to treat the disease. Three commonly prescribed antibiotics are ampicillin, trimethoprim-sulfamethoxazole, and ciprofloxacin. Persons given antibiotics usually begin to feel better within 2 to 3 days, and deaths rarely occur. However, persons who do not get treatment may continue to have fever for weeks or months, and as many as 20% may die from complications of the infection.

Typhoid Fever's Danger Doesn't End When Symptoms Disappear

Even if your symptoms seem to go away, you may still be carrying *S. typhi*. If so, the illness could return, or you could pass the disease to other people. In fact, if you work at a job where you handle food or care for small children, you may be barred legally from going back to work until a doctor has determined that you no longer carry any typhoid bacteria.

If you are being treated for typhoid fever, it is important to do the following:

- Keep taking the prescribed antibiotics for as long as the doctor has asked you to take them.

- Wash your hands carefully with soap and water after using the bathroom, and do not prepare or serve food for other people. This will lower the chance that you will pass the infection on to someone else.

- Have your doctor perform a series of stool cultures to ensure that no *S. typhi* bacteria remain in your body.

Chapter 21

Vibrio Diseases

*Cholera (*Vibrio cholerae*)*

In January 1991, epidemic cholera appeared in South America and quickly spread to several countries. A few cases have occurred in the United States among persons who traveled to South America or ate contaminated food brought back by travelers.

Cholera has been very rare in industrialized nations for the last 100 years; however, the disease is still common today in other parts of the world, including the Indian subcontinent and sub-Saharan Africa.

Although cholera can be life-threatening, it is easily prevented and treated. In the United States, because of advanced water and sanitation systems, cholera is not a major threat; however, everyone, especially travelers, should be aware of how the disease is transmitted and what can be done to prevent it.

What is cholera?

Cholera is an acute, diarrheal illness caused by infection of the intestine with the bacterium *Vibrio cholerae*. The infection is often mild or without symptoms, but sometimes it can be severe. Approximately

"Cholera," reviewed June 20, 2001, "*Vibrio parahaemolyticus*," reviewed March 29, 2000, and "*Vibrio vulnificus*," reviewed March 29, 2000, Division for Bacterial and Mycotic Diseases, Centers for Disease Control and Prevention (CDC).

one in 20 infected persons has severe disease characterized by profuse watery diarrhea, vomiting, and leg cramps. In these persons, rapid loss of body fluids leads to dehydration and shock. Without treatment, death can occur within hours.

How does a person get cholera?

A person may get cholera by drinking water or eating food contaminated with the cholera bacterium. In an epidemic, the source of the contamination is usually the feces of an infected person. The disease can spread rapidly in areas with inadequate treatment of sewage and drinking water.

The cholera bacterium may also live in the environment in brackish rivers and coastal waters. Shellfish eaten raw have been a source of cholera, and a few persons in the United States have contracted cholera after eating raw or undercooked shellfish from the Gulf of Mexico. The disease is not likely to spread directly from one person to another; therefore, casual contact with an infected person is not a risk for becoming ill.

What is the risk for cholera in the United States?

In the United States, cholera was prevalent in the 1800s but has been virtually eliminated by modern sewage and water treatment systems. However, as a result of improved transportation, more persons from the United States travel to parts of Latin America, Africa, or Asia where epidemic cholera is occurring. U.S. travelers to areas with epidemic cholera may be exposed to the cholera bacterium. In addition, travelers may bring contaminated seafood back to the United States; foodborne outbreaks have been caused by contaminated seafood brought into this country by travelers.

What should travelers do to avoid getting cholera?

The risk for cholera is very low for U.S. travelers visiting areas with epidemic cholera. When simple precautions are observed, contracting the disease is unlikely.

All travelers to areas where cholera has occurred should observe the following recommendations:

- Drink only water that you have boiled or treated with chlorine or iodine. Other safe beverages include tea and coffee made with boiled water and carbonated, bottled beverages with no ice.

- Eat only foods that have been thoroughly cooked and are still hot, or fruit that you have peeled yourself.

- Avoid undercooked or raw fish or shellfish, including ceviche.

- Make sure all vegetables are cooked, avoid salads.

- Avoid foods and beverages from street vendors.

- Do not bring perishable seafood back to the United States.

A simple rule of thumb is "Boil it, cook it, peel it, or forget it."

Is a vaccine available to prevent cholera?

At the present time, the manufacture and sale of the only licensed cholera vaccine in the United States (Wyeth-Ayerst) has been discontinued. It has not been recommended for travelers because of the brief and incomplete immunity if offers. No cholera vaccination requirements exist for entry or exit in any country.

Two recently developed vaccines for cholera are licensed and available in other countries (Dukoral® from Biotec AB and Mutacol® from Berna). Both vaccines appear to provide a somewhat better immunity and fewer side-effects than the previously available vaccine. However, neither of these two vaccines is recommended for travelers nor are they available in the United States

Can cholera be treated?

Cholera can be simply and successfully treated by immediate replacement of the fluid and salts lost through diarrhea. Patients can be treated with oral rehydration solution, a prepackaged mixture of sugar and salts to be mixed with water and drunk in large amounts. This solution is used throughout the world to treat diarrhea. Severe cases also require intravenous fluid replacement. With prompt rehydration, fewer than 1% of cholera patients die.

Antibiotics shorten the course and diminish the severity of the illness, but they are not as important as rehydration. Persons who develop severe diarrhea and vomiting in countries where cholera occurs should seek medical attention promptly.

How long will the current epidemic last?

Predicting how long the epidemic in Latin America will last is difficult. The cholera epidemic in Africa has lasted more than 20 years.

In areas with inadequate sanitation, a cholera epidemic cannot be stopped immediately, and there are no signs that the epidemic in the Americas will end soon. Latin American countries that have not yet reported cases are still at risk for cholera in the coming months and years. Major improvements in sewage and water treatment systems are needed in many of these countries to prevent future epidemic cholera.

What is the U.S. government doing to combat cholera?

U.S. and international public health authorities are working to enhance surveillance for cholera, investigate cholera outbreaks, and design and implement preventive measures. The Centers for Disease Control is investigating epidemic cholera wherever it occurs and is training laboratory workers in proper techniques for identification of *V. cholerae*. In addition, the Centers for Disease Control is providing information on diagnosis, treatment, and prevention of cholera to public health officials and is educating the public about effective preventive measures.

The U.S. Agency for International Development is sponsoring some of the international government activities and is providing medical supplies to affected countries.

The Environmental Protection Agency is working with water and sewage treatment operators in the United States to prevent contamination of water with the cholera bacterium.

The Food and Drug Administration is testing imported and domestic shellfish for *V. cholerae* and monitoring the safety of U.S. shellfish beds through the shellfish sanitation program.

With cooperation at the state and local, national, and international levels, assistance will be provided to countries where cholera is present, and the risk to U.S. residents will remain small.

Where can a traveler get information about cholera?

The global picture of cholera changes periodically, so travelers should seek updated information on countries of interest. The Centers for Disease Control maintains a travelers' information telephone line on which callers can receive recent information on cholera and other diseases of concern to travelers. Data for this service are obtained from the World Health Organization. The number is 877-FYI-TRIP (394-8747) or check out http://www.cdc.gov/travel.

Vibrio parahaemolyticus

What is Vibrio parahaemolyticus?

Vibrio parahaemolyticus is a bacterium in the same family as those that cause cholera. It lives in brackish saltwater and causes gastrointestinal illness in humans. *V. parahaemolyticus* naturally inhabits coastal waters in the United States and Canada and is present in higher concentrations during summer; it is a halophilic, or salt-requiring organism.

What type of illness is caused by V. parahaemolyticus?

When ingested, *V. parahaemolyticus* causes watery diarrhea often with abdominal cramping, nausea, vomiting fever, and chills. Usually these symptoms occur within 24 hours of ingestion. Illness is usually self-limited and lasts 3 days. Severe disease is rare and occurs more commonly in persons with weakened immune systems. *V. parahaemolyticus* can also cause an infection of the skin when an open wound is exposed to warm seawater.

How does infection with V. parahaemolyticus *occur?*

Most people become infected by eating raw or undercooked shellfish, particularly oysters. Less commonly, this organism can cause an infection in the skin when an open wound is exposed to warm seawater.

How common is infection with V. parahaemolyticus?

In Asia, *V. parahaemolyticus* is a common cause of foodborne disease. In the United States, it is less commonly recognized as a cause of illness, partly because clinical laboratories rarely use the selective medium that is necessary to identify this organism. Not all states require that *V. parahaemolyticus* infections be reported to the state health department, but CDC collaborates with the Gulf Coast states of Alabama, Florida, Louisiana, and Texas to monitor the number of cases of Vibrio infection in this region. From those states, about 30–40 cases of *V. parahaemolyticus* infections are reported each year. The Foodborne Diseases Active Surveillance Network, Food Net, also tracks *V. parahaemolyticus* in regions outside the Gulf Coast. In 1997, the incidence of diagnosed *V. parahaemolyticus* infection in Food Net sites was 0.25/100,000.

How is V. parahaemolyticus *infection diagnosed?*

Vibrio organisms can be isolated from cultures of stool, wound, or blood. For isolation from stool, use of a selective medium that has thiosulfate, citrate, bile salts, and sucrose (TCBS agar) is recommended. If there is clinical suspicion for infection with this organism, the microbiology laboratory should be notified so that they will perform cultures using this medium. A physician should suspect *V. parahaemolyticus* infection if a patient has watery diarrhea and has eaten raw or undercooked seafood, especially oysters, or when a wound infection occurs after exposure to seawater.

How is V. parahaemolyticus *treated?*

Treatment is not necessary in most cases of *V. parahaemolyticus* infection. There is no evidence that antibiotic treatment decreases the severity or the length of the illness. Patients should drink plenty of liquids to replace fluids lost through diarrhea. In severe or prolonged illnesses, antibiotics such as tetracycline, ampicillin or ciprofloxacin can be used. The choice of antibiotics should be based on antimicrobial susceptibilities of the organism.

How do oysters get contaminated with V. parahaemolyticus?

Vibrio is a naturally occurring organism commonly found in waters where oysters are cultivated. When the appropriate conditions occur with regard to salt content and temperature, *V. parahaemolyticus* thrives.

How is V. parahaemolyticus *infection prevented?*

Most infections caused by *V. parahaemolyticus* in the United States can be prevented by thoroughly cooking seafood, especially oysters. Wound infections can be prevented by avoiding exposure of open wounds to warm seawater. When an outbreak is traced to an oyster bed, health officials recommend closing the oyster bed until conditions are less favorable for *V. parahaemolyticus*.

How can I learn more about Vibrio parahaemolyticus?

You can discuss your medical concerns with your doctor or other health care provider. Your local health department can provide information about this and other public health problems. Information about problems associated with raw seafood consumption can be obtained from the FDA's Center for Food Safety and Applied Nutrition (telephone 1-800-332-4010). At this number recorded information is available on many subjects including seafood consumption and handling. A public affairs specialist is available 12:00 p.m.–4:00 p.m. Eastern Standard Time. Seafood safety information is also available on the world wide web at http://vm.cfsan.fda.gov/, http://seafood.ucdavis.edu. There is more information about other Vibrio infections, such as *Vibrio vulnificus* at http://www.cdc.gov/ncidod/diseases/foodborn/vibrio.htm.

Vibrio vulnificus

What is Vibrio vulnificus?

Vibrio vulnificus is a bacterium in the same family as those that cause cholera. It normally lives in warm seawater and is part of a group of vibrios that are called "halophilic" because they require salt.

What type of illness does V. vulnificus *cause?*

V. vulnificus can cause disease in those who eat contaminated seafood or have an open wound that is exposed to seawater. Among healthy people, ingestion of *V. vulnificus* can cause vomiting, diarrhea, and abdominal pain. In immunocompromised persons, particularly those with chronic liver disease, *V. vulnificus* can infect the bloodstream, causing a severe and life-threatening illness characterized by fever and chills, decreased blood pressure (septic shock), and blistering skin lesions. *V. vulnificus* bloodstream infections are fatal about 50% of the time.

V. vulnificus can also cause an infection of the skin when open wounds are exposed to warm seawater; these infections may lead to skin breakdown and ulceration. Persons who are immunocompromised are at higher risk for invasion of the organism into the bloodstream and potentially fatal complications.

How common is V. vulnificus *infection?*

V. vulnificus is a rare cause of disease, but it is also underreported. Between 1988 and 1995, CDC received reports of over 300 *V. vulnificus* infections from the Gulf Coast states, where the majority of cases occur. There is no national surveillance system for *V. vulnificus*, but CDC collaborates with the states of Alabama, Florida, Louisiana, Texas, and

139

Mississippi to monitor the number of cases of *V. vulnificus* infection in the Gulf Coast region.

How do persons get infected with V. vulnificus?

Persons who are immunocompromised, especially those with chronic liver disease, are at risk for *V. vulnificus* when they eat raw seafood, particularly oysters. A recent study showed that people with these pre-existing medical conditions were 80 times more likely to develop *V. vulnificus* bloodstream infections than were healthy people. The bacterium is frequently isolated from oysters and other shellfish in warm coastal waters during the summer months. Since it is naturally found in warm marine waters, people with open wounds can be exposed to *V. vulnificus* through direct contact with seawater. There is no evidence for person-to-person transmission of *V. vulnificus*.

How can V. vulnificus *infection be diagnosed?*

V. vulnificus infection is diagnosed by routine stool, wound, or blood cultures; the laboratory should be notified when this infection is suspected by the physician, since a special growth medium can be used to increase the diagnostic yield. Doctors should have a high suspicion for this organism when patients present with gastrointestinal illness, fever, or shock following the ingestion of raw seafood, especially oysters, or with a wound infection after exposure to seawater.

How is V. vulnificus *infection treated?*

V. vulnificus infection is treated with antibiotics. Doxycycline or a third-generation cephalosporin (e.g., ceftazidime) is appropriate.

Are there long-term consequences of V. vulnificus *infection?*

V. vulnificus infection is an acute illness, and those who recover should not expect any long-term consequences.

What can be done to improve the safety of oysters?

Although oysters can be harvested legally only from waters free from fecal contamination, even legally harvested oysters can be contaminated with *V. vulnificus* because the bacterium is naturally present in marine environments. *V. vulnificus* does not alter the appearance, taste, or odor of oysters. Timely, voluntary reporting of *V. vulnificus* infections to CDC and to regional offices of the Food and Drug Administration (FDA) will help collaborative efforts to improve investigation of these infections. Regional FDA specialists with expert knowledge about shellfish assist state officials with tracebacks of shellfish and, when notified rapidly about cases, are able to sample harvest waters to discover possible sources of infection and to close oyster beds when problems are identified. Ongoing research may help us to predict environmental or other factors that increase the chance that oysters carry pathogens.

How can I learn more about V. vulnificus?

You can discuss your medical concerns with your doctor or other health care provider. Your local city or county health department can provide information about this and other public health problems that are occurring in your area. Information about the potential dangers of raw oyster consumption is available 24 hours a day from the FDA's Seafood Hotline (telephone 1-800-332-4010); FDA public affairs specialists are available at this number between 12 and 4 p.m. Monday through Friday. Information is also available on the world wide web at: http://vm.cfsan.fda.gov.

Some tips for preventing *V. vulnificus* infections, particularly among immunocompromised patients, including those with underlying liver disease:

- Do not eat raw oysters or other raw shellfish.
- Cook shellfish (oysters, clams, mussels) thoroughly:
  - For shellfish in the shell, either
  - boil until the shells open and continue boiling for 5 more minutes, or
  - steam until the shells open and then continue cooking for 9 more minutes. Do not eat those shellfish that do not open during cooking. Boil shucked oysters at least 3 minutes, or fry them in oil at least 10 minutes at 375°F.
- Avoid cross-contamination of cooked seafood and other foods with raw seafood and juices from raw seafood.
- Eat shellfish promptly after cooking and refrigerate leftovers.
- Avoid exposure of open wounds or broken skin to warm salt or brackish water, or to raw shellfish harvested from such waters.

- Wear protective clothing (e.g., gloves) when handling raw shell-fish.

Chapter 22

Yersinia Enterocolitica

What is yersiniosis?

Yersiniosis is an infectious disease caused by a bacterium of the genus *Yersinia*. In the United States, most human illness is caused by one species, *Y. enterocolitica*. Infection with *Y. enterocolitica* can cause a variety of symptoms depending on the age of the person infected. Infection with *Y. enterocolitica* occurs most often in young children. Common symptoms in children are fever, abdominal pain, and diarrhea, which is often bloody. Symptoms typically develop 4 to 7 days after exposure and may last 1 to 3 weeks or longer. In older children and adults, right-sided abdominal pain and fever may be the predominant symptoms, and may be confused with appendicitis. In a small proportion of cases, complications such as skin rash, joint pains, or spread of bacteria to the bloodstream can occur.

What sort of germ is Y. enterocolitica?

Y. enterocolitica belongs to a family of rod-shaped bacteria. Other species of bacteria in this family include *Y. pseudotuberculosis*, which causes an illness similar to *Y. enterocolitica*, and *Y. pestis*, which causes plague. Only a few strains of *Y. enterocolitica* cause illness in humans. The major animal reservoir for *Y. enterocolitica* strains that cause human illness is pigs, but other strains are also found in many other

"*Yersinia enterocolitica*," Division of Bacterial and Mycotic Diseases, Centers for Disease Control and Prevention (CDC), reviewed March 29, 2000.

animals including rodents, rabbits, sheep, cattle, horses, dogs, and cats. In pigs, the bacteria are most likely to be found on the tonsils.

How do people get infected with Y. enterocolitica?

Infection is most often acquired by eating contaminated food, especially raw or undercooked pork products. The preparation of raw pork intestines (chitterlings) may be particularly risky. Infants can be infected if their caretakers handle raw chitterlings and then do not adequately clean their hands before handling the infant or the infant's toys, bottles, or pacifiers. Drinking contaminated unpasteurized milk or untreated water can also transmit the infection. Occasionally *Y. enterocolitica* infection occurs after contact with infected animals. On rare occasions, it can be transmitted as a result of the bacterium passing from the stools or soiled fingers of one person to the mouth of another person. This may happen when basic hygiene and handwashing habits are inadequate. Rarely, the organism is transmitted through contaminated blood during a transfusion.

How common is infection with Y. enterocolitica?

Y. enterocolitica is a relatively infrequent cause of diarrhea and abdominal pain. Based on data from the Foodborne Diseases Active Surveillance Network (FoodNet), which measures the burden and sources of specific diseases over time, approximately one culture-confirmed *Y. enterocolitica* infection per 100,000 persons occurs each year. Children are infected more often than adults, and the infection is more common in the winter.

How can Y. enterocolitica infections be diagnosed?

Y. enterocolitica infections are generally diagnosed by detecting the organism in the stools. Many laboratories do not routinely test for *Y. enterocolitica*, so it is important to notify laboratory personnel when infection with this bacterium is suspected so that special tests can be done. The organism can also be recovered from other sites, including the throat, lymph nodes, joint fluid, urine, bile, and blood.

How can Y. enterocolitica infections be treated?

Uncomplicated cases of diarrhea due to *Y. enterocolitica* usually resolve on their own without antibiotic treatment. However, in more severe or complicated infections, antibiotics such as aminoglycosides, doxycycline, trimethoprim-sulfamethoxazole, or fluoroquinolones may be useful.

Are there long-term consequences of Y. enterocolitica infections?

Most infections are uncomplicated and resolve completely. Occasionally, some persons develop joint pain, most commonly in the knees, ankles or wrists. These joint pains usually develop about 1 month after the initial episode of diarrhea and generally resolve after 1 to 6 months. A skin rash, called "erythema nodosum," may also appear on the legs and trunk; this is more common in women. In most cases, erythema nodosum resolves spontaneously within a month.

What can be done to prevent the infection?

1. Avoid eating raw or undercooked pork.

2. Consume only pasteurized milk or milk products.

3. Wash hands with soap and water before eating and preparing food, after contact with animals, and after handling raw meat.

4. After handling raw chitterlings, clean hands and fingernails scrupulously with soap and water before touching infants or their toys, bottles, or pacifiers. Someone other than the food-handler should care for children while chitterlings are being prepared.

5. Prevent cross-contamination in the kitchen: Use separate cutting boards for meat and other foods. Carefully clean all cutting boards, counter-tops, and utensils with soap and hot water after preparing raw meat.

6. Dispose of animal feces in a sanitary manner.

What are public health agencies doing to prevent or control yersiniosis?

The Centers for Disease Control and Prevention (CDC) monitors the frequency of Y. enterocolitica infections through the foodborne disease active surveillance network (FoodNet). In addition, CDC conducts investigations of outbreaks of yersiniosis to control them and to learn more about how to prevent these infections. CDC has collaborated in an educational campaign to increase public awareness about prevention of *Y. enterocolitica* infections. The U.S. Food and Drug Administration inspects imported foods and milk pasteurization plants and promotes better food preparation techniques in restaurants and food processing plants. The U.S. Department of Agriculture monitors the health of food animals and is responsible for the quality of slaughtered and processed meat. The U.S. Environmental Protection Agency regulates and monitors the safety of our drinking water supplies.

Part Three

Insect and
Animal Borne Diseases

Chapter 23

Cat Scratch Disease and Other Diseases Pets Carry

What Is Cat Scratch Disease?

Cat scratch disease (CSD) is a bacterial disease caused by *Bartonella henselae*. Most people with CSD have been bitten or scratched by a cat and developed a mild infection at the point of injury. Lymph nodes, especially those around the head, neck, and upper limbs, become swollen. Additionally, a person with CSD may experience fever, headache, fatigue, and a poor appetite. Rare complications of *B. henselae* infection are bacillary angiomatosis and Parinaud's oculoglandular syndrome.

Cat Scratch Disease

You can get cat scratch disease from a cat bite or cat scratch. You can get the infection after a cat scratches you if the cat's paws have the

This chapter includes "What Is Cat Scratch Disease?" excerpted from "Cat Scratch Disease *Bartonella henselae* Infection," National Center for Infectious Diseases, Centers for Disease Control and Prevention (CDC), reviewed February 2003. Text beginning at "Cat-Scratch Disease" is reproduced from "Cat-Scratch Disease," used with permission of the American Academy of Family Physicians. Copyright © 2000 by the American Academy of Family Physicians (Updated July 2002). "Infections that Pets Carry," reviewed by Stephen Eppes, MD, was provided by KidsHealth, one of the largest resources online for medically reviewed health information written for parents, kids, and teens. For more articles like this one, visit www.kidsHealth.org, or www.TeensHealth.org. © 2003 The Nemours Center for Children's Health Media, a division of The Nemours Foundation.

bacteria on them. (A cat can get the bacteria on its paws when it licks itself.) With a cat bite, the cat can pass the bacteria to you in its saliva. You can also get the bacteria in your eyes if you pet a cat that has the bacteria on its fur and then rub your eyes. Many people who get cat scratch disease do not remember being scratched or bitten by a cat.

Cat scratch disease is not a severe illness in people who are healthy. But it can be a problem in people with weak immune systems. People with weak immune systems include those who are receiving chemotherapy for cancer, those who have diabetes or those who have acquired immunodeficiency syndrome (AIDS).

Should I call my doctor if I am bitten or scratched by a cat?

Call your family doctor if you notice any of the following problems:

- A cat scratch or bite that does not heal in the usual length of time.

- An area of redness around a cat scratch or bite that continues to get bigger for more than 2 days after the injury.

- Fever that lasts for several days after a cat scratch or bite.

- Painful and swollen lymph nodes for more than 2 or 3 weeks.

- Bone or joint pain, abdominal pain (without fever, vomiting or diarrhea) or an unusual degree of tiredness for more than 2 or 3 weeks.

What are the signs of cat scratch disease?

A sore may develop where a cat has bitten or scratched you. The sore might not happen right away. It may take 3 to 10 days for the sore to appear after the bite or scratch.

The sore may take a long time to heal. An infection of the lymph nodes (also called lymph glands) also develops, most often in the glands that are near the place where you got the cat scratch or cat bite. For example, if the infection is from a cat scratch on your arm, the glands in your armpit may become tender and swollen. The lymph nodes may swell to an inch or more in size.

What tests are needed to diagnose cat scratch disease?

If you remember that you were bitten or scratched by a cat, your doctor will probably be able to diagnose the illness based on the fact that you were bitten or scratched and then got painful, swollen lymph nodes. When the diagnosis is not clear, a blood test may help your doctor make the diagnosis.

How is cat scratch disease treated?

In most people, cat scratch disease clears up without treatment. However, antibiotics (medicines that kill bacteria) may be needed when infected lymph nodes stay painful and swollen for more than 2 or 3 months. Antibiotics may also help if you have a fever for a long time or if the infection is in your bones, liver or another organ.

If a lymph node is very large or painful, your doctor may drain it to help relieve the pain. The lymph node is drained by putting a needle through normal skin off to the side of the node and moving the needle to the swollen node. The needle is then inserted into the node and the fluid in the node is drained out.

Can cat scratch disease be prevented?

Avoiding cats is the simplest way to prevent the disease, but it is not usually necessary to get rid of your cat. Having your cat declawed helps lower your risk of getting the infection through a cat scratch. Washing your hands carefully after handling your cat is another way to prevent the infection. Getting rid of fleas on your cat will also keep you and your family members from catching the infection.

Cats only seem to be able to transmit this infection for a few weeks. Young cats seem to be more likely to carry the bacteria than older cats. Households with kittens have higher rates of infection. If the kittens have fleas, the infection rate is even higher.

Should cats be treated?

Cats require no treatment. The bacteria doesn't cause cats to get sick. They merely carry the bacteria that causes cat scratch disease in people.

Infections That Pets Carry

Caring for animals and pets offers a tremendous learning experience for children—it can teach them responsibility, gentleness, and respect for nature and other living beings. Like adults, children can benefit from the companionship, affection, and relationships they share with their pets.

But it's not uncommon for animals and pets to transmit infections to humans, especially children. Before you give in to your child's pleas at the pet store, keep reading for more information about how to protect your child from infections carried by pets and animals.

How Do Pets Spread Infections?

Zoonotic infections, also called zoonoses, are infections transmitted through or from animals to humans. Like people, all animals carry germs. Some illnesses that are common among house pets—such as distemper, canine parvovirus, and heartworms—can't be transmitted to humans. But pets also carry certain bacteria, viruses, parasites, and fungi that can cause illness if they are transmitted to humans. Humans get these animal-borne diseases when they are bitten or scratched or have contact with an animal's waste, saliva, or dander. Pets are also more likely to carry ticks and fleas in their fur, and these organisms can also carry disease.

"The most severe infections can be fatal, such as rabies; most infections won't kill you, but the severity can range depending on your age and overall health," says Grant Morrison, MD, a family practitioner. For example, he says, exposure to *Salmonella* from handling turtles or iguanas may cause a healthy adult to get severe but temporary diarrhea, but in infants or people with chronic illness, exposure to *Salmonella* could be life threatening. That's because zoonotic infections are particularly dangerous to infants and children, pregnant women, elderly people, and people whose immune systems have been compromised by illness or disease (such as cancer or AIDS).

Common Infections That Pets Carry

Dogs and cats. Dogs and cats are popular pets among children with families, but they may carry infections such as:

- *Campylobacter infection:* Household pets and animals can transmit *Campylobacter jejuni,* bacteria that cause diarrhea, abdominal pain, and fever in people. The *Campylobacter* bacteria may exist in the intestinal tract of an infected household or wild animal, and a person can become infected through contact with contaminated water, feces, or unpasteurized milk. More than 2 million cases of *Campylobacter* infection occur each year in the United States and *C. jejuni* is now the leading cause of bacterial gastroenteritis. *Campylobacter* infections are contagious, especially among members of the same family and children in day care or preschools. Children with *Campylobacter* infection are generally treated with antibiotics.

- **Cat scratch disease**: A person who is bitten or scratched from a feline with *Bartonella henselae* bacteria may develop swollen and tender lymph nodes, fever, headaches, and fatigue, a condition known as cat scratch disease. The symptoms of cat scratch disease usually resolve without treatment; however, a doctor may prescribe antibiotics if the infection is severe. Cat scratch disease rarely causes any long-term complications.

- **Rabies**: Rabies is a serious illness caused by a virus that enters a person's body through a bite or wound contaminated by the saliva from an infected animal. Animals that may carry the rabies virus include dogs, cats, raccoons, bats, skunks and foxes. Widespread immunization of dogs and cats has decreased the transmission of rabies in these animals and in people. Human rabies is rare in the United States: only five cases of rabies were reported in 2000. An effective vaccine is available for treatment following a bite with a potentially rabid animal.

- **Rocky Mountain spotted fever**: Rocky Mountain spotted fever (RMSF) is carried by ticks that attach themselves to animal skin, particularly dogs. The ticks that cause Rocky Mountain spotted fever are infected by the *Rickettsia* bacteria, which can cause high fever, chills, muscle aches, and headaches, as well as a rash that may spread across the wrists, ankles, palms, soles, and trunk of the body. Rocky Mountain spotted fever is not contagious and can be treated with antibiotics.

- **Lyme disease**: Like RMSF, Lyme disease is transmitted through the bite of an infected tick that may have hitchhiked into your home on your pet. Symptoms include a bull's-eye rash where the tick attached, followed by headache, fever, and joint or muscle pain. If treated with antibiotics during the rash stage, later complications can be prevented.

- **Dog tapeworm**: *Dipylidium caninum* is the most common tapeworm of dogs and cats in the United States. Most cases of dog tapeworm infection in humans occur in children; they become infected when they swallow an infected flea. Symptoms of tapeworm infestation include itching around the anus, vague abdominal pain, and diarrhea. Tapeworms may be seen stuck to the skin around the anal area or in the feces. Children infected with *Dipylidium caninum* are treated with oral medication to kill the tapeworm.

- **Ringworm:** Ringworm, also called tinea, is a skin infection caused by several types of fungi found in the soil and on the skin of humans and pets. Children can get ringworm from touching infected animals such as dogs and cats. Ringworm of the skin, or tinea corporis, usually is a dry, scaly round area with a raised red bumpy border and a clear center. When the scalp is affected, the area may be flaky, red, or swollen. Often there are bald patches. Ringworm is treated with antifungal medications including shampoo, cream, or oral medicine.

- **Toxocariasis:** Toxocariasis is an illness caused by the parasitic roundworm, *Toxocara*, which lives in the intestines of dogs and cats. The eggs from the worms are passed in the stools of dogs and cats, often contaminating soil where children play. When a child ingests the contaminated soil, the eggs hatch in the intestine and the larvae spread to other organs, an infection known as visceral larva migrans. Symptoms include fever, cough or wheezing, enlarged liver, rash, or swollen lymph nodes. Symptoms may resolve on their own, or a doctor may prescribe drugs to kill the larvae. When the larvae in the intestine make their way through the bloodstream to the eye, it is known as *ocular toxocariasis*, or *ocular larva migrans*, which may lead to a permanent loss of vision.

- **Toxoplasmosis:** A person can contract toxoplasmosis after contact with a parasite found in cat feces or undercooked meat. In most healthy people, toxoplasmosis infection is asymptomatic. When symptoms do occur they may include swollen glands, fatigue, muscle pain, fever, sore throat, and a rash. In pregnant women, toxoplasmosis can cause miscarriage, premature births, and severe illness and blindness in newborns. Pregnant women should avoid contact with litter boxes. People whose immune systems have been weakened by illnesses such as AIDS or cancer are at risk for severe complications from toxoplasmosis infection.

Birds. Pet birds, even if they are kept in a cage, may transmit the following diseases:

- **Cryptococcosis:** Cryptococcosis, like ringworm, is a fungal disease. People who inhale organisms found in bird droppings, especially from pigeons, may contract the disease, which can cause pneumonia. People with weakened immune systems from illnesses such as AIDS or cancer are at increased risk of contracting this disease and developing serious complications such as encephalitis (inflammation of the brain).

- *Psittacosis:* Psittacosis, also known as parrot fever, can occur when people have contact with infected bird feces or with the dust that accumulates in birdcages. Symptoms of this bacterial illness include coughing, high fever, and headache. Psittacosis is treated with antibiotics.

Reptiles. Reptiles include lizards, snakes, and turtles, and place children at risk for:

- *Salmonellosis:* Reptiles, such as lizards, snakes, and turtles, shed *Salmonella* in their feces. Touching the reptile's skin, cage, and other contaminated surfaces can lead to infection in people. Salmonellosis causes symptoms such as abdominal pain, diarrhea, vomiting, and fever. Young children are at risk for more serious illness, including dehydration, meningitis, and sepsis.

Other animals. Handling and caring for rodents, including hamsters and gerbils, as well as fish, may place children at risk for:

- *Lymphocytic choriomeningitis (LCM):* Lymphocytic choriomeningitis virus infects rodents, such as mice and hamsters, and people become infected by inhaling particles of rodent urine, feces, or saliva. LCM can cause flu-like symptoms such as fever, fatigue, headaches, muscle aches, nausea, and vomiting or the infection may lead to meningitis, an inflammation of the membrane that surrounds the brain and spinal cord, and encephalitis, an inflammation of the brain. Like most viruses, there is no specific treatment, but some patients may require hospitalization. Like toxoplasmosis, LCM may be passed from infected mother to fetus.

- *Mycobacteria marinum:* This mycobacterial infection may occur in people when they are exposed to contaminated water in aquariums or pools. Although mycobacteria marinum infections are generally mild and limited to the skin, they can be more severe in people with AIDS or with weakened immune systems.

Keeping Your Family and Your Pet Healthy

Being informed about the diseases pets can carry doesn't mean you have to give up your family's furry friends altogether. Pets can enrich your family life, and with a few precautions you can help to protect your child from contracting zoonoses.

Protecting your family from pet-related infections begins before bringing a pet home. Some animals are not recommended for homes with children and may increase the likelihood that your child may contract a zoonotic infection. Reptiles should not be allowed as pets in any household with young children.

You should also consider any health conditions your child has before bringing a pet into your home. "The health and age of the child would be the most important considerations. I would not recommend a pet that would require frequent handling to any immunocompromised child (such as a child with HIV, cancer undergoing chemotherapy, or frequent or chronic prednisone use). Children with eczema or atopic dermatitis should probably avoid aquariums," Dr. Morrison says.

If you're adopting or purchasing a pet make sure the breeder, shelter, or store is reputable and vaccinates all of their animals. A reputable breeder should belong to a national or local breeding club, such as the American Kennel Club. Contact the Humane Society of the United States or your veterinarian for information about animal shelters in your area.

As soon as you choose a family pet, take it to a local veterinarian for vaccinations and a physical examination. Don't forget to routinely vaccinate your pet on a schedule recommended by your vet—this will keep your pet healthy and will reduce the risk that infections will be transmitted to your child. You'll also want to regularly feed your pet nutritious animal food (ask your veterinarian for suggestions) and provide plenty of fresh water. Avoid feeding your pet raw meat because this can be a source of infection, and you should also not allow your pet to drink toilet water because infections can be spread through saliva, urine, and feces. Limit your young child's contact with outdoor pets that hunt and kill for food because a pet that ingests infected meat may contract an infection that can be passed to your child.

Teach your child these tips for caring for a pet safely:

- Always wash your hands, especially after touching your pet, handling your pet's food, or cleaning your pet's cage, tank, or litter box. Wear gloves when cleaning up after an animal's waste, and if you have a bird, wear a dust mask over your nose and mouth to prevent inhaling urine or fecal particles. "Don't have children clean cages or litter boxes unless there is supervision or until they have demonstrated they can do this safely and responsibly (and again, wash their hands afterwards)," Dr. Morrison says.

- Avoid kissing or touching your pet with your mouth because infections can be transmitted by saliva. Also, avoid sharing food with your pet.

- Keep your pet's living area clean and free of waste. If your pet eliminates waste outdoors, don't allow your child to play in that area and pick up waste regularly.

- Don't allow pets in areas where food is prepared or handled, and don't bathe your pet or clean aquariums in the kitchen sink or bathtub. Wash your pet outdoors or talk to your veterinarian about professional pet grooming.

- Avoid strange animals or those that appear sick. Never adopt a wild animal as a pet.

Watch your child carefully around pets. Small children are more likely to catch infections from pets because they crawl around on the floor with the animals, kiss them or share food with them, or put their fingers in the pets' mouths and then put their dirty fingers in their own mouths. Also, if your child visits a petting zoo, farm, or a friend's house where there are animals, make sure your child knows the importance of hand washing.

For your pet's comfort and for your family's safety, control flea and tick problems in your pet. Fleas and ticks can carry diseases, and they may be easily passed to children. Oral and topical medications are available for flea and tick control; avoid using flea collars because children can handle these collars and may become sick from the chemicals they contain. Check your pet regularly for fleas and ticks, as well as bites and scratches that may make them more susceptible to infection. Keep your pet leashed when outdoors and keep it away from animals that look sick or may be unvaccinated.

And, finally, spay or neuter your pet. Spaying and neutering may reduce your pet's contact with other animals that may be infected, especially if your pet goes outdoors.

Chapter 24

Encephalitis

Questions and Answers about Encephalitis

What is encephalitis?

Encephalitis is an inflammation of the brain. There are many types of encephalitis, most of which are caused by viral infection. Symptoms include sudden fever, headache, vomiting, photophobia (abnormal visual sensitivity to light), stiff neck and back, confusion, drowsiness, clumsiness, unsteady gait, and irritability. Symptoms that require emergency treatment include loss of consciousness, poor responsiveness, seizures, muscle weakness, sudden severe dementia, memory loss, withdrawal from social interaction, and impaired judgment.

How is encephalitis different from meningitis?

Meningitis is an infection of the membranes (called meninges) that surround the brain and spinal cord. Symptoms, which may appear suddenly, often include high fever, severe and persistent headache, stiff

---

This chapter includes excerpts from "Encephalitis and Meningitis Information Page," National Institute of Neurological Disorders and Stroke, reviewed April 2001 and "Eastern Equine Encephalitis," "Japanese Encephalitis Fact Sheet," "La Crosse Encephalitis," "Fact Sheet: St. Louis Encephalitis," "CDC Answers Your Questions about St. Louis Encephalitis," "Western Equine Encephalitis," "Arboviral Encephalitis" and "Information on Arboviral Encephalitides" Division of Vector-Borne Infectious Diseases, Centers for Disease Control and Prevention, July 2001.

neck, nausea, and vomiting. Changes in behavior such as confusion, sleepiness, and difficulty waking up are extremely important symptoms and may require emergency treatment. In infants symptoms of meningitis may include irritability or tiredness, poor feeding and fever. Meningitis may be caused by many different viruses and bacteria. Viral meningitis cases are usually self-limited to 10 days or less. Some types of meningitis can be deadly if not treated promptly. Anyone experiencing symptoms of meningitis or encephalitis should see a doctor immediately.

Are there any treatments for encephalitis?

Antiviral medications may be prescribed for herpes encephalitis or other severe viral infections. Antibiotics may be prescribed for bacterial infections. Anticonvulsants are used to prevent or treat seizures. Corticosteroids are used to reduce brain swelling and inflammation. Sedatives may be needed for irritability or restlessness. Over-the-counter medications may be used for fever and headache. Individuals with encephalitis are usually hospitalized for treatment.

What is the prognosis?

The prognosis for encephalitis varies. Some cases are mild, short and relatively benign and patients have full recovery. Other cases are severe, and permanent impairment or death is possible. The acute phase of encephalitis may last for 1 to 2 weeks, with gradual or sudden resolution of fever and neurological symptoms. Neurological symptoms may require many months before full recovery. With early diagnosis and prompt treatment, most patients recover from meningitis. However, in some cases, the disease progresses so rapidly that death occurs during the first 48 hours, despite early treatment.

Eastern Equine Encephalitis

Eastern equine encephalitis (EEE) is caused by a virus transmitted to humans and equines by the bite of an infected mosquito. EEE virus is an alphavirus that was first identified in the 1930's and currently occurs in focal locations along the eastern seaboard, the Gulf Coast, and some inland Midwestern locations of the United States. While small outbreaks of human disease have occurred in the United States, equine epizootics can be a common occurrence during the summer and fall.

It takes from 4–10 days after the bite of an infected mosquito for an individual to develop symptoms of EEE. These symptoms begin with a sudden onset of fever, general muscle pains, and a headache of increasing severity. Many individuals will progress to more severe symptoms such as seizures and coma. Approximately one-third of all people with clinical encephalitis caused by EEE will die from the disease and of those who recover, many will suffer permanent brain damage with many of those requiring permanent institutional care.

In addition to humans, EEE virus can produce severe disease in: horses, some birds such as pheasants, quail, ostriches and emus, and even puppies. Because horses are outdoors and attract hordes of biting mosquitoes, they are at high risk of contracting EEE when the virus is present in mosquitoes. Human cases are usually preceded by those in horses and exceeded in numbers by horse cases which may be used as a surveillance tool.

EEE virus occurs in natural cycles involving birds and *Culiseta melanura*, in some swampy areas nearly every year during the warm months. Where the virus resides or how it survives in the winter is unknown. It may be introduced by migratory birds in the spring or it may remain dormant in some yet undiscovered part of its life cycle. With the onset of spring, the virus reappears in the birds (native bird species do not seem to be affected by the virus) and mosquitoes of the swamp. In this usual cycle of transmission, the virus does not escape from these areas because the mosquito involved prefers to feed upon birds and does not usually bite humans or other mammals.

For reasons not fully understood, the virus may escape from enzootic foci in swamp areas in birds or bridge vectors such as *Coquilletidia perturbans* and *Aedes sollicitans*. These species feed on both birds and mammals and can transmit the virus to humans, horses, and other hosts. Other mosquito species such as *Ae. vexans* and *Culex nigripalpus* can also transmit EEE virus. When health officials maintain surveillance for EEE virus activity, this movement out of the swamp can be detected, and if the level of activity is sufficiently high, can recommend and undertake measures to reduce the risk to humans.

Clinical Features

- Symptoms range from mild flu-like illness to frank encephalitis, coma, and death

Etiologic Agent

- Eastern equine encephalitis virus, member of the family *Togaviridae*, genus *Alphavirus*

- Closely related to western and Venezuelan equine encephalitis viruses

Incidence

- 153 confirmed cases in the U.S. since 1964

Sequelae

- Mild to severe neurologic deficits in survivors

Costs

- Total case costs range from $21,000 for transiently infected individuals to $3 million for severely infected individuals
- Insecticide applications can cost as much as $1.4 million depending on the size of area treated

Transmission

- Mosquito-borne

Risk Groups

- Residents of endemic areas and visitors
- Persons with outdoor work and recreational activities

Trends

- Risk exposure increases as population expands into endemic areas

Challenges

- No licensed vaccine for human use
- No effective therapeutic drug
- Unknown overwintering cycle
- Control measures expensive
- Limited financial support of surveillance and prevention

Japanese Encephalitis

Japanese encephalitis (JE) virus is a flavivirus, related to St. Louis encephalitis, and is widespread throughout Asia. Worldwide, it is the most important cause of arboviral encephalitis with over 45,000 cases reported annually. In recent years, JE virus has expanded its geographic distribution with outbreaks in the Pacific. Epidemics occur in late summer in temperate regions, but the infection is enzootic and occurs throughout the year in many tropical areas of Asia. The virus is maintained in a cycle involving culicine mosquitoes and waterbirds. The virus is transmitted to man by *Culex mosquitoes*, primarily *Cx. tritaeniorhynchus*, which breed in rice fields. Pigs are the main amplifying hosts of JE virus in peridomestic environments.

The incubation period of JE is 5 to 14 days. Onset of symptoms is usually sudden, with fever, headache, and vomiting. The illness resolves in 5 to 7 days if there is no CNS involvement. The mortality in most outbreaks is less than 10%, but is higher in children and can exceed 30%. Neurologic sequelae in patients who recover are reported in up to 30% of cases. A formalin-inactivated vaccine prepared in mice is used widely in Japan, China, India, Korea, Taiwan, and Thailand. This vaccine is currently available for human use in the United States, for individuals who might be traveling to endemic countries.

Clinical Features

- Acute encephalitis; can progress to paralysis, seizures, coma, and death
- The majority of infections are subclinical

Etiologic Agent

- Japanese encephalitis (JE) virus: flavivirus antigenically related to St. Louis encephalitis virus

Incidence

- Leading cause of viral encephalitis in Asia with 30–50,000 cases reported annually
- Fewer than one case/year in U.S. civilians and military personnel traveling to and living in Asia
- Rare outbreaks in U.S. territories in Western Pacific

Sequelae

- Case-fatality ratio: 30%
- Serious neurologic sequela: 30%

Cost

- Domestic: less than $1 million/year—largely cost of immunizing travelers and military personnel
- International: no data, probably tens of millions of dollars

Transmission

- Mosquito-borne *Culex tritaeniorhynchus* group

Risk Groups

- Residents of rural areas in endemic locations
- Active duty military deployed to endemic areas
- Expatriates in rural areas
- Disease risk extremely low in travelers

Challenges

- Currently available killed vaccine expensive and occasionally reactogenic

La Crosse Encephalitis

La Crosse (LAC) encephalitis was discovered in La Crosse, Wisconsin in 1963. Since then, the virus has been identified in several Midwestern and Mid-Atlantic states. During an average year, about 75 cases of LAC encephalitis are reported to the CDC. Most cases of LAC encephalitis occur in children under 16 years of age. LAC virus is a Bunyavirus and is a zoonotic pathogen cycled between the daytime-biting treehole mosquito, *Aedes triseriatus*, and vertebrate amplifier hosts (chipmunks, tree squirrels) in deciduous forest habitats. The virus is maintained over the winter by transovarial transmission in mosquito eggs. If the female mosquito is infected, she may lay eggs that carry the virus, and the adults coming from those eggs may be able to transmit the virus to chipmunks and to humans.

Historically, most cases of LAC encephalitis occur in the upper Midwestern states (Minnesota, Wisconsin, Iowa, Illinois, Indiana, and Ohio). Recently, more cases are being reported from states in the mid-Atlantic (West Virginia, Virginia, and North Carolina) and southeastern (Alabama and Mississippi) regions of the country. It has long been suspected that LAC encephalitis has a broader distribution and a higher incidence in the eastern United States, but is under-reported because the etiologic agent is often not specifically identified.

LAC encephalitis initially presents as a nonspecific summertime illness with fever, headache, nausea, vomiting, and lethargy. Severe disease occurs most commonly in children under the age of 16 and is characterized by seizures, coma, paralysis, and a variety of neurological sequelae after recovery. Death from LAC encephalitis occurs in less than 1% of clinical cases. In many clinical settings, pediatric cases presenting with CNS involvement are routinely screened for herpes or enteroviral etiologies. Since there is no specific treatment for LAC encephalitis, physicians often do not request the tests required to specifically identify LAC virus, and the cases are reported as aseptic meningitis or viral encephalitis of unknown etiology.

Also found in the United States, Jamestown Canyon and Cache Valley viruses are related to LAC, but rarely cause encephalitis.

Clinical Features

- Frank encephalitis progressing to seizures, coma; majority of infections are subclinical or result in mild illness

Etiologic Agent

- La Crosse virus—California serogroup virus in the family *Bunyaviridae*

Incidence

- Approximately 70 cases reported per year

Sequelae

- Case-fatality ratio less than 1%
- Hospitalization for CNS infection
- Neurological sequelae that resolve within several years

Costs

- Short-term hospitalization to long-term care exceeding $450,000
- Social costs from adverse effects on IQ and school performance

Transmission

- Virus cycles in woodland habitats between the treehole mosquito (*Aedes triseriatus*) and vertebrate hosts (chipmunks, squirrels)
- Virus survives winter in mosquito
- Vector uses artificial containers (tires, buckets, etc.) in addition to treeholes

Risk Groups

- Children less than 16 years old: biological risk factor
- Residence in woodland habitats environmental risk factor
- Containers at residence environmental risk factor
- Outdoor activities: behavioral risk factor

Trends

- Traditional endemic foci in the great-Lakes states
- Increased case incidence in mid-Atlantic states
- Rural poor most affected

Challenges

- Multiple environmental, biological, and social factors contributing to disease occurrence
- Disease is considerably under-reported
- No vaccine available

St. Louis Encephalitis

In the United States, the leading cause of epidemic flaviviral encephalitis is St. Louis encephalitis (SLE) virus. SLE is the most common mosquito-transmitted human pathogen in the U.S. While periodic SLE epidemics have occurred only in the Midwest and southeast, SLE virus is distributed throughout the lower 48 states. Since 1964, there have been 4,437 confirmed cases of SLE with an average of 193 cases per year (range 4–1,967). However, less than 1% of SLE viral infections are clinically apparent and the vast majority of infections remain undiagnosed. Illness ranges in severity from a simple febrile headache to meningoencephalitis, with an overall case-fatality ratio of 5–15 %. The disease is generally milder in children than in adults, but in those children who do have disease, there is a high rate of encephalitis. The elderly are at highest risk for severe disease and death. During the summer season, SLE virus is maintained in a mosquito-bird-mosquito cycle, with periodic amplification by peri-domestic birds *and Culex mosquitoes.* In Florida, the principal vector is *Cx. nigripalpus,* in the Midwest, *Cx. pipiens pipiens* and *Cx. p. quinquefasciatus* and in the western United States, *Cx. tarsalis* and members of the *Cx. pipiens complex.*

Questions and Answers about St. Louis Encephalitis

How do people get St. Louis encephalitis?

People are infected by the bite of a mosquito (primarily the *Culex species*) that has become infected with St. Louis encephalitis virus (a flavivirus antigenically related to Japanese encephalitis virus).

What is the basic transmission cycle?

Mosquitoes become infected by feeding on birds infected with the St. Louis encephalitis virus. Infected mosquitoes then transmit the St. Louis encephalitis virus to humans and animals during the feeding process. The St. Louis encephalitis virus grows both in the infected mosquito and the infected bird, but does not make either one sick.

Could you get the St. Louis encephalitis from another person?

No. St. Louis encephalitis virus is not transmitted from person-to-person. For example, you cannot get the virus from touching or kissing a person who has the disease, or from a health care worker who has treated someone with the disease.

Could you get St. Louis encephalitis directly from birds or from insects other than mosquitoes?

No. Only infected mosquitoes can transmit St. Louis encephalitis virus.

What are the symptoms of St. Louis encephalitis?

Mild infections occur without apparent symptoms other than fever with headache. More severe infection is marked by headache, high fever, neck stiffness, stupor, disorientation, coma, tremors, occasional convulsions (especially in infants), and spastic (but rarely flaccid) paralysis.

What is the incubation period for St. Louis encephalitis?

The incubation period is usually 5 to 15 days.

What is the mortality rate of St. Louis encephalitis?

Case-fatality rates range from 3% to 30% (especially in the aged).

How many cases of St. Louis encephalitis occur in the U.S.?

Since 1964 there have been 4,478 reported human cases of St. Louis encephalitis, with an average of 128 cases reported annually.

How is St. Louis encephalitis treated?

There is no specific therapy. Intensive supportive therapy is indicated.

Is the disease seasonal in its occurrence?

In temperate areas of the United States, St. Louis encephalitis cases occur primarily in the late summer or early fall. In the southern United States where the climate is milder St. Louis encephalitis can occur year round.

Who is at risk for getting St. Louis encephalitis?

All residents of areas where active cases have been identified are at risk of getting St. Louis encephalitis.

Where does St. Louis encephalitis occur?

St. Louis encephalitis outbreaks can occur throughout most of the United States. The last major epidemic of St. Louis encephalitis occurred in the Midwest from 1974–1977. During that outbreak, over 2,500 cases in 35 states were reported to the Centers for Disease Control and Prevention (CDC). Currently, outbreaks of St. Louis encephalitis have been limited in size (usually fewer than 30 cases), although the potential still exists for epidemic St. Louis encephalitis. The most recent outbreak of St. Louis encephalitis occurred in New Orleans, Louisiana in 1999, with 20 reported cases.

Is there a vaccine against St. Louis encephalitis?

No.

Clinical Features

- Aseptic meningitis or encephalitis
- The majority of infections are subclinical or result in mild illness

Etiologic Agent

- St. Louis encephalitis virus—flavivirus related to Japanese encephalitis virus

Incidence

- Intermittent epidemic transmission—up to 3,000 cases per year (1975)

Sequelae

- Hospitalization for CNS (Central Nervous System) infection— 95% of recognized cases

Costs

- National expenditures for mosquito control activities—$150 million, SLE surveillance and control activities 0–70% of total; varies by state

Transmission

- Mosquito-borne
- Specific mosquito vectors vary regionally:
- Gulf Coast, Ohio and Mississippi Valley: *Culex pipiens, Cx. quinquefasciatus*; Florida: *Cx. nigripalpus*; Western States: *Cx. tarsalis*

Risk Groups

- Elderly—biological risk factor
- Low SES (socio-economic status) areas—environmental risk factor

- Outdoor occupation—exposure risk factor

Trends

- Largest outbreaks in 15 years occurred in 1990
- Urban transmission in west first recognized in 1987
- Deterioration of inner cities, global warming may increase vector abundance and transmission
- Unpredictable and intermittent occurrences of outbreaks
- Multiple environmental, biological and social factors contributing to disease occurrence
- Virus maintenance and overwintering cycle
- Develop more effective disease prevention and treatment
- No vaccine available

Western Equine Encephalitis

The alphavirus western equine encephalitis (WEE) was first isolated in California in 1930 from the brain of a horse with encephalitis, and remains an important cause of encephalitis in horses and humans in North America, mainly in western parts of the U.S. and Canada. In the western United States, the enzootic cycle of WEE involves passerine birds, in which the infection is inapparent, and culicine mosquitoes, principally *Cx. tarsalis*, a species that is associated with irrigated agriculture and stream drainages. The virus has also been isolated from a variety of mammal species. Other important mosquito vector species include *Aedes melanimon* in California, *Ae. dorsalis* in Utah and New Mexico and *Ae. campestris* in New Mexico. WEE virus was isolated from field collected larvae of *Ae. dorsalis*, providing evidence that vertical transmission may play an important role in the maintenance cycle of an alphavirus.

Expansion of irrigated agriculture in the North Platte River Valley during the past several decades has created habitats and conditions favorable for increases in populations of granivorous birds such as the house sparrow, *Passer domesticus*, and mosquitoes such as *Cx. tarsalis*, *Aedes dorsalis*, *and Aedes melanimon*. All of these species may play a role in WEE virus transmission in irrigated areas. In addition to *Cx. tarsalis*, *Ae. Dorsalis*, and *Ae. melanimon*, WEE virus also has been isolated occasionally from some other mosquito species present in the area. Two confirmed and several suspect cases of WEE were reported from Wyoming in 1994. In 1995, two strains of WEE virus were isolated from *Culex tarsalis* and neutralizing antibody to WEE virus was demonstrated in sera from pheasants and house sparrows. During 1997, 35 strains of WEE virus were isolated from mosquitoes collected in Scotts Bluff County, Nebraska.

Human WEE cases are usually first seen in June or July. Most WEE infections are asymptomatic or present as mild, nonspecific illness. Patients with clinically apparent illness usually have a sudden onset with fever, headache, nausea, vomiting, anorexia, and malaise, followed by altered mental status, weakness, and signs of meningeal irritation. Children, especially those under 1 year old, are affected more severely than adults and may be left with permanent sequelae, which is seen in 5 to 30% of young patients. The mortality rate is about 3%.

Clinical Features

- Symptoms range from mild flu-like illness to frank encephalitis, coma and death

Etiologic Agent

- Western equine encephalitis virus, member of the family *Togaviridae*, genus *Alphavirus*. Closely related to eastern and Venezuelan equine encephalitis viruses

Incidence

- 639 confirmed cases in the U.S. since 1964

Sequelae

- Mild to severe neurologic deficits in survivors

Costs

- Total case costs range from $21,000 for transiently infected individuals to $3 million for severely infected individuals
- Insecticide applications can cost as much as $1.4 million depending on the size of area treated

Transmission

- Mosquito-borne

Risk Groups

- Residents of endemic areas and visitors
- Persons with outdoor work and recreational activities

Trends

- Epidemic disease that is difficult to predict
- Risk exposure increases as population expands into endemic areas

Challenges

- No licensed vaccine for human use
- No effective therapeutic drug
- Unknown overwintering cycle
- Control measures expensive
- Limited financial support of surveillance and prevention

Other Arboviral Encephalitides

Powassan Encephalitis

Powassan (POW) virus is a flavivirus and currently the only well documented tick-borne transmitted arbovirus occurring in the United States and Canada. Recently a Powassan-like virus was isolated from the deer tick, *Ixodes scapularis*. Its relationship to POW and its ability to cause human disease has not been fully elucidated. POW's range in the United States is primarily in the upper tier states. In addition to isolations from man, the virus has been recovered from ticks (*Ixodes marxi, I. cookie*, and *Dermacentor andersoni*) and from the tissues of a skunk (*Spiligale putorius*). It is a rare cause of acute viral encephalitis. POW virus was first isolated from the brain of a 5-year-old child who died in Ontario in 1958. Patients who recover may have residual neurological problems.

Venezuelan Equine Encephalitis

Like EEE and WEE viruses, Venezuelan equine encephalitis (VEE) is an alphavirus and causes encephalitis in horses and humans and is an important veterinary and public health problem in Central and South America. Occasionally, large regional epizootics and epidemics

172

can occur resulting in thousands of equine and human infections. Epizootic strains of VEE virus can infect and be transmitted by a large number of mosquito species. The natural reservoir host for the epizootic strains is not known. A large epizootic that began in South America in 1969 reached Texas in 1971. It was estimated that over 200,000 horses died in that outbreak, which was controlled by a massive equine vaccination program using an experimental live attenuated VEE vaccine. There were several thousand human infections. A more recent VEE epidemic occurred in the fall of 1995 in Venezuela and Colombia with an estimated 90,000 human infections. Infection of man with VEE virus is less severe than with EEE and WEE viruses, and fatalities are rare. Adults usually develop only an influenza-like illness, and overt encephalitis is usually confined to children. Effective VEE virus vaccines are available for equines.

Enzootic strains of VEE virus have a wide geographic distribution in the Americas. These viruses are maintained in cycles involving forest dwelling rodents and mosquito vectors, mainly *Culex* (*Melanoconion*) species. Occasional cases or small outbreaks of human disease are associated with there viruses, the most recent outbreaks were in Venezuela in 1992, Peru in 1994 and Mexico in 1995–96.

Tick-Borne Encephalitis

Tick-borne encephalitis (TBE) is caused by two closely related flaviviruses which are distinct biologically. The eastern subtype causes Russian spring-summer encephalitis (RSSE) and is transmitted by *Ixodes persulcatus*, whereas the western subtype is transmitted by *Ixodes ricinus* and causes Central European encephalitis (CEE). The name CEE is somewhat misleading, since the condition can occur throughout much of Europe. Of the two subtypes, RSSE is the more severe infection, having a mortality of up to 25% in some outbreaks, whereas mortality in CEE seldom exceeds 5%.

The incubation period is 7 to 14 days. Infection usually presents as a mild, influenza-type illness or as benign, aseptic meningitis, but may result in fatal meningoencephalitis. Fever is often biphasic, and there may be severe headache and neck rigidity, with transient paralysis of the limbs, shoulders, or less commonly, the respiratory musculature. A few patients are left with residual paralysis. Although the great majority of TBE infections follow exposure to ticks, infection has occurred through the ingestion of infected cows' or goats' milk. An inactivated TBE vaccine is currently available in Europe and Russia.

Murray Valley Encephalitis

Murray Valley encephalitis (MVE) is endemic in New Guinea and in parts of Australia; and is related to SLE, WN (West Nile), and JE viruses. Unapparent infections are common, and the small number of fatalities have mostly been in children.

Chapter 25

Ehrlichiosis

Tick species that transmit ehrlichiosis are Deer tick, American dog tick, and Lone Star tick.

What Is Ehrlichiosis?

Ehrlichiosis is a tick-associated disease caused by bacteria in the genus *Ehrlichia*. To date, two types of ehrlichiosis have been identified in humans in the United States; HME, or human monocytic ehrlichiosis, caused by *Ehrlichia chaffeensis*, and HGE, or human granulocytic ehrlichiosis, caused by a yet unnamed species. It is possible that additional forms of ehrlichiosis in humans may be identified in the future.

Unlike Lyme disease, ehrlichiosis is considered an acute infection without chronic long-term consequences. Its severity varies from person to person. Many people exposed to the disease agent remain asymptomatic, while others suffer mild symptoms that resolve without treatment. In a minority of cases, however, ehrlichiosis produces severe symptoms requiring immediate antibiotic treatment. These cases can be life-threatening and even fatal for elderly patients and others with compromised immune systems.

Like Lyme disease, transmission of the ehrlichiosis bacterium is delayed an average of 36 hours or more after an infected tick begins to feed. Although Lyme disease and HGE infection rates in deer ticks are thought to be comparable in endemic areas of the northeast, evidence indicates that the transmission of *Ehrlichia* bacteria to humans may be less efficient than that of the Lyme disease bacteria *Borrelia burgdorferi*. This, combined with the characteristics of the disease itself, may account for the relatively few reported cases of HGE compared to Lyme disease. Nevertheless, the value of frequent tick checks while spending time outdoors cannot be overemphasized as a precaution against contracting this potentially severe disease.

Where Is Ehrlichiosis Prevalent?

First identified in 1987, the HME bacterium *E. chaffeensis* is primarily transmitted by the Lone Star tick. Ticks infected with *E. chaffeensis* occur mostly south of the line connecting southern New Jersey and western Texas, and throughout the high plains states north of Texas to the Canadian border.

The HGE bacterium, identified in 1994 but not yet named, is primarily transmitted by the deer tick. Found mostly in the upper midwest and along the eastern seaboard from New Jersey to Massachusetts, this bacterium, like *E. chaffeensis*, is also expanding its range. Both forms of ehrlichiosis are being diagnosed more widely as awareness of the disease increases and laboratory tests are improved.

Symptoms

Clinical manifestations of both HME and HGE are similar, and can range from mild to life-threatening depending on the patient's age and general health.

Onset of ehrlichiosis generally begins within a week of a tick bite, and often includes fever, severe headaches, malaise, muscle pains, and chills. Other symptoms may include nausea, vomiting, confusion and joint pain. A rash may appear in some HME cases but rarely with HGE unless the patient has also contracted Lyme disease.

Diagnosis

An initial diagnosis is based on the patient's symptoms and laboratory tests. Routine laboratory results include a low white blood cell count, low platelet count and elevated liver enzymes (ALT, AST, LDH). A confirmed diagnosis can be made using the PCR (polymerase chain reaction) test within the first ten days of infection, or an antibody IFA (immuno-fluorescent assay) after 21 days of suspected infection. In severe cases, blood smears can be taken and examined for the presence of either inclusions or morulae in affected blood cells.

Treatment

Patients suspected of having ehrlichiosis can be treated immediately with doxycycline or tetracycline for 7–10 days. Some physicians may treat for up to 28 days if the patient lives in an area endemic to Lyme disease on the chance that both disease agents have been transmitted. Ehrlichiosis symptoms usually subside within 24–48 hours of treatment; if not, the physician should consider other diagnoses.

Prevention and Control

Deer ticks, the primary transmitters of both HGE and Lyme disease, are generally found underneath leaf litter or clinging to low vegetation in shady, moist areas. They may also inhabit lawns and gardens, especially at the edges of woodlands and old stone walls. Within the endemic ranges of the *Ehrlichia* bacteria known to cause HGE, no natural, vegetated area can be considered completely free of infected ticks.

Ticks cannot jump or fly, and will not drop from above onto a passing animal. Potential hosts (which include all wild birds and mammals, domestic animals, and humans) acquire ticks only by direct contact with them. Once a tick gains access to human skin it generally climbs upward until it reaches a more protected area, often the back of the knee, groin, navel, armpit, ears, or nape of the neck. It then begins the process of inserting its mouthparts into the skin until it reaches the blood supply.

In tick-infested areas, the best precaution against ehrlichiosis is to avoid contact with soil, leaf litter and vegetation as much as possible. However, if you garden, hike, camp, hunt, work outdoors or otherwise spend time in woods, brushy areas or overgrown fields, you should use the following personal precautions to avoid exposure to ticks:

- Wear enclosed shoes and light-colored clothing with a tight weave to spot ticks easily.

- Scan clothes and any exposed skin frequently for ticks while outdoors.

- Stay on cleared, well-traveled trails.

177

- Use insect repellent containing DEET (Diethyl-meta-toluamide) on skin or clothes if you intend to go off-trail or into overgrown areas.

- Avoid sitting directly on the ground or on stone walls that harbor mice, chipmunks and other small mammals.

- Keep long hair pulled back, especially when gardening.

- Do a final, head-to-toe tick check at the end of the day; check your children and pets, too.

When taking the above precautions, consider these important facts:

- If you tuck long pants into socks and shirts into pants, be aware that ticks that contact your clothes will climb upward in search of exposed skin. This means they may climb to hidden areas of the head and neck if not intercepted first. Spot-check clothes frequently.

- Never use DEET in high concentrations, follow the manufacturers directions. Formulations containing 30% DEET are recommended for adults, 10% for children.

- After an outing, clothes can be spun in the dryer for 20 minutes to kill any unseen ticks.

- A shower and shampoo are only somewhat effective in dislodging crawling ticks. Inspect yourself and your children carefully after a shower or bath. Keep in mind that deer tick nymphs are the size of poppy seeds; deer tick adults are the size of sesame seeds.

Any contact with vegetation, even playing in the yard, can bring you into contract with ticks, so thorough, daily self-inspection is necessary whenever you engage in outdoor activities and the temperature exceeds 40 degrees F (the temperature above which deer ticks are active). Frequent tick checks should include a systematic, whole-body examination each night before going to bed. Performed consistently, this ritual is perhaps the single most effective current method for prevention of ehrlichiosis.

If you do find a tick attached to your skin, there is no need to panic. Not all ticks are infected with *Ehrlichia* bacteria, and studies of infected feeding ticks suggest that the time required for disease transmission is similar to that for Lyme disease—an average of 36 or more hours. Therefore, your chances of contracting ehrlichiosis are greatly reduced if you remove a tick within the first 24 hours.

To remove a tick, follow these steps:

1. Using a pair of fine-pointed tweezers, grasp the tick by its mouthparts right where they enter the skin. ***Do not*** grasp the tick by the body. Keep in mind that certain types of fine-pointed tweezers, especially those that are etched, or rasped, at the tips, may not be effective in removing nymphal deer ticks. Choose unrasped fine-pointed tweezers whose tips align tightly when pressed firmly together.

2. Without jerking, pull firmly and steadily directly outward. ***Do not*** twist the tick out or apply petroleum jelly, a hot match, alcohol or any other irritant to the tick in an attempt to get it to back out. These methods can backfire and even increase the chances of the tick transmitting the disease.

3. Place the tick in a vial or jar of alcohol to kill it.

4. Clean the bite wound with disinfectant.

Then, monitor the site of the bite for the appearance of a rash beginning 3 to 30 days after the bite. At the same time, learn about the other early symptoms of Lyme disease and watch to see if they appear in about the same timeframe. If a rash or other early symptoms develop, see a physician immediately.

Finally, prevention is not limited to personal precautions. Those who enjoy spending time in their yards can reduce the tick population around the home by:

- keeping lawns mowed and edges trimmed
- clearing brush, leaf litter and tall grass around houses and at the edges of gardens and stone walls
- stacking woodpiles neatly in a dry location and preferably off the ground
- clearing all leaf litter (including the remains of perennials) out of the garden in the fall
- keeping the ground under bird feeders clean so as not to attract small mammals
- having a licensed professional spray the yard with an insecticide in late May (to control nymphs) and optionally in September (to control adults).

Chapter 26

Hantavirus

Tracking a Mystery Disease

The "First" Outbreak

In May 1993, an outbreak of an unexplained pulmonary illness occurred in the southwestern United States, in an area shared by Arizona, New Mexico, Colorado and Utah known as "The Four Corners." A young, physically fit Navajo man suffering from shortness of breath was rushed to a hospital in New Mexico and died very rapidly.

While reviewing the results of the case, medical personnel discovered that the young man's fiancee had died a few days before after showing similar symptoms, a piece of information that proved key to discovering the disease. As Dr. James Cheek of the Indian Health Service (IHS) noted, "I think if it hadn't been for that initial pair of people that became sick within a week of each other, we never would have discovered the illness at all."

An investigation combing the entire Four Corners region was launched by the New Mexico Office of Medical Investigations (OMI) to find any other people who had a similar case history. Within a few hours, Dr. Bruce Tempest of IHS, working with OMI, had located five young, healthy people who had all died after acute respiratory failure.

A series of laboratory tests had failed to identify any of the deaths as caused by a known disease, such as bubonic plague. At this point,

"All About Hantavirus," Centers for Disease Control and Prevention (CDC), National Center for Infectious Diseases, Special Pathogens Branch, June 1999. Reviewed and revised by David A. Cooke, M.D., on January 26, 2004.

the CDC Special Pathogens Branch was notified. CDC, the state health departments of New Mexico, Colorado and Utah, the Indian Health Service, the Navajo Nation, and the University of New Mexico all joined together to confront the outbreak.

During the next few weeks, as additional cases of the disease were reported in the Four Corners area, physicians and other scientific experts worked intensively to narrow down the list of possible causes. The particular mixture of symptoms and clinical findings pointed researchers away from possible causes, such as exposure to a herbicide or a new type of influenza, and toward some type of virus. Samples of tissue from patients who had gotten the disease were sent to CDC for exhaustive analysis. Virologists at CDC used several tests, including new methods to pinpoint virus genes at the molecular level, and were able to link the pulmonary syndrome with a virus, in particular a previously unknown type of hantavirus.

Researchers Launch Investigations to Pin Down the Carrier of the New Virus

Researchers knew that all other known hantaviruses were transmitted to people by rodents, such as mice and rats. Therefore, an important part of their mission was to trap as many different species of rodents living in the Four Corners region as possible to find the particular type of rodent that carried the virus. From June through mid-August of 1993, all types of rodents were trapped inside and outside homes where people who had hantavirus pulmonary syndrome had lived, as well as in piñon groves and summer sheep camps where they had worked. Additional rodents were trapped for comparison in and around nearby households as well. Taking a calculated risk, researchers decided not to wear protective clothing or masks during the trapping process. "We didn't want to go in wearing respirators, scaring...everybody," John Sarisky, an Indian Health Service environmental disease specialist said. However, when the almost 1,700 rodents trapped were dissected to prepare samples for analysis at CDC, protective clothing and respirators were worn.

Among rodents trapped, the deer mouse (*Peromyscus maniculatus*) was found to be the main host to a previously unknown type of hantavirus. Since the deer mouse often lives near people in rural and semirural areas—in barns and outbuildings, woodpiles, and inside people's homes—researchers suspected that the deer mouse might be transmitting the virus to humans. About 30% of the deer mice tested showed evidence of infection with hantavirus. Tests also showed that several other types of rodents were infected, although in lesser numbers.

The next step was to pin down the connection between the infected deer mice and households where people who had gotten the disease lived. Therefore, investigators launched a case-control investigation. They compared "case" households, where people who had gotten the disease lived, with nearby "control" households. Control households were similar to those where the case-patients lived, except for one factor: no one in the control households had gotten the disease.

The results? First, investigators trapped more rodents in case households than in control households, so more rodents may have been living in close contact with people in case households. Second, people in case households were more likely than those in control households to do cleaning around the house or to plant in or hand-plow soil outdoors in fields or gardens. However, it was unclear if the risk for contracting HPS was due to performing these tasks, or with entering closed-up rooms or closets to get tools needed for these tasks.

In November 1993, the specific hantavirus that caused the Four Corners outbreak was isolated. The Special Pathogens Branch at CDC used tissue from a deer mouse that had been trapped near the New Mexico home of a person who had gotten the disease and grew the virus from it in the laboratory. Shortly afterwards and independently, the U.S. Army Medical Research Institute of Infectious Diseases (USAMRIID) also grew the virus, from a person in New Mexico who had gotten the disease as well as from a mouse trapped in California.

The new virus was called Muerto Canyon virus—later changed to Sin Nombre virus (SNV)—and the new disease caused by the virus was named hantavirus pulmonary syndrome, or HPS.

The isolation of the virus in a matter of months was remarkable. This success was based on close cooperation of all the agencies and individuals involved in investigating the outbreak, years of basic research on other hantaviruses that had been conducted at CDC and USAMRIID, and on the continuing development of modern molecular virologic tests. To put the rapid isolation of the Sin Nombre virus in perspective, it took several decades for the first hantavirus discovered, the Hantaan virus, to be isolated.

HPS Not Really a New Disease

As part of the effort to locate the source of the virus, researchers located and examined stored samples of lung tissue from people who had died of unexplained lung disease. Some of these samples showed evidence of previous infection with Sin Nombre virus—indicating that the disease had existed before the "first" known outbreak—it simply had not been recognized.

Other early cases of HPS have been discovered by examining samples of tissue belonging to people who had died of unexplained adult respiratory distress syndrome. By this method, the earliest known case of HPS that has been confirmed has been the case of a 38-year-old Utah man in 1959.

Interestingly, while HPS was not known to the epidemiologic and medical communities, there is evidence that it was recognized elsewhere. The Navajo Indians, a number of whom contracted HPS during the 1993 outbreak, recognize a similar disease in their medical traditions, and actually associate its occurrence with mice. As strikingly, Navajo medical beliefs concur with public health recommendations for preventing the disease.

Why Did the Outbreak Occur in the Four Corners Area?

But why this sudden cluster of cases? The key answer to this question is that, during this period, there were suddenly many more mice than usual. The Four Corners area had been in a drought for several years. Then, in early 1993, heavy snows and rainfall helped drought-stricken plants and animals to revive and grow in larger-than-usual numbers. The area's deer mice had plenty to eat, and as a result they reproduced so rapidly that there were ten times more mice in May 1993 than there had been in May of 1992. With so many mice, it was more likely that mice and humans would come into contact with one another, and thus more likely that the hantavirus carried by the mice would be transmitted to humans.

Person-to-Person Spread of HPS Decided Unlikely

"Although person-to-person spread [of HPS] has not been documented with any of the other known hantaviruses, we were concerned [during this outbreak] because we were dealing with a new agent," said Charles Vitek, a CDC medical investigator.

Researchers and clinicians investigating the ongoing outbreak were not the only groups concerned about the disease. Shortly after the first few HPS patients died and it became clear that a new disease was affecting people in the area, and that no one knew how it was transmitted, the news media began extensive reporting on the out-break. Widespread concern among the public ensued.

Unfortunately, the first victims of the outbreak were Navajo. News reports focused on this fact, and the misperception grew that the un-known disease was somehow linked to Navajos. As a consequence, Navajos found themselves at the center of intense media attention and the objects of the some people's fears.

By later in the summer of 1993, the media frenzy had quieted some-what, and the source of the disease was pinpointed. Researchers de-termined that, like other hantaviruses, the virus that causes HPS is not transmitted from person to person the way other infections, such as the common cold, may be.

To date, no cases of HPS have been reported in the United States in which the virus was transmitted from one person to another. In fact, in a study of health care workers who were exposed to either patients or specimens infected with related types of hantaviruses (which cause a different disease in humans), none of the workers showed evidence of infection or illness.

HPS Since the First Outbreak

After the initial outbreak, the medical community nationwide was asked to report any cases of illness with symptoms similar to those of HPS that could not be explained by any other cause. As a result, additional cases have been reported.

Since 1993, researchers have discovered that there is not just one hantavirus that causes HPS, but several. In June 1993, a Louisiana bridge inspector who had not traveled to the Four Corners area de-veloped HPS. An investigation was begun. The patient's tissues were tested for the presence of antibodies to hantavirus. The results led to the discovery of another hantavirus, named Bayou virus, which was linked to a carrier, the rice rat (*Oryzomys palustris*). In late 1993, a 33-year-old Florida man came down with HPS symptoms; he later recovered. This person also had not traveled to the Four Corners area. A similar investigation revealed yet another hantavirus, named the Black Creek Canal virus, and its carrier, the cotton rat (*Sigmodon hispidus*). Another case occurred in New York. This time, the Sin Nombre-like virus was named New York-1, and the white-footed mouse, *Peromyscus leucopus*, was implicated as the carrier.

More recently, cases of HPS stemming from related hantaviruses have been documented in Argentina, Brazil, Canada, Chile, Paraguay, and Uruguay, making HPS a pan-hemispheric disease.

How Is Hantavirus Transmitted?

So just how do people get hantavirus pulmonary syndrome (HPS)? It all starts with rodents, like the deer mouse and cotton rat, which carry hantaviruses.

The Basic Transmission Cycle

The short story is that some rodents are infected with a type of hantavirus that causes HPS. In the United States, deer mice (plus cotton rats and rice rats in the southeastern states and the white-footed mouse in the Northeast) are the rodents carrying hantaviruses that cause hantavirus pulmonary syndrome.

These rodents shed the virus in their urine, droppings and saliva. The virus is mainly transmitted to people when they breathe in air contaminated with the virus.

This happens when fresh rodent urine, droppings or nesting materials are stirred up. When tiny droplets containing the virus get into the air, this process is known as "aerosolization."

There are several other ways rodents may spread hantavirus to people:

- If a rodent with the virus bites someone, the virus may be spread to that person—but this is very rare.

- Researchers believe that you may be able to get the virus if you touch something that has been contaminated with rodent urine, droppings or saliva, and then touch your nose or mouth.

- Researchers also suspect that if virus-infected rodent urine, droppings or saliva contaminates food that you eat, you could also become sick.

These possibilities demonstrate why disinfecting rodent-infested areas is so important in preventing transmission of the virus.

Transmission can happen any place that infected rodents have infested. (Remember, by "carrier rodent" we mean deer mice plus cotton rats and rice rats in the Southeast, and the white-footed mouse in the Northeast. Common house mice do not carry hantavirus.) This could be barns or sheds or other outbuildings, warehouses or summer cottages closed up for the season. But carrier rodents infest homes as well.

Therefore, the most sensible way to avoid contact with rodents is to prevent rodents from infesting the places where you live and work, and to follow safety precautions if you do stumble into a rodent-infested area.

Rodents That Carry the Types of Hantavirus Which Cause HPS in the United States

Deer mouse. The Deer Mouse (*Peromyscus maniculatus*) is a deceptively cute animal, with big eyes and big ears. Its head and body are normally about 2–3 inches long, and the tail adds another 2–3 inches in length. You may see it in a variety of colors, from gray to reddish brown, depending on its age. The underbelly is always white and the tail has sharply defined white sides. The deer mouse is found almost everywhere in North America. Usually, the deer mouse likes woodlands, but also turns up in desert areas.

Cotton rat. The Cotton Rat (*Sigmodon hispidus*), which you'll find in the southeastern United States (and way down into Central and South America), has a bigger body than the deer mouse—head and body about 5–7 inches, and another 3–4 inches for the tail. The hair is longer and coarser, of a grayish brown color, even grayish black. The cotton rat prefers overgrown areas with shrubs and tall grasses.

Rice rat. The Rice Rat (*Oryzomys palustris*) is slightly smaller than the cotton rat, having a head and body 5–6 inches long, plus a very long, 4- to 7-inch tail. Rice rats sport short, soft, grayish brown fur on top, and gray or tawny underbellies. Their feet are whitish. As you might expect from the name, this rat likes marshy areas and is semiaquatic. It's found in the southeastern United States and in Central America.

White-footed mouse. The White-footed Mouse (*Peromyscus leucopus*) is hard to distinguish from the deer mouse. The head and body together are about four inches long. Note that its tail is normally shorter than its body (about 2–4 inches long). Topside, its fur ranges from pale brown to reddish brown, while its underside and feet are white. The white-footed mouse is found through southern New England, the Mid-Atlantic and southern states, the midwestern and western states, and Mexico. It prefers wooded and brushy areas, although sometimes it will live in more open ground.

Sometimes, a "Country Mouse" Becomes a "City Mouse"

Both the deer mouse and the cotton rat usually live in rural areas, but can also be found in cities when conditions are right, such as easy availability of food, water and shelter. (Remember this point when it comes to "discouraging" rodents, which is discussed under "How Do I Prevent HPS").

Other Rodents May Also Carry Hantavirus

Other rodents carry strains of hantavirus that cause HPS, but they have not yet been identified. In addition, other rodent species may play host to other types of hantaviruses that cause a different type of infection, hemorrhagic fever with renal syndrome, or HFRS.

It is wise, therefore, to avoid close contact with rodents in general.

Can You Get Hantavirus from Another Person?

The types of hantavirus that cause HPS in the United States cannot be transmitted from one person to another. For example, you cannot get the virus from touching or kissing a person who has HPS, or from a health care worker who has treated someone with the disease. Finally, you cannot get the virus from a blood transfusion in which the blood came from a person who became ill with HPS and survived.

Can You Get Hantavirus from Animals Other Than Rodents, or from Insects? What About Pets?

No— the hantaviruses that cause HPS in the United States are not known to be transmitted by any types of animals other than certain species of rodents. You cannot get hantavirus farm animals, such as cows, chickens or sheep, or from insects, such as mosquitoes. Dogs and cats are not known to carry hantavirus. However, they may bring infected rodents into contact with people if they catch such animals and carry them home. Guinea pigs, hamsters, gerbils and other such pets are not known to carry hantavirus.

Transmission Details: So How Does "Aerosolization" Really Work?

For a hantavirus to cause HPS, the virus must travel from the rodents that carry it to a person. A common way this happens is when a person breathes in the hantavirus from the air.

Let's create an imaginary scenario and go through the process step by step. Say you have a storage room in your home that you hardly ever enter. You keep old furniture there, old newspapers and magazines, and so on. At some point, a group of deer mice find their way into the room, looking for places to build nests. They found their way into the room through a crack—deer mice can squeeze through holes as small as a shirt button! Some mice chew through the fabric of an old armchair and build a nest inside it. Other mice shred bits of magazines and build nests under the shredded pieces.

A few of these mice are infected with the hantavirus. The infected mice don't show any signs of being sick. In fact, the virus does not seem to make them ill at all; it simply lives in their bodies. However, the virus is shed continuously from them: into the droppings and urine they leave around the room, and into their saliva, which dries on anything they have chewed, such as nesting material. Out in the environment like this, the virus can live for several days.

Meanwhile, you decide to clean up your storage room. You go inside, spend a few minutes moving boxes and furniture. The mice hear you coming and scurry away, leaving a trail of fresh urine! Because you find mouse droppings and some of the furniture stuffing the mice have used as nesting material, you get a broom and sweep up the mess. As you move around and sweep, tiny particles of fresh urine, droppings and saliva, with the virus in them, get kicked up into the air. This is the aerosolization. It is these tiny particles that you breathe in—and this is the beginning of becoming sick with HPS.

Because the virus is spread when virus-containing particles are stirred up into the air, an essential HPS tactic in areas showing signs of rodents is to avoid actions that raise dust and to carefully wet the area down with disinfectant. The less chance the virus has to get into the air, the less chance it will be breathed in.

Summing Up: How Hantavirus is Transmitted

- exposure to infected rodent (deer mouse, white-footed mouse, cotton rat, rice rat)

- rodent saliva/droppings dry up, are "aerosolized" and breathed in

- no transmission from one person to another, in the United States

- no known transmission from other animals or insects

Who Is at Risk of Getting HPS, and Why?

Anyone who comes into contact with rodents that carry hantavirus is at risk of HPS. Rodent infestation in and around the home remains the primary risk for hantavirus exposure. Even healthy individuals are at risk for HPS infection if exposed to the virus.

What Kind of Activities Are Risky?

Any activity that puts you in contact with rodent droppings, urine, saliva, or nesting materials can place you at risk for infection. Hantavirus is spread when virus-containing particles from rodent urine, droppings, or saliva are stirred into the air. It is important to avoid actions that raise dust, such as sweeping or vacuuming. Infection occurs when you breathe in virus particles.

Opening and cleaning previously unused buildings. Opening or cleaning cabins, sheds, and outbuildings, including barns, garages and storage facilities, that have been closed during the winter is a potential risk for hantavirus infections, especially in rural settings.

Housecleaning activities. Cleaning in and around your own home can put you at risk if rodents have made it their home too. Many homes can expect to shelter rodents, especially as the weather turns cold.

Work-related exposure. Construction, utility and pest control workers can be exposed when they work in crawl spaces, under houses, or in vacant buildings that may have a rodent population.

Campers and hikers. Campers and hikers can also be exposed when they use infested trail shelters or camp in other rodent habitats.

The chance of being exposed to hantavirus is greatest when people work, play, or live in closed spaces where rodents are actively living. However, recent research results show that many people who have become ill with HPS were infected with the disease after continued contact with rodents and/or their droppings. In addition, many people who have contracted HPS reported that they had not seen rodents or their droppings before becoming ill. Therefore, if you live in an area where the carrier rodents, such as the deer mouse, are known to live, take sensible precautions—even if you do not see rodents or their droppings.

What Are The Symptoms of HPS?

Early Symptoms

Early symptoms include fatigue, fever and muscle aches, especially in the large muscle groups—thighs, hips, back, and sometimes shoulders. These symptoms are universal.

There may also be headaches, dizziness, chills, and abdominal problems, such as nausea, vomiting, diarrhea, and abdominal pain. About half of all HPS patients experience these symptoms.

Late Symptoms

Four to 10 days after the initial phase of illness, the late symptoms of HPS appear. These include coughing and shortness of breath, with the sensation of, as one survivor put it, a "...tight band around my chest and a pillow over my face" as the lungs fill with fluid.

Uncommon Symptoms

Earache, sore throat, runny nose, and rash are very uncommon symptoms of HPS.

How long after contracting the virus do symptoms appear?

Due to the small number of HPS cases, the "incubation time" is not positively known. However, on the basis of limited information, it appears that symptoms may develop between 1 and 5 weeks after exposure to urine, droppings, or saliva of infected rodents.

Another important point to remember from the data that the CDC Special Pathogens Branch keeps on all reported cases of HPS, is that it appears many people who have become ill were in a situation where they did not see rodents or rodent droppings. Other people have had frequent contact with rodents and their droppings before becoming ill. This apparent inconsistency makes it very difficult to pin down the precise time when the virus was transmitted.

What Is the Treatment for HPS?

At the present time, there is no specific treatment or "cure" for hantavirus infection. However, we do know that if the infected individuals are recognized early and are taken to an intensive care unit, some patients may do better. In intensive care, patients are intubated and given oxygen therapy to help them through the period of severe respiratory distress. An antiviral medication, ribavirin, may be effective against the hantavirus, but its use in HPS is still experimental.

The earlier the patient is brought in to intensive care, the better. If a patient is experiencing full distress, it is less likely the treatment will be effective.

Therefore, if you have been around rodents and have symptoms of fever, deep muscle aches and severe shortness of breath, see your doctor *immediately*. Very strong suspicion for hantavirus infection is required to make the diagnosis. Be sure to tell your doctor that you have been around rodents—this will alert your physician to look closely for any rodent-carried disease such as HPS.

How Do I Prevent HPS?

Eliminate or minimize contact with rodents in your home, workplace, or campsite. If rodents don't find that where you are is a good place for them to be, then you're less likely to come into contact with them. Seal up holes and gaps in your home or garage. Place traps in and around your home to decrease rodent infestation. Clean up any easy-to-get food.

Recent research results show that many people who became ill with HPS developed the disease after having been in frequent contact with rodents and/or their droppings around a home or a workplace. On the other hand, many people who became ill reported that they had not seen rodents or rodent droppings at all. Therefore, if you live in an area where the carrier rodents are known to live, try to keep your home, vacation place, workplace, or campsite clean.

Prevention Indoors and Outdoors

Indoors:

- Keep a clean home, especially kitchen (wash dishes, clean counters and floor, keep food covered in rodent-proof containers).

- Keep a tight-fitting lid on garbage, discard uneaten pet food at the end of the day.

- Set and keep spring-loaded rodent traps. Set traps near baseboards because rodents tend to run along walls and in tight spaces rather than out in the open.

- Set Environmental Protection Agency-approved rodenticide with bait under plywood or plastic shelter along baseboards. These are sometimes known as "covered bait stations." Remember to follow product use instructions carefully, since rodenticides are poisonous to pets and people, too.

- Seal all entry holes 1/4 inch wide or wider with lath screen or lath metal, cement, wire screening or other patching materials, inside and out.

If bubonic plague is a problem in your area, spray flea killer or spread flea powder in the area before setting traps. This is important. If you control rodents but do not control fleas as well, you may increase the risk of infection with bubonic plague, since fleas will leave rodents once the rodents die and will seek out other food sources, including humans.

Outdoors:

- Clear brush, grass and junk from around house foundations to eliminate a source of nesting materials.

- Use metal flashing around the base of wooden, earthen or adobe homes to provide a strong metal barrier. Install so that the flashing reaches 12 inches above the ground and six inches down into the ground.

- Elevate hay, woodpiles and garbage cans to eliminate possible nesting sites. If possible, locate them 100 feet or more from your house.

- Trap rodents outside, too. Poisons or rodenticides may be used as well, but be sure to keep them out of the reach of children or pets.

- Encourage the presence of natural predators, such as non-poisonous snakes, owls and hawks.

- Remember, getting rid of all rodents isn't feasible, but with on-going effort you can keep the population very low.

Some Common Signs of Rodent Infestation

- **Rodent droppings.** This is one of the most reliable signs that you have a rodent problem. You may find droppings in places where you store your food or your pet/animal food, such as in cupboards and drawers or in bins. Because mice like to run in places that offer them some protection from predators, you may find droppings in cupboards or under the sink, along walls, or on top of wall studs or beams. Mice will leave droppings near their nests as well. Storage rooms, sheds, barns, or cabins loaded with boxes, bags, old furniture, and other objects make an ideal home for rodents, so you may find droppings there, even inside boxes and other containers.

  Workplaces can also make good rodent homes. Warehouses, res-taurants, and the like are obvious places to look because food may be plentiful there. However, rodents can infest office buildings, too. Once again, look for droppings in protected places, such as closets, storage rooms, or inside boxes.

- **Signs of rodent nests.** Rodents tend to build their nests from materials that are soft, fuzzy, or warm. Among common rodent nest materials are shredded paper, bunches of dry grass or small twigs, fabric, and furniture stuffing. Rodents will nest wherever safety from enemies can be found close enough to food and water, and they prefer places that are relatively quiet. Inside buildings, here are some places to look:
  - inside cabinets
  - under or inside dressers
  - in and among boxes
  - behind and inside machinery and appliances (kitchen appliances such as stoves or refrigerator drip pans; water coolers; and electric motor cases or computer cases)
  - inside upholstered furniture
  - inside double walls or the space between floors and ceilings.

- **Food boxes, containers, or food itself that appears to be nibbled.** Look for droppings nearby. Rodents can chew through plastic, so plastic bags do not make safe food storage containers.

- **Signs of rodent "feeding stations."** These are semi-hidden spots where rodents eat food they have collected. At these stations, rodents may leave larger-than-normal amounts of droppings/urine, plus remnants of a variety of foods (such as nut shells), bits of plastic or paper, and cockroach carcasses.

- **Evidence of gnawing.** To get to food, rodents will gnaw on almost anything that is softer than the enamel of their teeth. This includes such things as wood, paper board, cloth sacks, and materials even harder than these. Because rodents' teeth grow continuously, they must gnaw to keep them short. That may help to explain why chair legs or similar surfaces show gnawed spots or tooth marks in rodent-infested places.

- **An odd, stale smell.** In closed-up rooms infested by rodents, you will commonly smell an unusual, musky odor.

- **You see a mouse in your house.** However, this doesn't happen very frequently. Why? Rodents are normally active at night, and generally avoid humans. If you have rodents, unless the infestation is large, you may never see one.

Remember that not all types of rodents carry hantavirus. Neither common house mice nor common rats have been associated with HPS in humans, for example. Yet because it can be tough to tell just what kind of rodents you have, play it safe—clean up the infestation and rodent-proof your home or workplace.

Clean Up Infested Areas, Using Safety Precautions

Put on latex rubber gloves before cleaning up.

Don't stir up dust by sweeping up or vacuuming up droppings, urine or nesting materials.

Instead, thoroughly wet contaminated areas with detergent or liquid to deactivate the virus. Most general purpose disinfectants and household detergents are effective. However, a hypochlorite solution prepared by mixing 1 and 1/2 cups of household bleach in 1 gallon of water may be used in place of commercial disinfectant. When using the chlorine solution, avoid spilling the mixture on clothing or other items that may be damaged.

Once everything is wet, take up contaminated materials with a damp towel, then mop or sponge the area with disinfectant.

Spray dead rodents with disinfectant, then double-bag along with all cleaning materials and bury or burn—or throw out in an appropriate waste disposal system. If burning or burying isn't feasible, contact your local or state health department about other disposal methods.

Finally, disinfect gloves before taking them off with disinfectant or soap and water. After taking off the clean gloves, thoroughly wash hands with soap and warm water.

When going into cabins or outbuildings (or work areas) that have been closed for awhile, open them up and air out before cleaning.

Hantaviruses and disinfectants. Hantaviruses are surrounded by a lipid (fatty) envelope, so they are somewhat fragile. The lipid envelope can be destroyed and the virus killed by fat solvents, such as alcohol, ordinary disinfectants and household bleach. That is why one of the most important ways to prevent transmitting the disease is to carefully wet down dead rodents and areas where rodents have been with disinfectant and/or bleach. When you do this, you are killing the virus itself and reducing the chance that the virus will get into the air.

Special Pathogens Branch recommends a 10% bleach solution be used to inactivate hantaviruses. A 10% solution corresponds to 1 and a half cups of household bleach per gallon of water, or 1 part bleach to nine parts water.

What If My House or Workplace Is Heavily Infested with Rodents?

You should get help from a professional exterminator if you see lots of droppings or rodents—you may have a bad infestation problem. Or you can contact your local health authorities for advice.

CDC has recommendations for how heavy infestations may most safely be handled. Read "Special Precautions for Homes of Persons with Confirmed Hantavirus Infection or Buildings with Heavy Rodent Infestations" below for more information.

Special Precautions for Homes of Persons with Confirmed Hantavirus Infection or Buildings with Heavy Rodent Infestations

Special precautions should be used for cleaning homes or buildings with heavy rodent infestations in areas where HPS has been reported. If you are attempting to deal with such an infestation, it is recommended that you contact the responsible local, state, or federal public health agency for guidance.

The special precautions may also apply to vacant dwellings that have attracted numbers of rodents while unoccupied and to dwellings and other structures that have been occupied by persons with confirmed hantavirus infection.

Workers who are either hired specifically to perform the clean-up or asked to do so as part of their work activities should receive a thorough orientation from the responsible health agency about hantavirus transmission and should be trained to perform the required activities safely.

Precautions to be used:

- Persons involved in the clean-up should wear coveralls (disposable, if possible), rubber boots or disposable shoe covers, rubber or plastic gloves, protective goggles, and an appropriate respiratory protection device, such as a half-mask air-purifying (or negative-pressure) respirator with a high-efficiency particulate air (HEPA) filter or a powered air-purifying respirator (PAPR) with HEPA filters.

Note: The HEPA classification has been discontinued. Please read "Update On the Nomenclature and Use of Respirators as a Precaution for Hantavirus Infection" for details.

- Personal protective gear should be decontaminated upon removal at the end of the day. If the coveralls are not disposable, they should be laundered on site. If no laundry facilities are available, the coveralls should be immersed in liquid disinfectant until they can be washed.

- All potentially infective waste material (including respirator filters) from clean-up operations that cannot be burned or deep buried on site should be double bagged in appropriate plastic bags. The bagged material should then be labeled as infectious (if it is to be transported) and disposed of in accordance with local requirements for infectious waste.

- Workers who develop symptoms suggestive of HPS within 45 days of the last potential exposure should immediately seek medical attention. The physician should contact local health authorities promptly if hantavirus-associated illness is suspected. A blood sample should be obtained and forwarded with the baseline serum through the state health department to CDC for hantavirus antibody testing.

Precautions for Workers in Affected Areas Who are Regularly Exposed to Rodents

Persons who frequently handle or are exposed to rodents (e.g., mammalogists, pest-control workers) in the affected area are probably at higher risk for hantavirus infection than the general public because of their frequency of exposure. Therefore, enhanced precautions are warranted to protect them against hantavirus infection.

Precautions to be used:

- Workers in potentially high-risk settings should be informed about the symptoms of the disease and be given detailed guidance on prevention measures.

- Workers who develop a febrile or respiratory illness within 45 days of the last potential exposure should immediately seek medical attention and inform the attending physician of the potential occupational risk of hantavirus infection. The physician should contact local health authorities promptly if hantavirus-associated illness is suspected. A blood sample should be obtained and forwarded with the baseline serum through the state health department to CDC for hantavirus antibody testing.

- Workers should wear a half-face air-purifying (or negative-pressure) respirator or PAPR equipped with HEPA filters when removing rodents from traps or handling rodents in the affected area. (Please note: the HEPA classification recently has been discontinued. Under the new classification system, the N-100 filter type is recommended. Read the Federal Occupational Safety and Health Administration (OSHA) directive online, at "OSHA Directives: CPL 2-0.120 - Inspection procedures for the Respiratory Protection Standard".), at http://www.osha.gov/pls/oshaweb/owadisp.show_document?p_table=DIRECTIVES&p_id=2275

- Respirators (including positive-pressure types) are not considered protective if facial hair interferes with the face seal, since proper fit cannot be assured. Respirator use practices should be in accord with a comprehensive user program and should be supervised by a knowledgeable person.

- Workers should wear rubber or plastic gloves when handling rodents or handling traps containing rodents. Gloves should be washed and disinfected before removing them, as described above.

- Traps contaminated by rodent urine or feces or in which a rodent was captured should be disinfected with a commercial disinfectant or bleach solution.

- Spray dead rodents with disinfectant, then double-bag along with all cleaning materials and bury or burn—or throw out in an appropriate waste disposal system. If burning or burying isn't feasible, contact your local or state health department about other disposal methods.

- Persons removing organs or obtaining blood from rodents in affected areas should contact the Special Pathogens Branch, Division of Viral and Rickettsial Diseases, National Center for Infectious Diseases, Centers for Disease Control and Prevention, [telephone (404) 639-1115] for detailed safety precautions.

Precautions for Other Occupational Groups Who Have Potential Rodent Contact

Insufficient information is available at this time to allow general recommendations regarding risks or precautions for persons in the

affected areas who work in occupations with unpredictable or incidental contact with rodents or their habitations. Examples of such occupations include telephone installers, maintenance workers, plumbers,
electricians, and certain construction workers. Workers in these jobs
may have to enter various buildings, crawl spaces, or other sites that
may be rodent infested. Recommendations for such circumstances
must be made on a case-by-case basis after the specific working environment has been assessed and state or local health departments
have been consulted.

Precautions for Campers and Hikers in the Affected Areas

There is no evidence to suggest that travel into areas where HPS
has been reported should be restricted. Most usual tourist activities
pose little or no risk that travelers will be exposed to rodents or their
urine and/or droppings.

However, persons who do outdoor activities such as camping or
hiking in areas where the disease has been reported should take precautions to reduce the likelihood of their exposure to potentially infectious materials.

Useful precautions:

- Avoid coming into contact with rodents and rodent burrows or
  disturbing dens (such as pack rat nests).

- Air out, then disinfect cabins or shelters before using them.
  These places often shelter rodents.

- Do not pitch tents or place sleeping bags in areas in proximity
  to rodent droppings or burrows or near areas that may shelter
  rodents or provide food for them (e.g., garbage dumps or woodpiles).

- If possible, do not sleep on the bare ground. In shelters, use a cot
  with the sleeping surface at least 12 inches above the ground. Use
  tents with floors or a ground cloth if sleeping in the open air.

- Keep food in rodent-proof containers.

- Promptly bury (or—preferably—burn followed by burying, when
  in accordance with local requirements) all garbage and trash, or
  discard in covered trash containers.

- Use only bottled water or water that has been disinfected by filtration, boiling, chlorination, or iodination for drinking, cooking,
  washing dishes, and brushing teeth.

- And last but not least, do not play with or handle any rodents that show up at the camping or hiking site, even if they appear friendly.

Update On the Nomenclature and Use of Respirators as a Precaution for Hantavirus Infection

The CDC Interim Recommendations for Risk Reduction for Hantavirus Infection describe precautions for persons who are involved in the cleanup of homes of confirmed cases of hantavirus infection or of areas with heavy rodent infestation and for workers in affected areas who are regularly exposed to rodents. Among these precautions is the wearing of one of the following types of respirators equipped with a high-efficiency particulate air (HEPA) filter:

- half-mask air-purifying (or negative-pressure) respirator

- powered air-purifying respirator (PAPR)

Table 26.1. New Classes of Filters for Respiratory Protection Devices As described in NIOSH 42, CFR 84.

New classes of filters ††		Equivalent to HEPA	Characteristics
N-95	N-99	N-100 (99.97)	Not resistant to oil
R-95	R-99	R-100 (99.97)	Resistant to oil
P-95	P-99	P-100 (99.97)	Oil Proof

†† number indicates % efficiency in removing monodispersed particles 0.3 micrometers in diameter.

Authority for testing and certifying these respirators has been given exclusively to NIOSH. For additional information:

- Contact the Industrial Hygiene Section, Office of Health & Safety, CDC at 404 639-3112.

- Read the NIOSH directive online, at "OSHA Directives: CPL 2-0.120 - Inspection procedures for the Respiratory Protection Standard", at http://www. osha.gov/pls/oshaweb/owadisp.show_document?p_table= DIRECTIVES&p_id=2275

Changes (made in February 1999) in the nomenclature and certification of the type of filters used in these respirators include the discontinuation of the HEPA designation and the designation of new classes of filters. As shown on the Table 26.1, the N-100 (99.97) is equivalent to the previous HEPA filter.

Use of an N-100 filter should provide the same protection as the HEPA filter. Due to the nature of the virus, no studies have been able to test the efficacy of either the HEPA or N-100 filters in protecting against HPS transmission. Available evidence suggests that HPS is transmitted by inspiring small (less than 5 micron) viral particles in aerosols which the N-100 is the most effective in removing.

Cautions: All negative-pressure respirators are fit-dependent. Anything that interferes with the respirator's face seal, such as facial hair, will allow ambient air to bypass the filter medium in the respirator. Ideally, users should be fit-tested with the same make, model, style, and size of respirator that will be actually used. Respirator practices should follow a comprehensive user program and be supervised by a knowledgeable person.

Chapter 27

Leishmaniasis

Leishmania Infection (Leishmaniasis)

What is leishmaniasis?

Leishmaniasis (LEASH-ma-NIGH-a-sis) is a parasitic disease spread by the bite of infected sand flies. There are several different forms of leishmaniasis. The most common forms are cutaneous (cue-TAY-knee-us) leishmaniasis, which causes skin sores, and visceral (VIS-er-al) leishmaniasis, which affects some of the internal organs of the body (for example, spleen, liver, bone marrow).

What are the signs and symptoms of cutaneous leishmaniasis?

People who have cutaneous leishmaniasis have one or more sores on their skin. The sores can change in size and appearance over time. They often end up looking somewhat like a volcano, with a raised edge and central crater. Some sores are covered by a scab. The sores can be painless or painful. Some people have swollen glands near the sores (for example, under the arm if the sores are on the arm or hand).

What are the signs and symptoms of visceral leishmaniasis?

People who have visceral leishmaniasis usually have fever, weight loss, and an enlarged spleen and liver (usually the spleen is bigger

"Leishmania Infection," Division of Parasitic Diseases (DPD), Centers for Disease Control and Prevention (CDC), reviewed June 9, 2000.

than the liver). Some patients have swollen glands. Certain blood tests are abnormal. For example, patients usually have low blood counts, including a low red blood cell count (anemia), low white blood cell count, and low platelet count.

How common is leishmaniasis?

The number of new cases of cutaneous leishmaniasis each year in the world is thought to be about 1.5 million. The number of new cases of visceral leishmaniasis is thought to be about 500,000.

In what parts of the world is leishmaniasis found?

Leishmaniasis is found in parts of about 88 countries. Approximately 350 million people live in these areas. Most of the affected countries are in the tropics and subtropics. The settings in which leishmaniasis is found range from rain forests in Central and South America to deserts in West Asia. More than 90 percent of the world's cases of visceral leishmaniasis are in India, Bangladesh, Nepal, Sudan, and Brazil.

Leishmaniasis is found in some parts of the following areas:

- In Mexico, Central America, and South America—from northern Argentina to southern Texas (not in Uruguay, Chile, or Canada)
- Southern Europe (leishmaniasis is not common in travelers to southern Europe)
- Asia (not Southeast Asia)
- The Middle East
- Africa (particularly East and North Africa, with some cases elsewhere)

Leishmaniasis is not found in Australia or Oceania (that is, islands in the Pacific, including Melanesia, Micronesia, and Polynesia).

Could I get leishmaniasis in the United States?

Probably not. It is possible but very unlikely that you would get leishmaniasis in the United States. Very rarely, people living in rural southern Texas have developed skin sores from cutaneous leishmaniasis.

No cases of visceral leishmaniasis are known to have been acquired in the United States.

How is leishmaniasis spread?

Leishmaniasis is spread by the bite of some types of phlebotomine sand flies. Sand flies become infected by biting an infected animal (for example, a rodent or dog) or person. Since sand flies do not make noise when they fly, people may not realize they are present. Sand flies are very small and may be hard to see; they are only about one-third the size of typical mosquitoes. Sand flies usually are most active in twilight, evening, and night-time hours (from dusk to dawn). Sand flies are less active during the hottest time of the day. However, they will bite if they are disturbed, such as when a person brushes up against the trunk of a tree where sand flies are resting. Rarely, leishmaniasis is spread from a pregnant woman to her baby. Leishmaniasis also can be spread by blood transfusions or contaminated needles.

Who is at risk for leishmaniasis?

People of all ages are at risk for leishmaniasis if they live or travel where leishmaniasis is found. Leishmaniasis usually is more common in rural than urban areas; but it is found in the outskirts of some cities. The risk for leishmaniasis is highest from dusk to dawn because this is when sand flies are the most active. All it takes to get infected is to be bitten by one infected sand fly. This is more likely to happen the more people are bitten, that is, the more time they spend outside in rural areas from dusk to dawn. Adventure travelers, Peace Corps volunteers, missionaries, ornithologists (people who study birds), other people who do research outdoors at night, and soldiers are examples of people who may have an increased risk for leishmaniasis (especially cutaneous leishmaniasis).

If I were bitten by an infected sand fly, how quickly would I become sick?

People with cutaneous leishmaniasis usually develop skin sores within a few weeks (sometimes as long as months) of when they were bitten.

People with visceral leishmaniasis usually become sick within several months (rarely as long as years) of when they were bitten.

Can leishmaniasis be a serious disease if not treated?

Yes, it can be. The skin sores of cutaneous leishmaniasis will heal on their own, but this can take months or even years. The sores can leave ugly scars. If not treated, infection that started in the skin rarely spreads to the nose or mouth and causes sores there (mucosal leishmaniasis). This can happen with some of the types of the parasite found in Central and South America. Mucosal leishmaniasis might not be noticed until years after the original skin sores healed. The best way to prevent mucosal leishmaniasis is to treat the cutaneous infection before it spreads.

If not treated, visceral leishmaniasis can cause death.

What should I do if I think I might have leishmaniasis?

See your health care provider, particularly if you have traveled to an area where leishmaniasis is found and you have developed skin sores that aren't healing. Be sure to tell your health care provider where you have traveled and that you might be at risk for leishmaniasis.

It is very rare for travelers to get visceral leishmaniasis.

How will my health care provider know if I have leishmaniasis?

The first step is to find out if you have traveled to a part of the world where leishmaniasis is found. Your health care provider will ask you about any signs or symptoms of leishmaniasis you may have, such as skin sores that have not healed. If you have skin sores, your health care provider will likely want to take some samples directly from the sores. These samples can be examined for the parasite under a microscope, in cultures, and through other means. A blood test for detecting antibody (immune response) to the parasite can be helpful, particularly for cases of visceral leishmaniasis. However, tests to look for the parasite itself should also be done. CDC staff can help with the laboratory testing. Diagnosing leishmaniasis can be difficult. Sometimes the laboratory tests are negative even if a person has leishmaniasis.

How is leishmaniasis treated?

Your health care provider can talk with CDC staff about whether your case of leishmaniasis should be treated, and, if so, how. Most people who have cutaneous leishmaniasis do not need to be hospitalized during their treatment.

How is leishmaniasis prevented?

The best way for travelers to prevent leishmaniasis is by protecting themselves from sand fly bites. Vaccines and drugs for preventing infection are not yet available. To decrease their risk of being bitten, travelers should:

- Stay in well-screened or air-conditioned areas as much as possible. Avoid outdoor activities, especially from dusk to dawn, when sand flies are the most active.

- When outside, wear long-sleeved shirts, long pants, and socks. Tuck your shirt into your pants.

- Apply insect repellent on uncovered skin and under the ends of sleeves and pant legs. Follow the instructions on the label of the repellent. The most effective repellents are those that contain the chemical DEET (N,N-diethyl-meta-toluamide). The concentration of DEET varies among repellents. Repellents with DEET concentrations of 30–35% are quite effective, and the effect should last about 4 hours. Lower concentrations should be used for children (no more than 10% DEET). Repellents with DEET should be used sparingly on children from 2 to 6 years old and not at all on children less than 2 years old.

- Spray clothing with permethrin-containing insecticides. The insecticide should be reapplied after every five washings.

- Spray living and sleeping areas with an insecticide to kill insects.

- If you are not sleeping in an area that is well screened or air-conditioned, use a bed net and tuck it under your mattress. If possible, use a bed net that has been soaked in or sprayed with permethrin. The permethrin will be effective for several months if the bed net is not washed. Keep in mind that sand flies are much smaller than mosquitoes and therefore can get through smaller holes. Fine-mesh netting (at least 18 holes to the inch; some sources say even finer) is needed for an effective barrier against sand flies. This is particularly important if the bed net has not been treated with permethrin. However, it may be uncomfortable to sleep under such a closely woven bed net when it is hot.

Note: Bed nets, repellents containing DEET, and permethrin should be purchased before traveling and can be found in hardware, camping, and military surplus stores.

If I have already had leishmaniasis, could I get it again?

Yes. Some people have had cutaneous leishmaniasis more than once. Therefore, you should follow the preventive measures listed above whenever you are in an area where leishmaniasis is found.

For More Information:

Herwaldt BL. Leishmaniasis. *Lancet* 1999;354:1191–9.

Herwaldt BL, Stokes SL, Juranek DD. American cutaneous leishmaniasis in U.S. travelers. *Ann Intern Med* 1993;118:779–84.

Berman JD. Human leishmaniasis: clinical, diagnostic, and chemotherapeutic developments in the last 10 years. *Clin Infect Dis* 1997;24: 684–703.

Desjeux P. Leishmaniasis: public health aspects and control. *Clin Dermatol* 1996;14:417–23.

Chapter 28

Lyme Disease

Tick species that transmit Lyme Disease are the Black-legged tick (Deer tick), and the western black-legged tick.

What Is Lyme Disease?

Lyme disease (LD) is an infection caused by *Borrelia burgdorferi*, a type of bacterium called a spirochete (pronounced spy-ro-keet) that is carried by deer ticks. An infected tick can transmit the spirochete to the humans and animals it bites. Untreated, the bacterium travels through the bloodstream, establishes itself in various body tissues, and can cause a number of symptoms, some of which are severe.

LD manifests itself as a multisystem inflammatory disease that affects the skin in its early, localized stage, and spreads to the joints, nervous system and, to a lesser extent, other organ systems in its later, disseminated stages. If diagnosed and treated early with antibiotics, LD is almost always readily cured. Generally, LD in its later stages can also be treated effectively, but because the rate of disease progression and individual response to treatment varies from one patient to the next, some patients may have symptoms that linger for months or even years following treatment. In rare instances, LD causes permanent damage.

Although LD is now the most common arthropod-borne illness in the U.S. (more than 100,000 cases have been reported to the Centers for Disease Control and Prevention [CDC] since 1982), its diagnosis and treatment can be challenging for clinicians due to its diverse manifestations and the unreliability of currently available serological (blood) tests.

The prevalence of LD in the northeast is due to the presence of large numbers of the deer tick's preferred hosts—white-footed mice and deer—and their proximity to humans. White-footed mice serve as the principal "reservoirs of infection" on which many nymphal (juvenile) ticks feed and become infected with the LD spirochete. An infected tick can then transmit its store of spirochetes to its next host (e.g., an unsuspecting human).

The LD spirochete, *Borrelia burgdorferi*, infects other species of ticks but is known to be transmitted to humans and other animals only by the deer tick (also known as the black-legged tick) and the related Western black-legged tick. Studies have shown that an infected tick normally cannot begin transmitting the spirochete until it has been attached to its host about 36–48 hours; the best line of defense against LD, therefore, is to examine yourself at least once daily and remove any ticks before they become engorged (swollen) with blood.

Generally, if you discover a deer tick attached to your skin that has not yet become engorged, it has not been there long enough to transmit the LD spirochete. Nevertheless, it is advisable to be alert in case any symptoms do appear; a red rash (especially surrounding the tick bite), flu-like symptoms, or joint pains in the first month following any deer tick bite could signal the onset of LD.

Manifestations of what we now call Lyme disease were first reported in medical literature in Europe in 1883. Over the years, various clinical signs of this illness have been noted as separate medical conditions: acrodermatitis chronica atrophicans (ACA), lymphadenosis benigna cutis (LABC), erythema migrans (EM), and lymphocytic meningoradiculitis (Bannwarth's syndrome). However, these diverse manifestations were not recognized as indicators of a single infectious illness until 1975, when LD was described following an outbreak of apparent juvenile arthritis, preceded by a rash, among residents of Lyme, Connecticut.

Where Is Lyme Disease Prevalent?

LD is spreading slowly along and inland from the upper east coast, as well as in the upper midwest and the northern California and Oregon coast. The mode of spread is not entirely clear and is probably due to a number of factors such as bird migration, mobility of deer and other large mammals, and infected ticks dropping off of pets as people travel around the country.

In order to assess LD risk you should know whether infected deer ticks are active in your area or in places you may visit. The population density and percentage of infected ticks that may transmit LD vary markedly from one region of the country to another. There is even great variation from county to county within a state and from area to area within a county. For example, less than 5% of adult ticks south of Maryland are infected with *B. burgdorferi*, while up to 50% are infected in hyperendemic areas (areas with a high tick infection rate) of the northeast. The tick infection rate in Pacific coastal states is between 2% and 4%.

Symptoms

The early symptoms of LD can be mild and easily overlooked. People who are aware of the risk of LD in their communities and who don't ignore the sometimes subtle early symptoms are most likely to seek medical attention and treatment early enough to be assured of a full recovery.

The first symptom is usually an expanding rash (called erythema migrans, or EM, in medical terms) which is thought to occur in 80% to 90% of all LD cases. An EM rash generally has the following characteristics:

- Usually (but not always) radiates from the site of the tickbite.

- Appears either as a solid red expanding rash or blotch, *or* a central spot surrounded by clear skin that is in turn ringed by an expanding red rash (looks like a bull's-eye).

- Appears an average of 1 to 2 weeks (range = 3 to 30 days) after disease transmission.

- Has an average diameter of 5 to 6 inches (range = 2 inches to 2 feet).

- Persists for about 3 to 5 weeks.

- May or may not be warm to the touch.

- Is usually not painful or itchy.

EM rashes appearing on brown-skinned or sun-tanned patients may be more difficult to identify because of decreased contrast between normal skin tones and the red rash. A dark, bruise-like appearance is more common on dark-skinned patients.

Ticks will attach anywhere on the body, but prefer body creases such as the armpit, groin, back of the knee, and nape of the neck; rashes will therefore often appear in (but are not restricted to) these areas. Please note that multiple rashes may, in some cases, appear elsewhere on the body some time after the initial rash, or, in a few cases, in the absence of an initial rash.

Around the time the rash appears, other symptoms such as joint pains, chills, fever, and fatigue are common, but they may not seem serious enough to require medical attention. These symptoms may be brief, only to recur as a broader spectrum of symptoms as the disease progresses.

As the LD spirochete continues disseminating through the body, a number of other symptoms including severe fatigue, a stiff, aching neck, and peripheral nervous system (PNS) involvement such as tingling or numbness in the extremities or facial palsy (paralysis) can occur.

The more severe, potentially debilitating symptoms of later-stage LD may occur weeks, months, or, in a few cases, years after a tick bite. These can include severe headaches, painful arthritis and swelling of joints, cardiac abnormalities, and central nervous system (CNS) involvement leading to cognitive (mental) disorders.

The following is a checklist of common symptoms seen in various stages of LD:

Localized Early (Acute) Stage:

- Solid red or bull's-eye rash, usually at site of bite
- Swelling of lymph glands near tick bite
- Generalized achiness
- Headache

Early Disseminated Stage:

- Two or more rashes not at site of bite
- Migrating pains in joints/tendons
- Headache
- Stiff, aching neck
- Facial palsy (facial paralysis similar to Bell's palsy)
- Tingling or numbness in extremities
- Multiple enlarged lymph glands

212

- Abnormal pulse
- Sore throat
- Changes in vision
- Fever of 100° to 102° F
- Severe fatigue

Late Stage:

- Arthritis (pain/swelling) of one or two large joints
- Disabling neurological disorders (disorientation; confusion; dizziness; short-term memory loss; inability to concentrate, finish sentences or follow conversations; mental "fog")
- Numbness in arms/hands or legs/feet

Diagnosis

If you think you have LD symptoms you should see your physician immediately. The EM rash, which may occur in up to 90% of the reported cases, is a specific feature of LD, and treatment should begin immediately.

Even in the absence of an EM rash, diagnosis of early LD should be made solely on the basis of symptoms and evidence of a tick bite, not blood tests, which can often give false results if performed in the first month after initial infection (later on, the tests are considered more reliable). If you live in an endemic area, have symptoms consistent with early LD and suspect recent exposure to a tick, present your suspicion to your doctor so that he or she may make a more informed diagnosis.

If early symptoms are undetected or ignored, you may develop more severe symptoms weeks, months or perhaps years after you were infected. In this case, the CDC recommends using the ELISA and Western-blot blood tests to determine whether you are infected. These tests, as noted above, are considered more reliable and accurate when performed at least a month after initial infection, although no test is 100% accurate.

If you have neurological symptoms or swollen joints your doctor may, in addition, recommend a PCR (polymerase chain reaction) test via a spinal tap or withdrawal of synovial fluid from an affected joint. This test amplifies the DNA of the spirochete and will usually indicate its presence.

Treatment

Early treatment of LD (within the first few weeks after initial infection) is straightforward and almost always results in a full cure. Treatment begun after the first three weeks will also likely provide a cure, but the cure rate decreases the longer treatment is delayed.

Doxycycline, amoxicillin and Ceftin are the three oral antibiotics most highly recommended for treatment of all but a few symptoms of LD. A recent study of Lyme arthritis in the *New England Journal of Medicine* indicates that a four-week course of oral doxycycline is just as effective in treating late LD, and much less expensive, than a similar course of intravenous ceftriaxone (Rocephin®) unless neurological or severe cardiac abnormalities are present. If these symptoms are present, the study recommends immediate intravenous (IV) treatment.

Treatment of late-Lyme patients is, unfortunately, an inexact science. Often, LD in its later stages can be treated effectively, but individual variation in the rate of disease progression and response to treatment may, in some cases, render standard antibiotic treatment regimens ineffective. In a small percentage of late-Lyme patients, the disease becomes a treatment-resistant chronic condition with symptoms persisting for many months or even years. Conversely, a significant percentage of late-Lyme patients have reported a slow improvement in and ultimate resolution of their persisting symptoms months or even years following oral or IV treatment that apparently eliminated the infection.

Although treatment approaches for patients with late-stage LD have become a matter of considerable debate, many physicians and the CDC recognize that, in some cases, multiple courses of either oral or IV (depending on the symptoms presented) antibiotic treatment may be indicated. However, long-term IV treatment courses (longer than the recommended 4–6 weeks) are not usually advised due to possible adverse side effects, including auto-immune deficiencies. While there is some speculation that long-term courses may be more effective than the recommended 4–6 weeks in certain cases, there is currently no scientific evidence to support this assertion.

Prevention and Control

Deer ticks prefer to hide in shady, moist ground litter, but can often be found above the ground clinging to tall grass, brush, shrubs and low tree branches. They also inhabit lawns and gardens, especially at the edges of woodlands and around old stone walls where deer and white-footed mice, the ticks' preferred hosts, thrive. Within the endemic range of *B. burgdorferi* (the spirochete that infects the deer tick and causes LD), no natural, vegetated area can be considered completely free of infected ticks.

Deer ticks cannot jump or fly, and do not drop from above onto a passing animal. Potential hosts (which include all wild birds and mammals, domestic animals, and humans) acquire ticks only by direct contact with them. Once a tick latches onto human skin it generally climbs upward until it reaches a protected or creased area, often the back of the knee, groin, navel, armpit, ears, or nape of the neck. It then begins the process of inserting its mouthparts into the skin until it reaches the blood supply.

In tick-infested areas, the best precaution against LD is to avoid contact with soil, leaf litter and vegetation as much as possible. However, if you garden, hike, camp, hunt, work outdoors or otherwise spend time in woods, brush or overgrown fields, you should use a combination of precautions to dramatically reduce your chances of getting Lyme disease:

First, using color and size as indicators (see Figures 28.1 and 28.2), learn how to distinguish between:

- deer tick nymphs and adults—deer ticks are found east of the Rockies; their look-alike close relatives, the western black-legged ticks, are found and can transmit Lyme disease west of the Rockies.

- deer ticks and two other common tick species—dog ticks and Lone Star ticks (neither of which is known to transmit Lyme disease).

Then, when spending time outdoors, make these easy precautions part of your routine:

- Wear enclosed shoes and light-colored clothing with a tight weave to spot ticks easily

- Scan clothes and any exposed skin frequently for ticks while outdoors

- Stay on cleared, well-traveled trails

- Use insect repellant containing DEET (Diethyl-meta-toluamide) on skin or clothes if you intend to go off-trail or into overgrown areas

- Avoid sitting directly on the ground or on stone walls (havens for ticks and their hosts)

- Keep long hair tied back, especially when gardening

- Do a final, full-body tick-check at the end of the day (also check children and pets)

When taking the above precautions, consider these important facts:

- If you tuck long pants into socks and shirts into pants, be aware that ticks that contact your clothes will climb upward in search of exposed skin. This means they may climb to hidden areas of the head and neck if not intercepted first; spot-check clothes frequently.

- Clothes can be sprayed with either DEET or Permethrin. Only DEET can be used on exposed skin, but never in high concentrations; follow the manufacturer's directions.

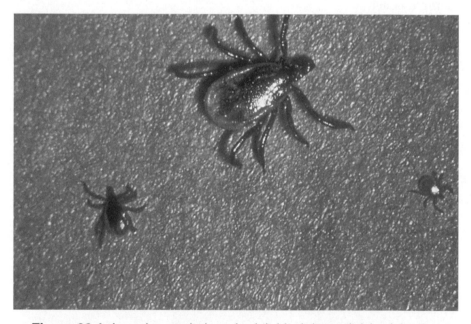

Figure 28.1. Larval, nymphal, and adult black-legged ticks (also known as deer ticks), Ixodes scapularis. The adult tick is approximately the same size as the letter "M" in the word DIME on the back of the U.S. coin. (From Public Health Image Library, Image #1205, provided by Michael L. Levin, Ph.D., Centers for Disease Control and Prevention),

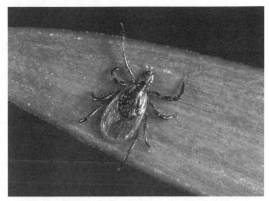

These "black-legged ticks" are known to transmit Lyme disease.

Figure 28.2. Black-legged ticks, Ixodes scapularis *(From Public Health Image Library, Image #1699 by Jim Gathany, provided by Michael L. Levin, Ph.D., Centers for Disease Control and Prevention); Female American brown dog tick,* Dermacentor variabilis *(From Public Health Image Library, Image #170, provided by Gary O. Maupin, Ph.D., Centers for Disease Control and Prevention); and Lone Star tick,* Amblyomma americanum *(From Public Health Image Library, Image #4407 by James Gathany, provided by Michael L. Levin, Ph.D., Centers for Disease Control and Prevention).*

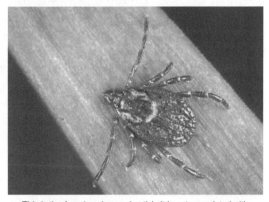

This is the American brown dog tick. It is not associated with Lyme disease transmission.

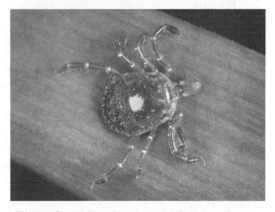

This Lone Star tick (brown) is not associated with Lyme disease transmission, but it is a vector for other diseases, including Rocky Mountain spotted fever.

217

- Upon returning home, clothes can be spun in the dryer for 20 minutes to kill any unseen ticks

- A shower and shampoo may help to dislodge crawling ticks, but is only somewhat effective. Inspect yourself and your children carefully after a shower. Keep in mind that nymphal deer ticks are the size of poppy seeds; adult deer ticks are the size of sesame seeds.

Any contact with vegetation, even playing in the yard, can result in exposure to ticks, so careful daily self-inspection is necessary whenever you engage in outdoor activities and the temperature exceeds 40 degrees F (the temperature above which deer ticks are active). Frequent tick checks should be followed by a systematic, whole-body examination each night before going to bed. Performed consistently, this ritual is perhaps the single most effective current method for prevention of Lyme disease.

If you *do* find a tick attached to your skin, there is no need to panic. Not all ticks are infected, and studies of infected deer ticks have shown that they begin transmitting Lyme disease an average of 36 to 48 hours after attachment. Therefore, your chances of contracting LD are greatly reduced if you remove a tick within the first 24 hours. Remember, too, that the majority of early Lyme disease cases are easily treated and cured.

To remove a tick, follow these steps:

1. Using a pair of pointed precision tweezers, grasp the tick by the head or mouthparts right where they enter the skin. *Do not* grasp the tick by the body. Keep in mind that certain types of fine-pointed tweezers, especially those that are etched, or rasped, at the tips, may not be effective in removing nymphal deer ticks. Choose unrasped fine-pointed tweezers whose tips align tightly when pressed firmly together.

2. Without jerking, pull firmly and steadily directly outward. *Do not* twist the tick out or apply petroleum jelly, a hot match, alcohol or any other irritant to the tick in an attempt to get it to back out. These methods can backfire and even increase the chances of the tick transmitting the disease.

3. Place the tick in a vial or jar of alcohol to kill it.

4. Clean the bite wound with disinfectant.

Then, monitor the site of the bite for the appearance of a rash beginning 3 to 30 days after the bite. At the same time, learn about the other early symptoms of Lyme disease and watch to see if they appear in about the same timeframe. If a rash or other early symptoms develop, see a physician immediately.

Finally, prevention is not limited to personal precautions. Those who enjoy spending time in their yards can reduce the tick population around the home by:

- keeping lawns mowed and edges trimmed.

- clearing brush, leaf litter and tall grass around houses and at the edges of gardens and open stone walls.

- stacking woodpiles neatly in a dry location and preferably off the ground.

- clearing all leaf litter (including the remains of perennials) out of the garden in the fall.

- keeping the ground under bird feeders clean so as not to attract small mammals.

- having a licensed professional spray the residential environment (only the areas frequented by humans) with an insecticide in late May (to control nymphs) and optionally in September (to control adults).

Chapter 29

Lymphatic Filariasis

What is lymphatic filariasis?

Lymphatic filariasis is a parasitic disease caused by microscopic, thread-like worms. The adult worms only live in the human lymph system. The lymph system maintains your body's fluid balance and fights infections.

Lymphatic filariasis affects over 120 million people in 80 countries throughout the tropics and sub-tropics of Asia, Africa, the Western Pacific, and parts of the Caribbean and South America. You cannot get the worms in the United States.

How does infection occur?

The disease spreads from person to person by mosquito bites. When a mosquito bites a person who has lymphatic filariasis, microscopic worms circulating in the person's blood enter and infect the mosquito. If the infected mosquito bites you, you can get lymphatic filariasis. The microscopic worms pass from the mosquito through your skin, and travel to your lymph vessels. In your lymph vessels they grow into adults. An adult worm lives for about 7 years. The adult worms mate and release millions of microscopic worms into your blood. Once you have the worms in your blood when a mosquito bites you, you can give the infection to others through mosquitoes.

"Lymphatic Filariasis," Division of Parasitic Diseases (DPD), Centers for Disease Control and Prevention (CDC), reviewed January 31, 2003.

Who is at risk for infection?

You need many mosquito bites over several months to years to get lymphatic filariasis. People living or staying for a long time in tropical or sub-tropical areas where the disease is common are at the greatest risk for infection. Short-term tourists have a very low risk. An infection will show up on a blood test.

What are the symptoms of lymphatic filariasis?

At first, most people don't know they have lymphatic filariasis. They usually don't feel any symptoms until after the adult worms die. The disease usually is not life threatening, but it can permanently damage your lymph system and kidneys. Because your lymph system does not work right, fluid collects and causes swelling in the arms, breasts, legs, and, for men, the genital area. The name for this swelling is lymphedema (limf-ah-DE-ma). The entire leg, arm, or genital area may swell to several times its normal size. Also, the swelling and the decreased function of the lymph system make it difficult for your body to fight germs and infections. You will have more bacterial infections in your skin and lymph system. This causes hardening and thickening of the skin, which is called elephantiasis (el-ah-fan-TIE-ah-sis).

What is the impact of this disease?

Lymphatic filariasis is a leading cause of permanent and long-term disability worldwide. People with the disease can suffer pain, disfigurement, and sexual disability. Communities frequently shun women and men disfigured by the disease. Many women with visible signs of the disease will never marry, or their spouses and families will reject them. Affected people frequently are unable to work because of their disability. This hurts their families and their communities. Poor sanitation and rapid population growth in tropical and subtropical areas of the world, where the disease is common, has created more places for mosquitoes to breed and has led to more people becoming infected.

How can I prevent infection?

Prevention includes giving entire communities medicine that kills the microscopic worms and controlling mosquitoes. Avoiding mosquito bites is another form of prevention. The mosquitoes that carry the microscopic worms usually bite between the hours of dusk and dawn. If you live in an area with lymphatic filariasis:

- Sleep under a mosquito net.

- Use mosquito repellant on your exposed skin between dusk and dawn.

- Take a yearly dose of medicine that kills the worms circulating in the blood. The medicine will kill all of the microscopic worms in the blood and some of the adult worms. It does not kill all of them.

What is the treatment for lymphatic filariasis?

If you have adult worms, you should take a yearly dose of medicine that kills the microscopic worms circulating in your blood. While this does not kill the adult worms, it does prevent you from giving the disease to someone else. Even after the adult worms die, you can have swelling of your arms, legs, breasts, or genitals. You can keep the swelling from getting worse.

- Carefully wash the swollen area with soap and water every day.

- Use anti-bacterial cream on any wounds. This stops bacterial infections and keeps the swelling from worsening.

- Elevate and exercise the swollen arm or leg to move the fluid and improve the lymph flow.

Chapter 30

Mad Cow Disease

Questions and Answers about Transmissible Spongiform Encephalopathies

What are transmissible spongiform encephalopathies?

Transmissible spongiform encephalopathies (TSEs), also known as prion diseases, are a group of rare degenerative brain disorders characterized by tiny holes that give the brain a "spongy" appearance. These holes can be seen when brain tissue is viewed under a microscope.

Creutzfeldt-Jakob disease (CJD) is the most well-known of the human TSEs. It is a rare type of dementia that affects about one in every one million people each year. Other human TSEs include kuru, fatal familial insomnia (FFI), and Gerstmann-Straussler-Scheinker disease (GSS). Kuru was identified in people of an isolated tribe in Papua New Guinea and has now almost disappeared. FFI and GSS are extremely rare hereditary diseases, found in just a few families around the world.

This chapter includes text from "NINDS Transmissible Spongiform Encephalopathies Information Page," National Institute of Neurological Disorders and Stroke (NINDS), reviewed December 2001, "Commonly Asked Questions about BSE in Products Regulated by FDA's Center for Food Safety and Applied Nutrition (CFSAN)," CFSAN, FDA, January 14, 2004, and "USDA Issues New Regulations to Address BSE," Food Safety and Inspection Service (FSIS), U.S. Department of Agriculture, January 2004.

How is mad cow disease related to TSEs?

A new type of CJD, called variant CJD (vCJD), was first described in 1996 and has been found in Great Britain and several other European countries. The initial symptoms of vCJD are different from those of classic CJD and the disorder typically occurs in younger patients. Research suggests that vCJD may have resulted from human consumption of beef from cattle with a TSE disease called bovine spongiform encephalopathy (BSE), also known as "mad cow disease." Other TSEs found in animals include scrapie, which affects sheep and goats; chronic wasting disease, which affects elk and deer; and transmissible mink encephalopathy. In a few rare cases, TSEs have occurred in other mammals such as zoo animals. These cases are probably caused by contaminated feed. CJD and other TSEs also can be transmitted experimentally to mice and other animals in the laboratory.

What are the symptoms of TSEs in humans?

Symptoms of TSEs vary, but they commonly include personality changes, psychiatric problems such as depression, lack of coordination, and/or an unsteady gait. Patients also may experience involuntary jerking movements called myoclonus, unusual sensations, insomnia, confusion, or memory problems. In the later stages of the disease, patients have severe mental impairment and lose the ability to move or speak.

Is there any treatment?

TSEs tend to progress rapidly and usually culminate in death over the course of a few months to a few years. There is currently no treatment that can halt progression of any of the TSEs. Treatment is aimed at alleviating symptoms and making the patient as comfortable as possible.

Commonly Asked Questions and Answers about BSE

What is "mad cow disease" (bovine spongiform encephalopathy/BSE)?

Mad cow disease is the commonly used name for bovine spongiform encephalopathy (BSE), a slowly progressive, degenerative, fatal disease affecting the central nervous system of adult cattle. Since 1990, the U.S. Department of Agriculture (USDA) has conducted aggressive surveillance of the highest risk cattle going to slaughter in the United

States, in which 10,000–20,000 animals per year have been tested. At the time this text was prepared (January 14, 2004), the only cow that has been found to be affected with BSE was the one diagnosed with BSE in December 2003.

What causes BSE?

The exact cause of BSE is not known but it is generally accepted by the scientific community that infectious forms of a type of protein which is normally found in animals causes BSE. These agents are called prions. In cattle with BSE, these abnormal prions initially occur in the small intestines and tonsils, and are found in central nervous tissues, such as the brain and spinal cord, and other tissues of infected animals experiencing later stages of the disease.

Was a case of BSE identified in the U.S. in December 2003?

Yes, the U.S. Department of Agriculture (USDA) surveillance program identified the first BSE case in the U.S. in a dairy cow in the state of Washington. The cow was bought from a farm in Canada.

Did meat and meat products from the BSE cow enter the food supply?

As soon as the BSE case was identified, both USDA and FDA activated their BSE Emergency Response Plans and USDA immediately recalled the meat. Meat that did enter the food supply was quickly traced and was removed from the marketplace. Moreover, all the organs in which infectious prions occur were removed at slaughter and did not enter the food supply. Muscle meat is not a source of infectious prions.

FDA and state inspectors located all other parts of the animal, and rendering plants that processed this material from the BSE cow voluntarily held the material. None of this material left the control of the companies and entered commercial distribution.

Will there be additional cases?

Regulatory measures to prevent introduction of BSE into U.S. cattle herds and contamination of U.S. foods and food products are being reviewed and updated. Since 1989, the USDA has banned imports of live ruminants, such as cattle, sheep, and goats, and most products from these animals from countries known to have BSE. This ban was extended to all Europe in 1997. The FDA prohibited the use of ruminant protein in the manufacture of animal feed intended for cows and other ruminants in 1997 and extended the prohibition in 2001 to forbid use of all mammalian protein in ruminant feed. See the FDA/CVM (Center for Veterinary Medicine) website at http://www.fda.gov/cvm/default.html for further information on the ruminant feed ban.

Under an Import Alert, FDA also prevents U.S. entry of cosmetic and dietary supplement ingredients containing high risk bovine materials from animals originating in BSE countries.

In 1998, the USDA commissioned the Harvard Center for Risk Analysis to conduct an analysis and evaluation of the U.S. regulatory measures to prevent the spread of BSE in the U.S. and to reduce the potential exposure of U.S. consumers to BSE. The Harvard study concluded that if introduced, due to the preventive measures currently in place in the U.S., BSE is extremely unlikely to become established in the United States. Should BSE enter the United States, the Harvard study concluded that only a small amount of potentially infective tissues would likely reach the human food supply.

Furthermore, on January 8, 2004, the USDA's Food Safety and Inspection Service issued four new rules to enhance safeguards against BSE. These rules are described below. Additional details may be found at the USDA website (http://www.usda.gov). FDA fully supports the safety policies announced by the USDA, which build on the principles and procedures that FDA and USDA have developed since 1989. These protective measures will add an additional layer of protection for the American public.

Does BSE affect people?

There is a disease similar to BSE called Creutzfeldt-Jacob Disease (CJD) that is found in people. A variant form of CJD (vCJD) is believed to be caused by eating contaminated beef products from BSE-affected cattle. To date, there have been 155 confirmed and probable cases of vCJD worldwide among the hundreds of thousands of people who may have consumed BSE-contaminated beef products. The one reported case of vCJD in the United States is in a young woman who contracted the disease while residing in the United Kingdom (UK) and developed symptoms after moving to the U.S.

Is cow's milk a source of BSE?

Scientific research indicates that BSE cannot be transmitted in cow's milk, even if the milk comes from a cow with BSE.

Is the food in the U.S. likely to be a BSE risk to consumers?

FDA and other federal agencies have had preventive measures in place to reduce the U.S. consumer's risk of exposure to any BSE-contaminated meat and food products. Since 1989, the USDA had prohibited the importation of live animals and animal products from BSE-positive countries. Since 1997 the FDA has prohibited the use of cattle and other ruminant protein in the manufacture of ruminant feed. This ban was expanded in 2001 to prohibit the use of all mammalian protein in ruminant feed. FDA continues to implement policies to keep safe all FDA-regulated products, including food, food ingredients, dietary supplements, drugs, vaccines, and cosmetics from risk of any BSE-contaminated bovine material.

When and how did BSE in cattle occur?

BSE in cattle was first reported in 1986 in the UK. The exact origins of BSE remain uncertain but it is thought that cattle initially may have become infected when fed feed contaminated with scrapie-infected sheep meat-and-bone meal (MBM). Scrapie is a prion disease in sheep similar to BSE in cattle. The scientific evidence suggests that the UK BSE outbreak in cattle then was expanded by feeding BSE-contaminated cattle protein (MBM) to calves. The definitive nature of the BSE agent is not completely known. The agent is thought to be a modified form of a protein, called a prion, which becomes infectious and accumulates in neural tissues causing a fatal, degenerative, neurological disease. These abnormal prions are resistant to common food disinfection treatments, such as heat, to reduce or eliminate their infectivity or presence. It is important for consumers to know that BSE, like other forms of transmissible spongiform encephalopathy (TSE), is not a communicable disease—most TSEs are not spread easily between animals or to humans. Research is ongoing to better understand TSE diseases and the nature of prion transmission.

Is BSE in cattle the same disease as chronic wasting disease (CWD) in deer and elk in the U.S.?

BSE is a transmissible spongiform encephalopathy (TSE), a family of similar diseases that may infect certain species of animals and people, such as scrapie in sheep and goats, bovine spongiform encephalopathy (BSE) in cattle, chronic wasting disease (CWD) in deer and elk, and Creutzfeldt-Jacob disease (CJD) in people.

To date, there is no scientific evidence that BSE in cattle is related to CWD in deer and elk. Research is continuing, but there is no evidence that either BSE or CWD can be transmitted between cattle, deer, or elk. FDA is working closely with other government agencies and the public health community to address CWD in wild and domesticated deer and elk herds. Wildlife and public health officials advise people not to harvest, handle, or consume any wild deer or elk that appear to be sick, regardless of the cause, especially in those states where CWD has been detected.

What countries have reported cases of BSE or are considered to have a substantial risk associated with BSE?

These countries are: Albania, Austria, Belgium, Bosnia-Herzegovina, Bulgaria, Croatia, Czech Republic, Denmark, Federal Republic of Yugoslavia, Finland, France, Germany, Greece, Hungary, Ireland, Israel, Italy, Liechtenstein, Luxembourg, former Yugoslavia Republic of Macedonia, The Netherlands, Norway, Oman, Poland, Portugal, Romania, Slovak Republic, Slovenia, Spain, Sweden, Switzerland, Japan, and United Kingdom (Great Britain including Northern Ireland and the Falkland Islands).

Canada (May 2003) and the U.S. (December 2003) each have recently reported one BSE-positive cow but remain countries considered to have a low risk. The U.S. BSE-positive cow reported in December 2003 was confirmed to have been imported from Canada in 2001.

USDA Issues New Regulations to Address BSE

On January 8, 2004 the U.S. Department of Agriculture's Food Safety and Inspection Service issued four new rules to further enhance safeguards against Bovine Spongiform Encephalopathy (BSE). These policies involve: requiring additional process controls for establishments using advanced meat recovery (AMR) systems; holding meat from cattle that have been tested for BSE until the test results are received and they are negative; and prohibiting the air-injection stunning of cattle. The new rules include:

Product Holding. USDA is publishing a notice announcing that Food Safety and Inspection Service (FSIS) inspectors are no longer marking cattle tested for BSE as "inspected and passed" until confirmation is received that the cattle have, in fact, tested negative for BSE. FSIS will be issuing a directive to inspection program personnel outlining this policy.

Specified Risk Material. With the filing of an interim final rule, FSIS is declaring that skull, brain, trigeminal ganglia, eyes, vertebral column, spinal cord and dorsal root ganglia of cattle 30 months of age or older and the small intestine of all cattle are specified risk materials, thus prohibiting their use in the human food supply. Tonsils from all cattle are already considered inedible and therefore do not enter the food supply. These enhancements are consistent with the actions taken by Canada after the discovery of BSE there in May 2003. These prohibitions are effective immediately upon publication in the *Federal Register*.

In this rule, FSIS is requiring federally inspected establishments that slaughter cattle remove, segregate and dispose of these specified risk materials so that they cannot possibly enter the food chain. To facilitate the enforcement of this rule, FSIS has developed procedures for verifying the approximate age of cattle that are slaughtered in official establishments. State inspected plants must have equivalent procedures in place to prevent these specified risk materials from entering the food supply.

Advanced Meat Recovery. AMR is a technology that removes muscle tissue from the bone of beef carcasses under high pressure without incorporating bone material. AMR product can be labeled as "meat." FSIS has previously established and enforced regulations that prohibit spinal cord from being included in products labeled as "meat."

This interim final rule expands that prohibition to include dorsal root ganglia, clusters of nerve cells connected to the spinal cord along the vertebral column, in addition to spinal cord tissue. In addition, because the vertebral column and skull in cattle 30 months and older will be considered inedible, they cannot be used for AMR.

Air-Injection Stunning. To ensure that portions of the brain are not dislocated into the tissues of the carcass as a consequence of humanely stunning cattle during the slaughter process, FSIS is issuing an interim final rule to ban the practice of air-injection stunning.

Additional Information

Updated information about BSE be obtained from the U.S. Food and Drug Administration through the following website: http://www.fda.gov/oc/opacom/hottopics/bse.html

News releases and other information from the FSIS can be accessed through the website at http://www.fsis.usda.gov or by contacting:

FSIS Congressional and Public Affairs Staff
Phone: 202-720-9113
Fax: 202-690-0460

Chapter 31

Malaria

Quick Facts

Incidence:

- Worldwide: Up to 2.7 million people die each year from malaria, most of them African children. Between 400 million and 900 million cases of acute malaria occur annually in African children alone.

- United States: According to the U.S. Centers for Disease Control and Prevention (CDC), more than 1,000 new cases are reported annually in travelers returning from malaria-endemic areas.

Cause:

- One-celled parasite, genus *Plasmodium*

- Four species infect humans: *Plasmodium falciparum, Plasmodium vivax, Plasmodium malariae,* and *Plasmodium ovale*

Transmission: Most commonly, from an infected *Anopheles* mosquito bite.

"Malaria," September 2002, NIH Pub. No. 02-7139, and "Malaria Research," October 2002, National Institutes of Health (NIH), National Institute of Allergy and Infectious Diseases (NIAID).

Symptoms: Flu-like, including chills, fever, and sweating accompanied by headache, nausea, and vomiting; attacks can recur. Life-threatening illnesses, such as severe anemia or cerebral malaria, may occur in some infected individuals.

Diagnosis: Based on symptoms and travel history; confirmed by blood smears that identify the parasite.

Treatment: Chloroquine, where parasite is not resistant to it; combination of antimalarial drugs where chloroquine is ineffective; treatment of symptoms as required.

Prevention: Chloroquine or other antimalarial drugs taken before and during travel to a malarious area and continued for several weeks after returning; mosquito repellants and sleeping under bed nets; no approved vaccine is currently available.

What is malaria?

Malaria is a disease caused by a parasite that lives part of its life in humans and part in mosquitoes. It remains one of the major killers of humans worldwide, threatening the lives of more than one-third of the world's population. Malaria thrives in the tropical areas of Asia, Africa, and South and Central America, where it strikes millions of people. Sadly, as many as 2.7 million of its victims, mostly infants and children, die yearly.

Although malaria has been virtually eradicated in the United States and other regions with temperate climates, it continues to affect hundreds of people in this country every year. In 2000, health care workers reported 1,400 cases of malaria to the U.S. Centers for Disease Control and Prevention (CDC). Malaria in the United States is typically acquired during trips to malaria-endemic areas of the world and therefore is often called travelers' malaria.

During the past 10 years, CDC has documented local cases of malaria in states as varied as California, Florida, Texas, Michigan, New Jersey, and New York. In the summer of 1999, one highly publicized case occurred at a Boy Scout camp on Long Island, New York, where two boys were infected by mosquitoes.

History of Malaria

Malaria has been around since ancient times. The early Egyptians wrote about it on papyrus, and the famous Greek physician Hippocrates

234

described it in detail. It devastated the invaders of the Roman Empire. In ancient Rome, as in other temperate climates, malaria lurked in marshes and swamps. People blamed the unhealthiness in these areas on rot and decay that wafted out on the foul air, or, as the Italians were to say, "mal aria" or bad air. In 1880, scientists discovered the real cause of malaria, the one-celled *Plasmodium* parasite, and 18 years later, they attributed the transmission of malaria to the *Anopheles* mosquito.

Historically, the United States is no stranger to the tragedy of malaria. The toll that this disease, commonly known as "fever and ague," took on early settlers is vividly depicted in the popular children's book *Little House on the Prairie* by Laura Ingalls Wilder. Historians believe that the incidence of malaria in this country peaked around 1875, but they estimate that by 1914 more than 600,000 new cases still occurred every year. Malaria has been a significant factor in virtually all of the military campaigns involving the United States. In both World War II and the Vietnam War, more personnel time was lost due to malaria than to bullets.

The malaria parasite typically is transmitted to humans by mosquitoes belonging to the genus *Anopheles*. In rare cases, a person may contract malaria through contaminated blood, or a fetus may become infected by its mother during pregnancy. The larval stage of the *Anopheles* mosquito thrives in still waters, such as swamps. The discovery by scientists that mosquitoes carried the disease unleashed a flurry of ambitious public health measures designed to stamp out malaria. These measures were targeted at both the larval and adult stages of the insect. In some areas, such as the southern United States, draining swamps and changing the way land was used was somewhat successful in eliminating mosquitoes.

The pace of the battle accelerated rapidly when the insecticide DDT and the drug chloroquine were introduced during World War II. DDT was remarkably effective and could be sprayed on the walls of houses where adult *Anopheles* mosquitoes rested after feeding. Chloroquine has been a highly effective medicine for preventing and treating malaria.

In the mid-1950s, the World Health Organization (WHO) launched a massive worldwide campaign to eliminate malaria. At the beginning, the WHO program, which combined insecticide spraying and drug treatment, had many successes, some spectacular. In some cases, malaria was conquered completely, benefiting more than 600 million people, and it was sharply curbed in the homelands of 300 million others.

Difficulties soon developed, however. Some stumbling blocks were administrative, others financial. Even worse, nature had begun to intervene. More and more strains of *Anopheles* mosquitoes were developing resistance to DDT and other insecticides. Meanwhile, the *Plasmodium* parasite was becoming resistant to chloroquine, the mainstay of antimalarial drug treatment in humans.

Researchers estimate that infection rates increased by 40 percent between 1970 and 1997 in sub-Saharan Africa. To cope with this dangerous resurgence, public health workers carefully select prevention methods best suited to a particular environment or area. In addition to medicines and insecticides, these include such standbys as draining swampy areas and filling them with dirt, and using window screens, mosquito netting, and insect repellents.

At the same time, scientists are intensively researching ways to develop better weapons against malaria, including

- Sophisticated techniques for tracking disease transmission worldwide

- More effective ways of treating malaria

- New ways, some quite ingenious, to control transmission of malaria by mosquitoes

- A vaccine for blocking its development and spread

Malaria Parasite

Malaria is caused by a one-celled parasite from the genus *Plasmodium*. More than 100 different species of *Plasmodium* exist, and they produce malaria in many types of animals and birds, as well as in people.

Four species of *Plasmodium* infect humans. Each one has a distinctive appearance under the microscope, and each one produces a somewhat different pattern of symptoms. Two or more species can live in the same area and can infect a single individual at the same time.

Plasmodium falciparum is responsible for most malaria deaths, especially in Africa. The infection can develop suddenly and produce several life-threatening complications. With prompt treatment, however, it is almost always curable.

Plasmodium vivax, the most geographically widespread of the species and the cause of most malaria cases diagnosed in the United States, produces less severe symptoms. Relapses, however, can occur for up to 3 years, and chronic disease is debilitating. Once common in temperate climates, *P. vivax* is now found mostly in the tropics, especially throughout Asia.

Plasmodium malariae infections not only produce typical malaria symptoms but they also can persist in the blood for very long periods, possibly decades, without ever producing symptoms. A person with asymptomatic (no symptoms) *P. malariae*, however, can infect others, either through blood donation or mosquito bites. *P. malariae* has been wiped out from temperate climates, but it persists in Africa.

Plasmodium ovale is rare, can cause relapses, and generally occurs in West Africa.

Life Cycle

The human malaria parasite has a complex life cycle that requires both a human host and an insect host. In *Anopheles* mosquitoes, *Plasmodium* reproduces sexually (by merging the parasite's sex cells). In people, the parasite reproduces asexually (by cell division), first in liver cells and then, repeatedly, in red blood cells.

When an infected female *Anopheles* mosquito bites a human, she takes in blood. At the same time, she injects saliva that contains the infectious form of the parasite, the sporozoite, into a person's bloodstream.

The thread-like sporozoite promptly invades a liver cell. There, during the next week or two (depending on the *Plasmodium* species), each sporozoite develops into a schizont, a structure that contains thousands of tiny rounded merozoites (another stage of the parasite). When the schizont matures, it ruptures and releases the merozoites into the bloodstream.

Alternatively, some *P. vivax* and *P. ovale* sporozoites turn into hypnozoites, a form that can remain dormant in the liver for months or years. If they become active again, the hypnozoites cause relapses in infected individuals.

Merozoites released from the liver rapidly invade red blood cells where they fuel their activities by consuming hemoglobin, the oxygen-carrying part of the blood. Within the red blood cell, most merozoites go through another round of asexual reproduction, again forming schizonts filled with yet more merozoites. When the schizont matures, the cell ruptures and merozoites burst out.

The newly released merozoites invade other red blood cells, and the infection continues its cycle until it is brought under control, either by medicine or the body's immune defenses.

The *Plasmodium* parasite can complete its life cycle through the mosquito because some of the merozoites that penetrate red blood cells do not develop asexually into schizonts. Rather, they change into male and female sexual forms known as gametocytes. These circulate in the person's bloodstream, awaiting the arrival of a blood-seeking female *Anopheles*.

When she bites an infected person, the female mosquito sucks up gametocytes along with blood. Once in the mosquito's stomach, the

Figure 31.1. *Parasite Life Cycle (on facing page)*

1. Female anopheline mosquito injects *Plasmodium* sporozoites into the bloodstream.

2. Sporozoites migrate to the liver and infect liver cells.

3. Sporozoites reproduce asexually to form thousands of merozoites, which ultimately rupture from the liver cells and re-enter the bloodstream.

4. Once in the bloodstream the merozoites invade red blood cells (RBCs). Parasites mature within those cells and are then released to infect even more RBCs. Disease and death in malaria is most commonly caused by this stage of infection. The common malaria drugs chloroquine and quinine also block the parasite's life cycle at this stage.

5. Some RBC parasites differentiate into male and female forms called gametocytes.

6. When a female mosquito feeds on an infected person, she ingests gametocytes from the blood.

7. Inside the mosquito midgut, the gametocytes differentiate into forms resembling sperm and eggs, allowing sexual reproduction to occur. The resulting parasites grow into sporozoites and migrate to the insect's salivary glands.

gametocytes develop into sperm-like male gametes or large, egg-like female gametes. Fertilization produces an oocyst filled with infectious sporozoites. When the oocyst matures, it ruptures and the thread-like sporozoites migrate, by the thousands, to the mosquito's salivary (saliva-producing) glands. And the cycle starts over again when she bites her next victim.

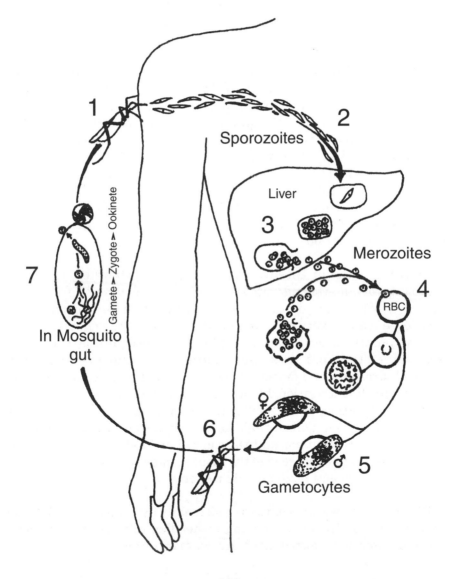

Spread of Malaria

Many biological and environmental factors shape the character of malaria in a given location. Nearly all the people who live in endemic areas are exposed to infection repeatedly. Those who survive malaria in childhood gradually build up some immunity. They may carry the infection, serving as reservoirs for transmission by mosquitoes without developing severe disease. In other areas, where the infection rate is low, people do not develop immunity because they rarely are exposed to the disease. This makes them more susceptible to the ravages of an epidemic. An epidemic can occur when conditions, such as those discussed below, allow the mosquito population to suddenly increase.

Effects of Climate: Climate affects both parasites and mosquitoes. Mosquitoes cannot survive in low humidity. Rainfall expands breeding grounds, and in many tropical areas, malaria cases increase during the rainy season. Mosquitoes must live long enough for the parasite to complete its development within them. Therefore, environmental factors that affect mosquito survival can influence malaria incidence. *Plasmodium* parasites are affected by temperature—their development slows as the temperature drops. *P. vivax* stops developing altogether when the temperature falls below 60° F. *P. falciparum* stops at somewhat higher temperatures. This explains why parasites can be found in various parts of temperate areas.

Effect of Human Intervention: People have worked for centuries to control malaria and were successful in eradicating it from most of the New World early in the 20th century. Certain human activities, however, have inadvertently worsened the spread of malaria.

City conditions can create new places for mosquito larvae to develop. Agricultural practices also can affect mosquito breeding areas. Although draining and drying of swamps gets rid of larval breeding sites, water-filled irrigation ditches may give mosquitoes another area to breed. In addition, because farmers use the same pesticides on their crops as those used against malaria vector mosquitoes, the problem of insecticide-resistant mosquitoes is growing. Modern transportation also contributes to the spread of the disease, moving travelers between malaria-endemic and non-endemic regions.

Blood: Malaria is transmitted occasionally by transfusions of blood from infected individuals, sharing of needles to inject intravenous drugs, or from an infected pregnant woman to her unborn child. In the United States, however, transmission rarely occurs through blood transfusions because blood donors are not allowed to donate for specified periods of time after traveling to or living in a malarious area.

Symptoms of Malaria

Malaria typically produces a string of recurrent attacks, or paroxysms, each of which has three stages—chills, followed by fever, and then sweating. Along with chills, the person is likely to have headache, nausea, and vomiting. Within an hour or two, the person's temperature rises, and the skin feels hot and dry. Then, as the body temperature falls, a drenching sweat begins. The person, feeling tired and weak, is likely to fall asleep.

The symptoms first appear some 10 to 16 days after the infectious mosquito bite and coincide with the bursting of infected red blood cells. When many red blood cells are infected and break at the same time, malaria attacks can recur at regular time periods—every 2 days for *P. vivax* malaria and *P. ovale*, and every 3 days for *P. malariae*.

With *P. vivax* malaria, the patient may feel fine between attacks. Even without treatment, the paroxysms subside in a few weeks. A person with *P. falciparum* malaria, however, is likely to feel miserable even between attacks and, without treatment, may die. One reason *P. falciparum* malaria is so virulent is that the parasite can infect red blood cells in all stages of development, leading to very high parasite levels in the blood. In contrast, *P. vivax* parasites infect only young red blood cells, which means the number of parasites in the blood does not reach the same high levels as seen in *P. falciparum* infection.

Diagnosing Malaria

A doctor or other health care worker should suspect malaria whenever a person who has been in the tropics recently or received a blood transfusion develops a fever and other signs that resemble the flu. A doctor will examine blood smears, taken from a finger prick, under a microscope. If parasites are present, the diagnosis is confirmed. A "thick" smear makes it possible for the health care worker to examine a large amount of blood. Then, the species of parasite can be identified by looking at a corresponding "thin" smear. This is important for deciding on the best treatment.

Mixed infections are possible. For example, a person can be infected with *P. vivax* as well as the more dangerous *P. falciparum*.

In the unusual event that parasites cannot be seen immediately in a blood smear, but the patient's condition and prior activities

241

strongly suggest malaria, the doctor may decide to start treatment before being sure the patient has malaria.

Treating Malaria

In most cases, malaria can be successfully treated, although the recuperating patient may find it takes several weeks to recover full strength. Before deciding on the best medicine to use, the doctor should try to identify the species of parasite responsible for the disease and where the patient got the infection. Up-to-date information on the geography of malaria, such as which species are present in which areas, whether chloroquine-resistant parasites are present, and which seasons of the year carry the greatest risk, is available at international travel clinics, CDC, and WHO.

In the United States, patients with *P. falciparum* malaria are usually hospitalized and treated as medical emergencies because their conditions may get worse quickly. Patients should talk with a doctor who specializes in infectious diseases and is knowledgeable about diagnosing and treating malaria and its complications.

Chloroquine, long considered the medicine of choice for treating malaria, is no longer considered the first-line antimalarial drug in many countries, and national malaria control programs are recommending alternatives. Because chloroquine-resistant parasites are becoming more widespread, doctors must carefully monitor patients who are treated with it.

If the number of parasites in the blood does not drop significantly during treatment, it may mean the parasites are resistant to the medicine. In addition, if a person develops any fever within a period of weeks to months after apparently successful treatment, the medicine may not have gotten rid of all the parasites. Additional treatment may then be required.

Health care workers should watch patients with *P. falciparum* malaria closely for potentially severe complications, including anemia, kidney failure, fluid imbalance, or respiratory distress. Brain damage can occur following cerebral malaria, which happens when large numbers of red blood cells containing parasites clog tiny blood vessels in the brain.

Preventing Malaria

Before leaving home, anyone traveling to a malarious area should consult CDC, WHO, a knowledgeable health care provider, an international travel clinic, or a local health department to get advice on what medicines to take before, during, and after the trip. Health risks for malaria vary with the destination and types of activities the traveler will undertake.

A traveler who spends even a single night in a malarious area risks getting infected. The first line of defense is to limit contact with mosquitoes by taking these measures.

- Use mosquito repellent

- Keep arms and legs covered

- Stay indoors beginning at dusk and throughout the night (when *Anopheles* mosquitoes like to feed)

- Sleep under mosquito netting

People traveling to malarious areas should also protect themselves by taking antimalarial medicines to prevent infection. CDC has current guidelines on antimalarial drugs.

Anyone who develops fever or other symptoms suggesting malaria, either while taking preventive medicines or after stopping them, should seek medical attention immediately.

Malaria and Pregnancy

Malaria poses a serious threat to both the pregnant woman and her unborn child. Women who live in malarious areas are much more likely to develop acute *P. falciparum* malaria when they become pregnant. Infants born to mothers with malaria often will have low birth weights.

If possible, pregnant women from non-malarious areas should postpone travel to those regions until after their babies are born. Pregnant women who cannot postpone travel until after delivery should protect themselves from mosquito bites and take antimalarial medicines, if recommended by their doctors.

Prospects of Conquering Malaria

Researchers in the fight against malaria have three major goals: new medicines, better methods of mosquito control, and a vaccine to prevent people from becoming infected.

Medicines: Medicines to treat malaria have been around for thousands of years. Perhaps the best known of the traditional remedies is quinine, which is derived from the bark of the *cinchona* tree. The Spanish learned about quinine from Peruvian Indians in the 1600s, and export of quinine to Europe, and later the United States, was a lucrative business until World War II cut off access to the world supply of cinchona bark. In the 1940s, an intensive research program to find alternatives to quinine gave rise to the manufacture of chloroquine and numerous other chemical compounds that became the forerunners of "modern" antimalarial drugs.

Chloroquine was the third most widely used drug in the world until the mid-1990s. It is cheap to manufacture, easy to give, and does not cause problems for most people. Unfortunately, chloroquine-resistant malaria parasites have developed and are increasing in numbers. From the 1950s to the present, chloroquine resistance gradually spread to nearly all *P. falciparum* malaria-endemic regions. In the 1960s, the U.S. Government, WHO, and other agencies launched a massive search for new antimalarial drugs. In addition, many doctors treating people in Asia are using yet another new family of drugs based on the parent drug artemisinin, an extract of the Chinese herbal remedy qinghaosu.

Unfortunately, malaria parasites in many geographic regions have become resistant to alternative drugs, many of which were discovered only in the last 30 years. Even quinine, the long-lived mainstay of malaria treatment, is losing its effectiveness in certain areas.

To address the problem of drug-resistant malaria, scientists are conducting research on the genetic devices that enable *Plasmodium* parasites to avoid the toxic effects of malaria drugs. Understanding how those devices work should enable scientists to develop new medicines or alter existing ones to make it more difficult for drug resistance to emerge. By knowing how the parasite survives and interacts with people during each distinct phase of its development, researchers also hope to develop drugs that attack the parasite at different stages.

Mosquito Control: The appearance and spread of insecticide-resistant mosquitoes, as well as stricter environmental regulations, now limit the effectiveness of the insecticide DDT, the mainstay of the 1950s and 1960s malaria eradication programs. More recently, researchers have found that mosquito netting soaked with other insecticides, which prevent mosquitoes from making contact with humans, significantly reduce malaria transmission. Therefore, as part of its Roll Back Malaria program, WHO is promoting widespread use of mosquito netting in endemic areas. Still, in some parts of Western Africa, mosquitoes have become resistant to the pyrethroid insecticide used to treat mosquito netting. Although scientists do not think this is a serious limitation yet, it points out the need to continue research to identify new tools for mosquito control.

Vaccines: Research studies conducted in the 1960s and 1970s showed that experimental vaccination of people with attenuated malaria parasites can effectively immunize them against getting another malaria infection. Current methods to develop vaccines based on weakened or killed malaria parasites are technically difficult and do not readily lend themselves to commercialization. Therefore, much of the research on vaccines has focused on identifying specific components or antigens of the malaria parasite that can stimulate protective immunity.

In 1997, the National Institute of Allergy and Infectious Diseases (NIAID) launched a 10-year Research Plan for Malaria Vaccine Development based on four cornerstones:

- Establishing a resource center to provide scientists worldwide with well-characterized research reagents

- Increasing support for discovery of new vaccine candidates

- Increasing capacity to produce vaccine candidates at the quality and quantity that will be required for clinical trials

- Establishing research and training centers in endemic areas where potential vaccines may undergo clinical trials

Under these and other programs, scientists are conducting research to understand the nature of protective immunity in humans and how to induce protective immune responses with malaria antigens.

Genome Sequencing: Genome sequencing, the process that allows scientists to determine an organism's genetic blueprint, is accelerating the discovery of new targets for drugs, vaccines, and diagnostic tests for malaria and other infectious diseases. By examining those blueprints, researchers can determine the genes that control a broad range of an organism's biological properties, such as feeding, reproducing, and adapting to its environment.

The complete genome sequences for the *Anopheles* mosquito and the *P. falciparum* parasite were published in 2002. Researchers are sequencing other *Plasmodium* species. These advances mark a milestone in malaria research. Combined with the recently completed human genome sequence, scientists have the complete genetic blueprints for the malaria parasite and both of its animal hosts. Researchers are now using that information to learn more about how *Plasmodium* survives within people and mosquitoes, and to discover new ways to diagnose, prevent, and treat the disease.

The conquest of malaria is a top priority for many international and government organizations, philanthropic foundations, and research institutions. In 2001, the NIAID published the *Global Health Research Plan for HIV/AIDS, Malaria, and Tuberculosis*. That plan highlighted the serious toll exacted by malaria and reinforced its position as one of the three biggest infectious global health problems. As the lessons of the past decades have so convincingly demonstrated, however, conquering malaria is difficult. No one anticipates a quick victory even if new malaria drugs hit the market or a vaccine proves highly successful. Rather, researchers and health planners expect their best chances lie in a many-sided attack, drawing upon a variety of weapons suited to local environments. Skillfully combining several approaches, both old and new, may at last make it possible to outmaneuver the persistent and deadly parasites.

As with all diseases of worldwide importance, a critical aspect of our future ability to control malaria will depend on the skills and expertise of scientists, health care providers, and public health specialists working in endemic regions. Therefore, strengthening the research capability of scientists in these areas is another major focus of these efforts. NIAID works closely with national and international organizations involved in malaria research and control. The Institute was also a founding member of the Multilateral Initiative on Malaria, which emphasizes strengthening research capacity in Africa.

Malaria Research

Basic Research

Basic research is the key to developing new ways to prevent and treat malaria. By researching the underlying biology of malaria parasites and how they interact with people and mosquitoes, scientists can identify new molecular targets for malaria drugs and vaccines. Researchers are also conducting studies on the specific human, mosquito and parasite factors that contribute to malaria, including serious complications such as cerebral malaria and anemia. Additional basic research is ongoing to learn how a person's immune system responds to malaria infection and fights off the disease.

In October 2002, researchers reported a major advancement in all areas of basic malaria research when they announced the complete genetic blueprints of the major malaria vector, the *Anopheles* mosquito, and of *Plasmodium falciparum*, the deadliest malaria parasite. Combined with the recently completed human genome sequence, scientists now have the complete set of human, parasite, and mosquito genes involved in malaria transmission. These accomplishments provide an unprecedented look at the underlying genetics of malaria and will enable scientists to use that information to develop new ways to treat and prevent the disease.

By mining the genome information for *P. falciparum* alone, NIAID scientists recently showed the parasite to be more genetically diverse and much older—at least 100,000 years old—than previously thought. Their research also showed that resistance to the malaria drug chloroquine arose independently on multiple continents and spread across the globe from at least four points of origin.

In 1998, NIAID funded and formed the Malaria Research and Reference Reagent Resource Center (MR4), which is managed by the Centers for Disease Control and Prevention and the American Type Culture Collection. The MR4, founded in response to the needs of researchers, provides reagents, materials, and protocols necessary for malaria research. All resources are provided free-of-charge, and more than 270 researchers have received assistance from MR4 to date. In collaboration with the World Health Organization and other agencies, MR4 also organizes workshops and training programs to help move potential products from the laboratory into clinical trials. Recently, MR4 has provided key reagents for a study of antimalarial drug resistance in Uganda, sponsored a drug-resistance workshop in Benin, and provided malaria research training in India and Cameroon.

Collaborating with the World to Combat Malaria

Malaria is a global health problem and therefore requires a global research approach. NIAID participates in many collaborative projects with other U.S. agencies, international organizations and foreign governments. Within the United States, NIAID participates in the Federal Malaria Vaccine Coordinating Committee, an interagency working group that provides for timely exchange of information and collaborative efforts to accelerate malaria vaccine research and development. The Institute also works with the U.S. Agency for International Development to support collaborative vaccine development research. NIAID also has joined with the Malaria Vaccine Initiative, administered by the Program for Appropriate Technology in Health (PATH), to support a promising vaccine candidate and to develop additional candidates for future testing. Within the National Institutes of Health (NIH), NIAID recently teamed with the National Institute of Child Health and Human Development and the Fogarty International Center (FIC) to fund research targeted at understanding malaria-associated anemia.

In 1997, NIAID joined with FIC, the World Health Organization, and other institutions to form the Multilateral Initiative on Malaria (MIM). MIM's mission is to increase and enhance worldwide research on malaria by facilitating multinational research cooperation. The Institute also has established malaria research facilities in Mali and Ghana and has trained local scientists and physicians to conduct

malaria research from within endemic countries. In addition to studies conducted by the Mali and Ghana laboratories, NIAID supports research on multiple aspects of malaria infection in Kenya, Cameroon, Indonesia, Malawi, The Gambia and Gabon.

Vaccine Research

An effective vaccine that will prevent malaria is a major goal of NIAID. In 2001, the Institute opened its Malaria Vaccine Development Unit (MVDU) at its Rockville, Maryland, research facility. The MVDU is an 8,000-square-foot, state-of-the-art biotechnology laboratory designed to develop and produce promising malaria vaccine candidate antigens. The facility is part of a joint effort by NIAID researchers and the Institute's administrative scientists who oversee NIAID-funded malaria research conducted at universities, private industries, and international research sites. The MVDU serves a vital function by moving potential vaccines through the pipeline for testing in people. The unit assists with production, scale-up, clinical-grade manufacturing, and clinical trials in the United States and malaria-endemic countries.

Scientists from the Institute's Laboratory of Parasitic Diseases are conducting exciting studies on malaria vaccines. Through the NIAID-sponsored Malaria Research and Training Center in Bamako, Mali, researchers are accelerating preparations and training for testing several vaccine candidates. Phase I clinical trials were expected to begin in early 2003. NIAID scientists also recently reported they could genetically modify mice to produce promising vaccine antigens in their milk. Once extracted from the milk, the experimental vaccine protected four out of five monkeys from an otherwise lethal dose of the malaria parasite. That research suggests that milk-giving animals such as goats may serve as inexpensive vaccine-manufacturing units.

NIAID also supports extensive research on malaria vaccines conducted by researchers from academia and industry. The Institute currently funds multiple studies aimed at developing vaccines against different stages of the malaria parasite and has conducted Phase I and Phase II clinical trials of several of the most promising candidates. Vaccines under study include those directed against the parasite both before and after it moves into red blood cells. Another promising approach under investigation is transmission-blocking vaccines. Those vaccines do not prevent a person from contracting malaria, but they prevent the malaria parasite from developing inside a mosquito that has bitten a vaccinated person. NIAID researchers and grantees from U.S. universities are working to develop such vaccines, which could reduce symptoms in infected people and slow the spread of malaria by breaking the cycle of mosquito transmission.

Research is also underway on combination vaccines derived from multiple parasite life stages, and early candidates are being prepared for use in Phase I human safety trials. DNA vaccines, one of the newest vaccine technologies, are an additional area under investigation by NIAID grantees, and several examples have been tested in animal models of malaria.

NIAID employs a number of mechanisms to generate corporate interest in malaria vaccines. Using grants, contracts, and other cooperative funding agreements, the Institute has enlisted the support of several pharmaceutical and biotechnology companies in producing an effective vaccine. Following the NIH lead, the European Union recently launched a small European Malaria Vaccine Initiative to try to develop links with industry and accelerate the movement of vaccine candidates through the development pipeline and into clinical trials.

Drug Research

New drugs to treat malaria, particularly those infections caused by forms of *Plasmodium* that are resistant to current medications, are greatly needed. Because the parasite has a complex life cycle, researchers are seeking to understand the molecular biology of the parasite and how it interacts with its human host at each stage in that cycle. Using that information, scientists hope to develop new drugs that block different molecular processes required for parasite survival.

NIAID researchers have made tremendous strides in elucidating *Plasmodium* biology, and they hope to use that information for developing new drugs. Scientists have identified key temperature-regulated genetic elements that switch on and off different phases of the parasite's life cycle. Other scientists have discovered additional genes or their regulatory elements that control the ability of the parasite to change its appearance and avoid immune detection, resist the effects of the malaria drug chloroquine, invade red blood cells via multiple ports of entry, bind to the human placenta, and invade the mosquito digestive tract. Scientists have also used studies of the three-dimensional structure and physical properties of human and mosquito cell membranes to learn more about how the parasites infect and grow inside red blood cells and the mosquito midgut. NIAID researchers have made seminal discoveries about how *Plasmodium* inserts a key channel in red blood cell membranes that enables the parasite to acquire nutrients and grow.

NIAID grantees are also hard at work identifying promising targets and compounds for new malaria drugs. Researchers have developed compounds that destroy a key reproductive stage of *Plasmodium* and others that appear to block the parasite's development within red blood cells. Other investigators are scanning the genes revealed by the *P. falciparum* genome project to identify new targets that exist in the malaria parasite but not in people. New drugs designed to attack those targets would therefore damage the parasite but not its human host.

Mosquito Research

Research on mosquito genetics, physiology, and ecology may lead to new ways to treat, prevent, or control malaria. NIAID funds many research projects at institutions in the United States and abroad aimed at developing a comprehensive understanding of the insect's biology.

One cutting-edge area of mosquito research is the development of genetically modified insects that are incapable of harboring and transmitting the malaria parasite. Researchers have identified small proteins that interfere with *Plasmodium* development within the mosquito; other scientists have shown that genes can be successfully introduced into the insects and maintained in future generations.

Because some mosquitoes support malaria parasites while others do not, researchers are attempting to understand the biological basis of that difference. Towards that end, some scientists are studying the fates of *Plasmodium* sexual stages in mosquitoes and the process by which the parasites may be encapsulated within the mosquito gut.

Other grantees are studying the genetic basis behind an insect's susceptibility or refractoriness to *Plasmodium* infection.

One NIAID scientist also has developed a new tool for studying how mosquitoes and parasites interact with one another. He recently developed a model of *Plasmodium* infection in fruit flies, which are well-studied laboratory animals whose genetic blueprints are known. Although those insects are not natural hosts of the malaria parasite, the new laboratory model allows scientists to study how insect physiology can affect the survivability of *Plasmodium*.

Investigators also are looking at the ecology of mosquitoes to determine the distribution of different species, their preferred ecological niches, the factors that affect where individual species and subspecies live, and how the partitioning of those species affects malaria transmission. Specifically, NIAID grantees are studying the relationship between vegetation and mosquito abundance in Belize and mosquito behavior and larval ecology in Kenya; the effect of rice irrigation on malaria prevalence in Mali; and how mining and deforestation are leading to the emergence of important new malaria vectors in Brazil.

For More Information

National Institute of Allergy and Infectious Diseases
National Institutes of Health
Bldg. 31, Room 7A50
31 Center Drive, MSC 2520
Bethesda, MD 20892-2520
Website: http://www.niaid.nih.gov

National Library of Medicine
Medline*plus*
8600 Rockville Pike
Bethesda, MD 20894
Phone: 301-496-6308
Website: http://www.medlineplus.gov

Centers for Disease Control and Prevention
National Center for Infectious Diseases
1600 Clifton Road, Mail Stop E-03
Atlanta, GA 30333
Phone: 1-888-232-3228
Website: http://www.cdc.gov

World Health Organization
Avenue Appia 20 1211
Geneva 27
Switzerland
Phone: 41-22-791-21-11 http://www.who.int

Chapter 32

Monkeypox

Overview: About Monkeypox

What is monkeypox?

Monkeypox is a rare viral disease that occurs mainly in the rain forest countries of central and west Africa. The disease was first discovered in laboratory monkeys in 1958. Blood tests of animals in Africa later found evidence of monkeypox infection in a number of African rodents. The virus that causes monkeypox was recovered from an African squirrel. Laboratory studies showed that the virus also could infect mice, rats, and rabbits. In 1970, monkeypox was reported in humans for the first time. In June 2003, monkeypox was reported in prairie dogs and humans in the United States.

What is the cause of monkeypox?

Monkeypox is caused by Monkeypox virus, which belongs to the orthopoxvirus group of viruses. Other orthopoxviruses that cause infections in humans include variola (smallpox), vaccinia (used for smallpox vaccine), and cowpox viruses.

What are the clinical features of monkeypox?

In humans, monkeypox is similar to smallpox, although it is often milder. Unlike smallpox, monkeypox causes lymph nodes to swell

"Questions and Answers about Monkeypox," Centers for Disease Control and Prevention (CDC), reviewed July 7, 2003.

(lymphadenopathy). The incubation period for monkeypox is about 12 days (range 7 to 17 days). The illness begins with fever, headache, muscle aches, backache, swollen lymph nodes, a general feeling of discomfort, and exhaustion. Within 1 to 3 days (sometimes longer) after the appearance of fever, the patient develops a papular rash (i.e., raised bumps), often first on the face but sometimes initially on other parts of the body. The lesions usually develop through several stages before crusting and falling off.

How long does monkeypox last?

The illness typically lasts for 2 to 4 weeks.

Is monkeypox fatal?

Studies of human monkeypox in rural central and west Africa—where people live in remote areas and are medically underserved—have reported case-fatality ratios of 1% to 10%.

How do people get monkeypox?

Monkeypox can spread to humans from an infected animal through an animal bite or direct contact with the animal's lesions or body fluids. The disease also can be spread from person to person, although it is much less infectious than smallpox. The virus is thought to be transmitted by respiratory droplets during direct and prolonged face-to-face contact. In addition, it is possible monkeypox can be spread by direct contact with body fluids of an infected person or with virus-contaminated objects, such as bedding or clothing.

Is there a treatment or vaccine for monkeypox?

Currently, there is no proven, safe treatment for monkeypox. Smallpox vaccine has been reported to reduce the risk of monkeypox among previously vaccinated persons in Africa. Centers for Disease Control and Prevention (CDC) is recommending that persons investigating monkeypox outbreaks and involved in caring for infected individuals or animals should receive a smallpox vaccination to protect against monkeypox. Persons who have had close or intimate contact with individuals or animals confirmed to have monkeypox should also be vaccinated. These persons can be vaccinated up to 14 days after exposure. CDC is not recommending preexposure vaccination for unexposed veterinarians, veterinary staff, or animal control officers, unless such persons are involved in field investigations.

Monkeypox in the United States

How did people in the U.S. become infected with monkeypox virus?

On the basis of preliminary investigations, it appears that most of the patients became ill after having close contact with infected prairie dogs that had been purchased as pets. Some patients also had contact with other persons with monkeypox in a household setting. No cases of monkeypox that could be attributed exclusively to person-to-person contact have been confirmed.

What evidence is there that monkeypox virus causes these illnesses?

The clinical features of the illness in U.S. patients—fever, headache, muscle aches, and rash—are consistent with those of monkeypox. There is also strong laboratory evidence of monkeypox. Scientists at the Marshfield Clinic in Marshfield, Wisconsin, recovered viral isolates from one of the first patients and a prairie dog. Using an electron microscope, they found that the virus had the size and appearance of a poxvirus. Laboratory tests at CDC—including several PCR [polymerase chain reaction]-based assays, serologic tests, electron microscopy, immunohistochemistry, and gene sequencing—confirmed these results and showed that the virus is Monkeypox virus. Many of the reported cases have had laboratory evidence of monkeypox virus.

Has monkeypox previously been reported in the United States?

No. Prior to the recent report of the disease in the United States, community-acquired monkeypox had never been reported outside of Africa.

How was monkeypox introduced in the United States?

Traceback investigations have implicated a shipment of animals from Ghana that was imported to Texas on April 9, 2003 as the probable source of introduction of monkeypox virus into the United States. The shipment contained approximately 800 small mammals of nine different species, including six genera of African rodents. These rodents included rope squirrels (*Funiscuirus* sp.), tree squirrels (*Helioscuirus* sp.), Gambian giant rats (*Cricetomys* sp.), brush-tailed porcupines (*Atherurus* sp.), dormice (*Graphiurus* sp.), and striped mice (*Hybomys* sp.).

Gambian rats from this shipment were kept in close proximity to prairie dogs at an Illinois animal vendor implicated in the sale of infected prairie dogs. CDC laboratory testing of some animals by using PCR and virus isolation demonstrated that one Gambian giant rat, three dormice, and two rope squirrels from the April 9, 2003 importation were infected with monkeypox virus. Evaluation of other animals associated with the shipment is ongoing. Evidence of infection was found in some animals that had been separated from the rest of the shipment on the day of their arrival into the United States, indicating early and possibly widespread infection among the remaining animals in the shipment. The laboratory investigation confirmed that multiple animal species are susceptible to infection with monkeypox virus.

What should people do if they think they have been exposed to an animal or person with monkeypox?

Persons who think they may have been exposed to a person or an animal (e.g., pet prairie dog) with monkeypox should contact their health care provider and their state or local health department.

Could I have monkeypox?

It appears that most people who are ill with monkeypox in the United States got sick after close contact with infected prairie dogs that had been purchased as pets. Some patients may have been infected through contact with other infected animals. If you have not had close contact with a wild or exotic animal, then the risk that you might have monkeypox is very low.

What measures have been taken to control the outbreak?

CDC and the public health departments in the affected states, together with the US Department of Agriculture, the Food and Drug Administration, and other agencies, are participating in a variety of activities to prevent further spread of monkeypox and identify the source of the outbreak. To assist with the investigation and outbreak response, CDC has taken the following steps:

- Activated its Emergency Operations Center.

- Deployed teams of medical officers, epidemiologists, and other experts to several states to assist with the investigation.

- Conducted extensive laboratory testing on specimens from humans and animals thought to have been exposed to monkeypox.

- Issued interim U.S. case definitions for human monkeypox and for animal monkeypox.

- Issued interim guidelines on infection control and exposure management for patients in the health care and community settings.

- Issued an immediate embargo and prohibition on the importation, interstate transportation, sale, and release into the environment of certain rodents and prairie dogs.

- Provided ongoing assistance to state and local health departments in investigating possible cases of monkeypox in both humans and animals the United States.

- Worked with state and federal agencies to trace the origin and distribution of potentially infected animals.

- Issued an interim guidance on the use of smallpox vaccine, cidofovir, and vaccinia immune globulin in the setting of an outbreak of monkeypox.

- Issued interim guidelines for veterinarians.

- Issued interim guidance for persons who have frequent contact with animals, including pet owners, pet shop employees, animal handlers, and animal control officers.

Additional information will be posted on CDC's website (www.cdc. gov) as it becomes available.

Pets and Monkeypox

How is monkeypox spread from animals to humans?

People can get monkeypox from an infected animal if they are bitten or touch the animal's blood, body fluids, or its rash. It is possible that the virus also might be spread through contact with respiratory droplets from an infected animal during close contact or with objects (for example, the animal's bedding) contaminated with the virus.

What kinds of animals can get monkeypox?

There is not enough information to determine all the types of animals that may become ill with monkeypox. Until more is known about this disease, it should be assumed that any mammal—including common household pets (e.g., dogs, cats) and "pocket pets" (e.g., hamsters or gerbils)—could get monkeypox if exposed to another animal that is infected.

What are the signs of monkeypox in animals?

In the current U.S. outbreak, illness in animals has been reported to include fever, cough, discharge from the eyes, and enlarged lymph nodes, followed by a bumpy or blister-like rash. Pets that have monkeypox also may appear to be very tired and may not be eating or drinking. It is possible that some animals may have only minimal signs of illness. Some animals have died and others have recovered.

Can my pet get the smallpox vaccine to protect it from monkeypox?

No, smallpox vaccination is not recommended for pets.

What should I do if I think my pet might have monkeypox?

If your pet could have been exposed to a sick animal and is showing the symptoms of monkeypox, follow these instructions:

- Separate the animal from people and other animals immediately. Lock it in a room or put it in a cage or cardboard box well apart from others, such as in the garage.

- Wash your hands well with soap and hot water after contact with the animal and any object that may be contaminated with virus.

- Clothing should be changed after feeding or caring for the animal. Laundry (e.g., towels, clothing) may be washed in a standard washing machine with hot water and detergent. The use of chlorine bleach during hot water washing can provide an added measure of safety. Care should be used when handling soiled laundry to avoid direct contact with contaminated material. Soiled laundry should not be shaken or moved around a lot. Infectious particles could be spread and breathed in.

- Inform your state or local health department that you think you have a pet with monkeypox. The health department may pick up the animal, or they may tell you to take the animal to a vet.

- Do **not** release your pet into the wild. If it is infected, this could spread the disease to other animals and people.

- Do **not** leave your pet at a shelter. Again, this could spread the disease.

- Do **not** take your pet to a vet without calling first. The vet must take precautions to receive your pet.

If my pet has monkeypox, what will happen to it?

If your vet determines that your pet has monkeypox, he or she will probably recommend that the animal be humanely euthanized to prevent further spread of this disease. This decision may be difficult for you, but it is the best step for the safety of family, friends, and community. If monkeypox were to establish itself in the United States, many animals and people could become ill.

Embargo and Prohibition of Certain Rodents and Prairie Dogs

What action have CDC and FDA taken?

On June 11, 2003, CDC and FDA issued a joint order announcing an immediate embargo on the importation of all rodents from Africa due to the potential that these rodents can spread monkeypox virus infection to other animal species and to humans. The joint order also banned within the United States any sale, offering for distribution, transport, or release into the environment, of prairie dogs and six specific genera of African rodents implicated in the current monkeypox outbreak.

What animals are subject to the order?

The joint order prohibits the importation of all rodents from Africa. In addition, prairie dogs and the following types of rodents from Africa may not be distributed, sold, transported, or released into the environment within the United States: tree squirrels (*Heliosciurus* sp.), rope squirrels (*Funisciurus* sp.), dormice (*Graphiurus* sp.), Gambian giant pouched rats (*Cricetomys* sp.), brush-tailed porcupines (*Atherurus* sp.), and striped mice (*Hybomys* sp.). The joint order applies to animals that are living or dead.

To what extent does this order apply to the import of these animals?

Until further notice, importation of all rodents from Africa is prohibited. This includes rodents in shipments originating in Africa and rodents in transshipments from Africa through other countries.

To what extent does this order apply to distribution of these animals in the United States?

The joint order bans within the United States any transportation, sale, offering for sale or distribution, including release into the environment, of prairie dogs and six specified genera of rodents from Africa. This ban includes any sale or offering for sale or distribution that occurs completely within one state.

May I take my animal to the veterinarian or animal control as directed by my state or local health department?

Individuals may transport prairie dogs and the six specified genera of rodents from Africa to veterinarians or animal control officials or other entities pursuant to guidance or instructions issued by Federal, state, or local government authorities. All other transports, distributions, or sales within the United States of prairie dogs and the six specified genera of rodents from Africa are prohibited.

May I release my prairie dog or one of the specified rodents from Africa into the wild?

No, under no circumstances may individuals release prairie dogs or one of the specified genera of rodents from Africa into the wild or any other public or private environment. This prohibition includes the wilderness, as well as any public or private lands, parks, prairies, or sanctuaries. Individuals who are apprehensive about retaining these animals should contact their state animal control office for information regarding appropriate disposition.

May I take my prairie dog or one of the specified rodents from Africa to a pet "swap meet" (pets for sale or exchange)?

No, individuals may not transport, sell, distribute, or offer for sale or distribution, prairie dogs and the six specified genera of rodents from Africa at pet "swap meets."

May I take my prairie dog or one of the specified rodents from Africa to a school "show and tell" or to a friend's house?

No. CDC and FDA have issued a joint order banning the transport of prairie dogs and six other types of animals, including tree squirrels, rope squirrels, dormice, Gambian giant pouched rats, brush-tailed porcupines, and striped mice. This ban includes all transport of any of these animals, even if the animal is healthy or acquired before April 15, 2003.

If you have a prairie dog, or one of the animals listed above, you can take it to the veterinarian or to animal control as instructed by your state or local health department. No other transport is allowed. Nor is the distribution, or sale of these animals allowed within the United States.

People who violate the joint order may be subject to criminal and/or civil penalties.

What is HHS' (U.S. Department of Health and Human Services) authority for taking this action?

These actions are based upon provisions in Title 42 United States Code Section 264 (Section 361 of the Public Health Service Act) which authorize HHS to make and enforce regulations necessary to prevent the introduction, transmission, or spread of communicable diseases from foreign countries into the United States, or from one State or possession into any other State or possession. CDC and FDA have implemented this statute through regulations, and those that specifically authorize the joint order can be found at 21 CFR 1240.30, 42 CFR 70.2, and 42 CFR 71.32(b).

How does this action affect the role of state and local health departments?

In order to implement and enforce the joint order, CDC, FDA, and other involved federal agencies will work collaboratively with state and local veterinary, agriculture, and public health authorities. HHS has authority to assist state and local authorities in the prevention and suppression of communicable diseases and to accept state and local assistance in the enforcement of federal communicable disease control regulations. In addition, the joint order does not supersede any action that may be lawfully undertaken by state or local authorities except to the extent that any such state or local action conflicts with the joint order. Some states involved in the outbreak, such as Wisconsin and Illinois, have already taken regulatory action. We expect that other states and local jurisdictions may do likewise.

Who will enforce the provisions of the order?

A number of federal agencies have authorities related to the animals involved. FDA will work with the Department of Agriculture,

State and local health authorities, and CDC to make sure that people who trade in prairie dogs and the listed rodent species as well as other people who may own these animals are aware of the ban and follow it. CDC and FDA will work with other appropriate federal agencies, such as the Bureau of Customs and Border Protection of the Department of Homeland Security, and the United States Fish and Wildlife Service of the Department of Interior, who have statutory responsibility for enforcing the importation embargoes.

What are the consequences of violating the joint order?

CDC and FDA are most concerned with bringing individuals into compliance with the joint order as a means of preventing the spread of monkeypox virus infection to humans and other animals. However, individuals who violate the joint order may be subject to criminal and/or civil penalties.

Chapter 33

Plague

Overview

Plague is an infectious disease caused by the bacterium *Yersinia pestis*. The bacterium is found mainly in rodents, particularly rats, and in the fleas that feed on them. Other animals and humans usually contract plague from rodent or flea bites.

Historically, plague decimated entire civilizations. In the 1300s, the "Black Death," as it was called, killed approximately one-third (20–30 million) of Europe's population. In the mid-1800s, it killed 12 million people in China. Today, thanks to better living conditions, antibiotics, and improved sanitation, there are only about 1,000 to 3,000 cases a year worldwide.

Transmission

Yersinia pestis is found in animals throughout the world, most commonly in rats but occasionally in other wild animals, such as prairie dogs. Most cases of human plague are caused by bites of infected animals or the infected fleas that feed on them. In almost all cases, only the pneumonic form of plague (see below) can be passed from person to person.

"Plague," National Institute of Allergy and Infectious Diseases (NIAID), February 2003.

Forms of Plague

Only one plague bacterium causes plague, but it can infect people in three different ways.

Bubonic plague

In bubonic plague, the most common form, plague bacteria infect the lymph system.

How is it contracted?

Most people contract bubonic plague either by being bitten by an infected flea or rodent. In rare cases, *Y. pestis* bacteria enter through an opening in the person's skin, from a piece of contaminated clothing or other material used by a person with plague.

What are the symptoms?

Bubonic plague affects the lymph nodes. Within 2 to 6 days of exposure to the bacteria, an infected person develops fever, headache, chills, weakness, and swollen, tender lymph glands (called buboes-hence the name bubonic).

Is it contagious?

Bubonic plague is rarely spread from person to person.

Septicemic plague

This form of plague occurs when the bacteria multiply in the blood.

How is it contracted?

Septicemic plague is contracted the same way as bubonic plague—usually through a flea or rodent bite. Septicemic plague also can appear as a complication of untreated bubonic or pneumonic plague.

What are the symptoms?

Symptoms include fever, chills, weakness, abdominal pain, shock, and bleeding underneath the skin or other organs. Buboes, however, do not develop.

Is it contagious?

Septicemic plague is rarely spread from person to person.

Pneumonic plague

This is the most serious form of plague and occurs when *Y. pestis* bacteria infect the lungs and cause pneumonia.

How is it contracted?

Pneumonic plague occurs two ways.

- Primary pneumonic plague occurs when a person inhales the plague bacteria. This type of plague can be spread from person to person, or animal to person, through the air.

- Secondary pneumonic plague occurs when a person with untreated bubonic or septicemic plague develops pneumonic plague after the disease spreads internally to their lungs. At this point, the disease can be spread person to person.

What are the symptoms?

Within 1 to 3 days of exposure to airborne droplets of pneumonic plague, people develop fever, headache, weakness, and rapidly developing pneumonia with shortness of breath, chest pain, cough, and sometimes bloody or watery sputum.

Is it contagious?

Pneumonic plague is contagious. When someone with pneumonic plague coughs, they release *Y. pestis* bacteria suspended in respiratory droplets into the air. If an uninfected person breathes in the droplets, they can develop pneumonic plague.

Diagnosis

Health care workers can diagnosis plague by doing laboratory tests on blood or sputum or on fluid from a lymph node.

Treatment

When the disease is suspected and diagnosed early, health care workers can treat people with plague with specific antibiotics, generally streptomycin or gentamycin. Certain other antibiotics are also effective. Left untreated, bubonic plague bacteria can quickly multiply in the bloodstream, causing septicemic plague, or even progress to the lungs, causing pneumonic plague.

Prevention

Antibiotics

Health experts recommend antibiotics for people exposed to wild rodent fleas during a plague outbreak in animals, or to a possible plague-infected animal. Because there are so few cases of plague in the United States, experts do not recommend taking antibiotics unless the person is certain that he or she has been exposed to plague-infected fleas or animals.

Vaccine

Currently, there is no commercially available vaccine against plague.

How Common Is Plague?

Approximately 10 to 20 people in the United States develop plague each year from flea or rodent bites—primarily infected prairie dogs—in rural areas of the southwestern United States. About 1 in 7 of those infected die from the disease. There has not been a person-to-person infection in the United States since 1924.

Worldwide, there have been small plague outbreaks in Asia, Africa, and South America.

Plague and Bioterror

Bioterrorism is a real threat to the United States and around the world. Although the United States does not currently expect a plague attack, it is possible that pneumonic plague could occur via an aerosol distribution. The *Y. pestis* bacterium is widely available in microbiology banks around the world, and thousands of scientists have worked with plague, making a biological attack with the disease a serious concern.

NIAID Research

The National Institute of Allergy and Infectious Diseases (NIAID), is part of the National Institutes of Health, an agency of the U.S. Department of Health and Human Services. NIAID supports research on the diagnosis, prevention, and treatment of infections caused by microbes, including those that have the potential for use as biological weapons.

The research program to address biodefense includes both short- and long-term studies targeted at designing, developing, evaluating, and approving specific tools (diagnostics, therapies, and vaccines) needed to defend against possible bioterrorist-caused disease outbreaks.

Current research projects include

- Identifying genes in the *Y. pestis* bacterium that infect the digestive tract of fleas and researching how the bacterium is transferred to humans

- Studying the disease-causing proteins and genes of *Y. pestis* that allow the bacterium to grow in humans and how they function in human lungs

NIAID is also working with the Department of Defense, the Centers for Disease Control and Prevention, and the Department of Energy to

- Develop a vaccine that protects against inhalationally acquired pneumonic plague

- Develop promising antibiotics and intervention strategies to prevent and treat plague infection

For More Information

National Institute of Allergy and Infectious Diseases
National Institutes of Health
31 Center Drive, MSC 2520
Bethesda, MD 20892-2520
Website: http://www.niaid.nih.gov

National Library of Medicine
MEDLINEplus
8600 Rockville Pike
Bethesda, MD 20894
Phone: 1-800-338-7657
Website: http://www.nlm.nih.gov/medlineplus

U.S. Centers for Disease Control and Prevention
1600 Clifton Road
Atlanta, GA 30333
Phone: 1-888-232-3228
Website: http://www.bt.cdc.gov

Johns Hopkins University Center for Civilian Biodefense Studies Website:

http://www.hopkins-biodefense.org/pages/agents/agentplague.html

Chapter 34

Rabies

Introduction

Rabies is a preventable viral disease of mammals most often transmitted through the bite of a rabid animal. The vast majority of rabies cases reported to the Centers for Disease Control and Prevention (CDC) each year occur in wild animals like raccoons, skunks, bats, and foxes. Domestic animals account for less than 10% of the reported rabies cases, with cats, cattle, and dogs most often reported rabid.

Rabies virus infects the central nervous system, causing encephalopathy and ultimately death. Early symptoms of rabies in humans are nonspecific, consisting of fever, headache, and general malaise. As the disease progresses, neurological symptoms appear and may include insomnia, anxiety, confusion, slight or partial paralysis, excitation, hallucinations, agitation, hypersalivation, difficulty swallowing, and hydrophobia (fear of water). Death usually occurs within days of the onset of symptoms.

This chapter contains excerpts from "Rabies: Introduction," "Rabies: Natural History," "Rabies: Diagnosis," Rabies: Epidemiology," "Rabies: Prevention and Control," and "Rabies: Questions and Answers," National Center for Infectious Diseases, Centers for Disease Control and Prevention, updated December 2003. The full text of these documents, along with additional information and links to other resources, is available online at http://www.cdc.gov/ncidod/dvrd/rabies, updated December 2003.

Public Health Importance of Rabies

Over the last 100 years, rabies in the United States has changed dramatically. More than 90% of all animal cases reported annually to CDC now occur in wildlife; before 1960 the majority were in domestic animals. The principal rabies hosts today are wild carnivores and bats. The number of rabies-related human deaths in the United States has declined from more than 100 annually at the turn of the century to one or two per year in the 1990's. Modern day prophylaxis has proven nearly 100% successful. In the United States, human fatalities associated with rabies occur in people who fail to seek medical assistance, usually because they were unaware of their exposure.

Cost of Rabies Prevention

Although human rabies deaths are rare, the estimated public health costs associated with disease detection, prevention, and control have risen, exceeding $300 million annually. These costs include the vaccination of companion animals, animal control programs, maintenance of rabies laboratories, and medical costs, such as those incurred for rabies postexposure prophylaxis (PEP).

Accurate estimates of these expenditures are not available. Although the number of PEPs given in the United States each year is unknown, it is estimated to be about 40,000. When rabies becomes epizootic or enzootic in a region, the number of PEPs in that area increases. Although the cost varies, a course of rabies immune globulin and five doses of vaccine given over a 4-week period typically exceeds $1,000. The cost per human life saved from rabies ranges from approximately $10,000 to $100 million, depending on the nature of the exposure and the probability of rabies in a region.

The Cost of Rabies Worldwide

Customarily, the level of international resources committed to the control of an infectious disease is a response to the associated human morbidity and mortality. For most infectious diseases, these data adequately reflect the deserved public health attention. It is difficult, however, to estimate the global impact of rabies by using only human mortality data. Because vaccines to prevent human rabies have been available for more than 100 years, most deaths from rabies occur in countries with inadequate public health resources and limited access to preventive treatment. These countries also have few diagnostic facilities and almost no rabies surveillance.

Underreporting is a characteristic of almost every infectious disease in developing countries, and increasing the estimated human mortality does not in itself increase the relative public health importance of rabies. There is, however, one often neglected aspect of rabies that does affect perception of its importance. Rabies is not, in the natural sense, a disease of humans. Human infection is incidental to the reservoir of disease in wild and domestic animals; therefore, a more accurate projection of the impact of rabies on public health should include an estimate of the extent to which the animal population is affected and the expense involved in preventing transmission of rabies from animals to humans.

An additional figure is needed to complete the global picture of rabies. The best estimates of the impact of rabies on a country and the public health resources available within that country for rabies control are found in data for the number and distribution of cases of rabies in domestic animals. Despite evidence that control of dog rabies through programs of animal vaccination and elimination of stray dogs can reduce the incidence of human rabies, exposure to rabid dogs is still the cause of over 90% of human exposures to rabies and of over 99% of human deaths worldwide. The cost of these programs prohibits their full implementation in much of the developing world, and in even the most prosperous countries the cost of an effective dog rabies control program is a drain on public health resources. The estimated annual expenditure for rabies prevention in the United States is over $300 million, most of which is spent on dog vaccinations. An annual turnover of approximately 25% in the dog population necessitates revaccination of millions of animals each year, and reintroduction of rabies through transport of infected animals from outside a controlled area is always a possibility should control programs lapse. Reservoirs of wildlife rabies, virtually unknown in Asia and tropical regions, are also potential sources of rabies infection for dogs in Europe and North America.

Natural History of Rabies

Rabies virus causes an acute encephalitis in all warm-blooded hosts, including humans, and the outcome is almost always fatal. Although all species of mammals are susceptible to rabies virus infection, only a few species are important as reservoirs for the disease. In the United States, several distinct rabies virus variants have been identified in terrestrial mammals, including raccoons, skunks, foxes, and coyotes. In addition to these terrestrial reservoirs, several species of insectivorous bats are also reservoirs for rabies.

271

Transmission

Transmission of rabies virus usually begins when infected saliva of a host is passed to an uninfected animal. Various routes of transmission have been documented and include contamination of mucous membranes (i.e., eyes, nose, mouth), aerosol transmission, and corneal transplantations. The most common mode of rabies virus transmission is through the bite and virus-containing saliva of an infected host.

Following primary infection, the virus enters an eclipse phase in which it cannot be easily detected within the host. This phase may last for several days or months. Investigations have shown both direct entry of virus into peripheral nerves at the site of infection and indirect entry after viral replication in nonnervous tissue (i.e., muscle cells). During the eclipse phase, the host immune defenses may confer cell-mediated immunity against viral infection because rabies virus is a good antigen. The uptake of virus into peripheral nerves is important for progressive infection to occur.

After uptake into peripheral nerves, rabies virus is transported to the central nervous system (CNS) via retrograde axoplasmic flow. Typically this occurs via sensory and motor nerves at the initial site of infection. The incubation period is the time from exposure to onset of clinical signs of disease. The incubation period may vary from a few days to several years, but is typically 1 to 3 months. Dissemination of virus within the CNS is rapid, and includes early involvement of limbic system neurons. Active cerebral infection is followed by passive centrifugal spread of virus to peripheral nerves. The amplification of infection within the CNS occurs through cycles of viral replication and cell-to-cell transfer of progeny virus. Centrifugal spread of virus may lead to the invasion of highly innervated sites of various tissues, including the salivary glands. During this period of cerebral infection, the classic behavioral changes associated with rabies develop.

Signs and Symptoms

The first symptoms of rabies may be nonspecific flu-like signs—malaise, fever, or headache, which may last for days. There may be discomfort or paresthesia at the site of exposure (bite), progressing within days to symptoms of cerebral dysfunction, anxiety, confusion, agitation, progressing to delirium, abnormal behavior, hallucinations, and insomnia. The acute period of disease typically ends after 2 to 10 days. Once clinical signs of rabies appear, the disease is nearly always fatal, and treatment is typically supportive. Disease prevention is entirely prophylactic and includes both passive antibody (immune globulin) and vaccine. Non-lethal exceptions are extremely rare. To date only six documented cases of human survival from clinical rabies have been reported and each included a history of either pre- or postexposure prophylaxis.

Pathology

Pathology of rabies infection is typically defined by encephalitis and myelitis. Perivascular infiltration with lymphocytes, polymorpho-nuclear leukocytes, and plasma cells can occur throughout the entire CNS. Rabies infection frequently causes cytoplasmic eosinophilic inclusion bodies (Negri bodies) in neuronal cells, especially pyramidal cells of the hippocampus and Purkinje cells of the cerebellum. These inclusions have been identified as areas of active viral replication by the identification of rabies viral antigen.

Several factors may affect the outcome of rabies exposure. These include the virus variant, the dose of virus inoculum, the route and location of exposure, as well as individual host factors, such as age and host immune defenses.

Rabies Diagnosis

Rabies Diagnosis in Animals

The direct fluorescent antibody test (dFA) is the test most frequently used to diagnose rabies. This test requires brain tissue from animals suspected of being rabid. The test can only be performed post-mortem (after the animal is dead).

Rabies Diagnosis in Humans

Several tests are necessary to diagnose rabies ante-mortem (before death) in humans; no single test is sufficient. Tests are performed on samples of saliva, serum, spinal fluid, and skin biopsies of hair follicles at the nape of the neck. Saliva can be tested by virus isolation or reverse transcription followed by polymerase chain reaction (RT-PCR). Serum and spinal fluid are tested for antibodies to rabies virus. Skin biopsy specimens are examined for rabies antigen in the cutaneous nerves at the base of hair follicles.

The Importance of Routine Rabies Tests

Rapid and accurate laboratory diagnosis of rabies in humans and other animals are essential for timely administration of postexposure prophylaxis. Within a few hours, a diagnostic laboratory can determine whether or not an animal is rabid and inform the responsible medical personnel. The laboratory results may save a patient from unnecessary physical and psychological trauma, and financial burdens, if the animal is not rabid.

In addition, laboratory identification of positive rabies cases may aid in defining current epidemiologic patterns of disease and provide appropriate information for the development of rabies control programs.

Rabies Epidemiology

Epidemiology is the study of the distribution and causes of disease in populations. Epidemiologists study how many people or animals have a disease, the outcome of the disease (recovery, death, disability, etc.), and the factors that influence the distribution and outcome of the disease.

The epidemiology of rabies addresses several questions: what animals have rabies and in what regions of the country, how many people get rabies and from what animals, and what are the best strategies for preventing rabies in people and animals. Epidemiologic information is often presented as statistical data (e.g., numbers or percentages in graphs and on maps). For example, in 2001, 7,437 cases of rabies were reported in the United States. Raccoons accounted for almost 40% of reported cases.

United States Rabies Surveillance Data, 2001

Each year, scientists from the Centers for Disease Control and Prevention (CDC) collect information about cases of animal and human rabies from the state health departments and publish the information in a summary report.

In 2001, 49 states, the District of Columbia, and Puerto Rico reported 7,437 cases of rabies in animals and no cases in humans to CDC (Hawaii is the only state that has never reported an indigenously acquired rabies case in humans or animals). The total number of reported cases increased by 0.92% from those reported in 2000 (7,369 cases).

Wild animals. Wild animals accounted for 93% of reported cases of rabies in 2001. Raccoons continued to be the most frequently reported rabid wildlife species (37.2% of all animal cases during 2001), followed by skunks (30.7%), bats (17.2%), foxes (5.9%), and other wild

274

animals, including rodents and lagomorphs (0.7%). Reported cases in raccoons and foxes decreased 0.4% and 3.5% respectively from the totals reported in 2000. Reported cases in skunks, and bats increased 2.6%, and 3.3% respectively from the totals reported in 2000.

Outbreaks of rabies infections in terrestrial mammals like raccoons, skunks, foxes, and coyotes are found in broad geographic regions across the United States.

Domestic animals. Domestic species accounted for 6.8% of all rabid animals reported in the United States in 2001. The number of reported rabid domestic animals decreased 2.4% from the 509 cases reported in 2000 to 497 in 2001.

In 2001, cases of rabies in cats increased 8.4%, whereas those in dogs, cattle, horses, sheep and goats, and swine decreased 21.9%, 1.2%, 1.9% and 70.0% respectively compared with those reported in 2000. Rabies cases in cats continue to be more than twice as numerous as those in dogs or cattle. Pennsylvania reported the largest number of rabid domestic animals (46) for any state, followed by New York (43).

Successful vaccination programs that began in the 1940s caused a decline in dog rabies in this country. But, as the number of cases of rabies in dogs decreased, rabies in wild animals increased.

Human rabies. In this century, the number of human deaths in the United States attributed to rabies has declined from 100 or more each year to an average of 1 or 2 each year. Two programs have been responsible for this decline. First, animal control and vaccination programs begun in the 1940's have practically eliminated domestic dogs as reservoirs of rabies in the United States. Second, effective human rabies vaccines and immunoglobins have been developed.

Rabies Prevention and Control

Rabies vaccine and Immune Globulin

There is no treatment for rabies after symptoms of the disease appear. However, two decades ago scientists developed an extremely effective new rabies vaccine regimen that provides immunity to rabies when administered after an exposure (postexposure prophylaxis) or for protection before an exposure occurs (preexposure prophylaxis). Although rabies among humans is rare in the United States, every year an estimated 18,000 people receive rabies preexposure prophylaxis and an additional 40,000 receive postexposure prophylaxis.

Preexposure Prophylaxis

Preexposure vaccination is recommended for persons in high-risk groups, such as veterinarians, animal handlers, and certain laboratory workers. Other persons whose activities bring them into frequent contact with rabies virus or potentially rabid bats, raccoons, skunks, cats, dogs, or other species at risk of having rabies should also be considered for preexposure prophylaxis. In addition, international travelers likely to come in contact with animals in areas of enzootic dog rabies which lack immediate access to appropriate medical care, including biologics, should be considered for preexposure prophylaxis.

People who work with live rabies virus in research laboratories or vaccine production facilities are at the highest risk of inapparent exposures. Such persons should have a serum (blood) sample tested for antibody every 6 months and receive booster vaccine, when necessary. Routine preexposure prophylaxis for other situations may generally not be indicated.

Purpose of preexposure prophylaxis. Preexposure prophylaxis is given for several reasons. First, although preexposure vaccination does not eliminate the need for additional medical attention after a rabies exposure, it simplifies therapy by eliminating the need for human rabies immune globulin (HRIG) and decreasing the number of vaccine doses needed—a point of particular importance for persons at high risk of being exposed to rabies in areas where immunizing products may not be available, and it minimizes adverse reactions to multiple doses of vaccine. Second, it may enhance immunity in persons whose postexposure therapy might be delayed. Finally, it may provide protection to persons with inapparent exposures to rabies.

Preexposure prophylaxis regimen. Preexposure prophylaxis consists of three doses of rabies vaccine given on days 0, 7, and 21 or 28.

Postexposure Prophylaxis

Postexposure prophylaxis (PEP) is indicated for persons possibly exposed to a rabid animal. Possible exposures include animal bites, or mucous membrane contamination with infectious tissue, such as saliva. PEP should begin as soon as possible after an exposure. There have been no vaccine failures in the United States (i.e., someone developed rabies) when PEP was given promptly and appropriately after an exposure.

Administration of rabies PEP is a medical urgency, not a medical emergency. Physicians should evaluate each possible exposure to rabies and as necessary consult with local or state public health officials regarding the need for rabies prophylaxis.

Postexposure prophylaxis regimen. In the United States, PEP consists of a regimen of one dose of immune globulin and five doses of rabies vaccine over a 28-day period. Rabies immune globulin and the first dose of rabies vaccine should be given as soon as possible after exposure. Additional doses of rabies vaccine should be given on days 3, 7, 14, and 28 after the first vaccination. Current vaccines are relatively painless and are given in your arm, like a flu or tetanus vaccine.

What to Do After a Possible Exposure

If you are exposed to a potentially rabid animal, wash the wound thoroughly with soap and water, and seek medical attention immediately. A health care provider will care for the wound and will assess the risk for rabies exposure. The following information will help your health care provider assess your risk:

- the geographic location of the incident
- the type of animal that was involved
- how the exposure occurred (provoked or unprovoked)
- the vaccination status of animal
- whether the animal can be safely captured and tested for rabies

Steps taken by the health care practitioner will depend on the circumstances of the bite. Your health care practitioner should consult state or local health departments, veterinarians, or animal control officers to make an informed assessment of the incident and to request assistance. The important factor is that you seek care promptly after you are bitten by any animal.

What You Can Do to Help Prevent the Spread of Rabies

Be a responsible pet owner:

- Keep vaccinations up-to-date for all dogs, cats and ferrets. This requirement is important not only to keep your pets from getting rabies, but also to provide a barrier of protection to you, if your animal is bitten by a rabid wild animal.

277

- Keep your pets under direct supervision so they do not come in contact with wild animals. If your pet is bitten by a wild animal, seek veterinary assistance for the animal immediately.

- Call your local animal control agency to remove any stray animals from your neighborhood. They may be unvaccinated and could be infected by the disease.

- Spay or neuter your pets to help reduce the number of unwanted pets that may not be properly cared for or regularly vaccinated.

Avoid direct contact with unfamiliar animals:

- Enjoy wild animals (raccoons, skunks, foxes) from afar. Do not handle, feed, or unintentionally attract wild animals with open garbage cans or litter.

- Never adopt wild animals or bring them into your home. Do not try to nurse sick animals to health. Call animal control or an animal rescue agency for assistance.

- Teach children never to handle unfamiliar animals, wild or domestic, even if they appear friendly. "Love your own, leave other animals alone" is a good principle for children to learn.

- Prevent bats from entering living quarters or occupied spaces in homes, churches, schools, and other similar areas, where they might come in contact with people and pets.

- When traveling abroad, avoid direct contact with wild animals and be especially careful around dogs in developing countries. Rabies is common in developing countries in Asia, Africa, and Latin America where dogs are the major reservoir of rabies. Tens of thousands of people die of rabies each year in these countries. Before traveling abroad, consult with a health care provider, travel clinic, or your health department about the risk of exposure to rabies, preexposure prophylaxis, and how you should handle an exposure, should it arise.

Questions and Answers about Rabies

How can I protect my pet from rabies?

There are several things you can do to protect your pet from rabies. First, visit your veterinarian with your pet on a regular basis and keep rabies vaccinations up-to-date for all cats, ferrets, and dogs.

Second, maintain control of your pets by keeping cats and ferrets indoors and keeping dogs under direct supervision. Third, spay or neuter your pets to help reduce the number of unwanted pets that may not be properly cared for or vaccinated regularly. Lastly, call animal control to remove all stray animals from your neighborhood since these animals may be unvaccinated or ill.

Why does my pet need the rabies vaccine?

Although the majority of rabies cases occur in wildlife, most humans are given rabies vaccine as a result of exposure to domestic animals. This explains the tremendous cost of rabies prevention in domestic animals in the United States. While wildlife are more likely to be rabid than are domestic animals in the United States, the amount of human contact with domestic animals greatly exceeds the amount of contact with wildlife. Your pets and other domestic animals can be infected when they are bitten by rabid wild animals. When "spillover" rabies occurs in domestic animals, the risk to humans is increased. Pets are therefore vaccinated by your veterinarian to prevent them from acquiring the disease from wildlife, and thereby transmitting it to humans.

What happens if a neighborhood cat bites me?

You should seek medical evaluation for any animal bite. However, rabies is uncommon in dogs, cats, and ferrets in the United States. Very few bites by these animals carry a risk of rabies. If the cat (or dog or ferret) appeared healthy at the time you were bitten, it can be confined by its owner for 10 days and observed. No anti-rabies prophylaxis is needed. No person in the United States has ever contracted rabies from a dog, cat or ferret held in quarantine for 10 days.

If a dog, cat, or ferret appeared ill at the time it bit you or becomes ill during the 10 day quarantine, it should be evaluated by a veterinarian for signs of rabies and you should seek medical advice about the need for anti-rabies prophylaxis.

The quarantine period is a precaution against the remote possibility that an animal may appear healthy, but actually be sick with rabies. To understand this statement, you have to understand a few things about the pathogenesis of rabies (the way the rabies virus affects the animal it infects). From numerous studies conducted on rabid dogs, cats, and ferrets, we know that rabies virus inoculated into a muscle travels from the site of the inoculation to the brain by moving within nerves. The animal does not appear ill during this time, which is called the incubation period and which may last for weeks to months. A bite by the animal during the incubation period does not carry a risk of rabies because the virus is not in saliva. Only late in the disease, after the virus has reached the brain and multiplied there to cause an encephalitis (or inflammation of the brain), does the virus move from the brain to the salivary glands and saliva. Also at this time, after the virus has multiplied in the brain, almost all animals begin to show the first signs of rabies. Most of these signs are obvious to even an untrained observer, but within a short period of time, usually within 3 to 5 days, the virus has caused enough damage to the brain that the animal begins to show unmistakable signs of rabies. As an added precaution, the quarantine period is lengthened to 10 days.

What happens if my pet (cat, dog, ferret) is bitten by a wild animal?

Any animal bitten or scratched by either a wild, carnivorous mammal or a bat that is not available for testing should be regarded as having been exposed to rabies. Unvaccinated dogs, cats, and ferrets exposed to a rabid animal should be euthanized immediately. If the owner is unwilling to have this done, the animal should be placed in strict isolation for 6 months and vaccinated 1 month before being released. Animals with expired vaccinations need to be evaluated on a case-by-case basis. Dogs and cats that are currently vaccinated are kept under observation for 45 days.

I am moving to a rabies-free country and want to take my pets with me. Where can I get more information?

The details of regulation about importing pets into rabies-free countries vary by country. Check with the embassy of your destination country.

How do people get rabies?

People usually get rabies from the bite of a rabid animal. It is also possible, but quite rare, that people may get rabies if infectious material from a rabid animal, such as saliva, gets directly into their eyes, nose, mouth, or a wound.

Can I get rabies in any way other than an animal bite?

Non-bite exposures to rabies are very rare. Scratches, abrasions, open wounds, or mucous membranes contaminated with saliva or other potentially infectious material (such as brain tissue) from a rabid animal constitute non-bite exposures. Occasionally reports of non-bite exposure are such that postexposure prophylaxis is given.

Inhalation of aerosolized rabies virus is also a potential non-bite route of exposure, but other than laboratory workers, most people are unlikely to encounter an aerosol of rabies virus.

Other contact, such as petting a rabid animal or contact with the blood, urine or feces (e.g., guano) of a rabid animal, does not constitute an exposure and is not an indication for prophylaxis.

How soon after an exposure should I seek medical attention?

Medical assistance should be obtained as soon as possible after an exposure. There have been no vaccine failures in the United States (i.e., someone developed rabies) when postexposure prophylaxis (PEP) was given promptly and appropriately after an exposure.

What medical attention do I need if I am exposed to rabies?

One of the most effective methods to decrease the chances for infection involves thorough washing of the wound with soap and water. Specific medical attention for someone exposed to rabies is called postexposure prophylaxis or PEP. In the United States, postexposure prophylaxis consists of a regimen of one dose of immune globulin and five doses of rabies vaccine over a 28-day period. Rabies immune globulin and the first dose of rabies vaccine should be given by your health care provider as soon as possible after exposure. Additional doses or rabies vaccine should be given on days 3, 7, 14, and 28 after the first vaccination. Current vaccines are relatively painless and are given in your arm, like a flu or tetanus vaccine.

Will the rabies vaccine make me sick?

Adverse reactions to rabies vaccine and immune globulin are not common. Newer vaccines in use today cause fewer adverse reactions than previously available vaccines. Mild, local reactions to the rabies vaccine, such as pain, redness, swelling, or itching at the injection site, have been reported. Rarely, symptoms such as headache, nausea, abdominal pain, muscle aches, and dizziness have been reported. Local pain and low-grade fever may follow injection of rabies immune globulin.

What if I cannot get rabies vaccine on the day I am supposed to get my next dose?

Consult with your doctor or state or local public health officials for recommended times if there is going to be a change in the recommended schedule of shots. Rabies prevention is a serious matter and changes should not be made in the schedule of doses.

Can rabies be transmitted from one person to another?

The only documented cases of rabies caused by human-to-human transmission occurred among 8 recipients of transplanted corneas. Investigations revealed each of the donors had died of an illness compatible with or proven to be rabies. The 8 cases occurred in 5 countries: Thailand (2 cases), India (2 cases), Iran (2 cases) the United States (1 case), and France (1 case). Stringent guidelines for acceptance of donor corneas have reduced this risk.

In addition to transmission from corneal transplants, bite and non-bite exposures inflicted by infected humans could theoretically transmit rabies, but no such cases have been documented. Casual contact, such as touching a person with rabies or contact with non-infectious fluid or tissue (urine, blood, feces) does not constitute an exposure and does not require postexposure prophylaxis. In addition, contact with someone who is receiving rabies vaccination does not constitute rabies exposure and does not require postexposure prophylaxis.

What animals get rabies?

Any mammal can get rabies. The most common wild reservoirs of rabies are raccoons, skunks, bats, foxes, and coyotes. Domestic mammals can also get rabies. Cats, cattle, and dogs are the most frequently reported rabid domestic animals in the United States.

How can I find out what animals have rabies in my area?

Each state collects specific information about rabies, and is the best source for information on rabies in your area. In addition, the CDC publishes rabies surveillance data every year for the United States. The report, entitled "Rabies Surveillance in the United States," contains information about the number of cases of rabies reported to CDC during the year, the animals reported rabid, maps showing where cases were reported for wild and domestic animals, and distribution maps showing outbreaks of rabies associated with specific animals.

What is the risk of rabies from squirrels, mice, rats, and other rodents?

Small rodents (such as squirrels, rats, mice, hamsters, guinea pigs, gerbils, and chipmunks,) and lagomorphs (such as rabbits and hares) are almost never found to be infected with rabies and have not been known to cause rabies among humans in the United States. Bites by these animals are usually not considered a risk of rabies unless the animal was sick or behaving in any unusual manner and rabies is widespread in your area. However, from 1985 through 1994, wood-chucks accounted for 86% of the 368 cases of rabies among rodents reported to CDC. Woodchucks or groundhogs (*Marmota monax*) are the only rodents that may be frequently submitted to state health department because of a suspicion of rabies. In all cases involving rodents, the state or local health department should be consulted before a decision is made to initiate postexposure prophylaxis (PEP).

Do bats get rabies?

Yes. Bats are mammals and are susceptible to rabies, but most do not have the disease. You cannot tell if a bat has rabies just by looking at it; rabies can be confirmed only by having the animal tested in a laboratory. To minimize the risk for rabies, it is best never to handle any bat.

What should I do if I come in contact with a bat?

If you are bitten by a bat—or if infectious material (such as saliva) from a bat gets into your eyes, nose, mouth, or a wound—wash the affected area thoroughly and get medical attention immediately. Whenever possible, the bat should be captured and sent to a laboratory for rabies testing.

People usually know when they have been bitten by a bat. However, because bats have small teeth which may leave marks that are not easily seen, there are situations in which you should seek medical advice even in the absence of an obvious bite wound. For example, if you awaken and find a bat in your room, see a bat in the room of an unattended child, or see a bat near a mentally impaired or intoxicated person, seek medical advice and have the bat tested.

People cannot get rabies just from seeing a bat in an attic, in a cave, or at a distance. In addition, people cannot get rabies from having contact with bat guano (feces), blood, or urine, or from touching a bat on its fur (even though bats should never be handled).

283

What should I do if I find a bat in my home?

If you see a bat in your home and you are sure no human or pet exposure has occurred, confine the bat to a room by closing all doors and windows leading out of the room except those to the outside. The bat will probably leave soon. If not, it can be caught, as described below, and released outdoors away from people and pets.

However, if there is any question of exposure, leave the bat alone and call animal control or a wildlife conservation agency for assistance. If professional assistance is unavailable, use precautions to capture the bat safely, as described below.

What you will need:

- leather work gloves (put them on)
- small box or coffee can
- piece of cardboard
- tape

When the bat lands, approach it slowly and place a box or coffee can over it. Slide the cardboard under the container to trap the bat inside. Tape the cardboard to the container securely. Contact your health department or animal control authority to make arrangements for rabies testing.

How can I tell if a bat has rabies?

Rabies can be confirmed only in a laboratory. However, any bat that is active by day, is found in a place where bats are not usually seen (for example in rooms in your home or on the lawn), or is unable to fly, is far more likely than others to be rabid. Such bats are often the most easily approached. Therefore, it is best never to handle any bat.

Should I be concerned about rabies when I travel outside the United States?

Yes. Rabies and the rabies-like viruses can occur in animals anywhere in the world. In most countries, the risk of rabies in an encounter with an animal and the precautions necessary to prevent rabies are the same as they are in the United States. When traveling, it is always prudent to avoid approaching any wild or domestic animal.

The developing countries in Africa, Asia, and Latin America have additional problems in that dog rabies is common there and preventive treatment for human rabies may be difficult to obtain. The importance of rabid dogs in these countries, where tens of thousands of people die of the disease each year, cannot be overstated. Unlike programs in developed countries, dog rabies vaccination programs in developing countries have not always been successful. Rates of postexposure prophylaxis in some developing countries are about 10 times higher than in the United States, and rates of human rabies are sometimes 100 times higher. Before traveling abroad, consult a health care provider, travel clinic, or health department about your risk of exposure to rabies and how to handle an exposure should it arise.

Should I receive rabies preexposure vaccination before traveling to other countries?

In most countries, the risk of rabies and the precautions for preventing rabies are the same as they are in the United States. However, in some developing countries in Africa, Asia, and Latin America, dog rabies may be common and preventive treatment for rabies may be difficult to obtain. If you are traveling to a rabies-endemic country, you should consult your health care provider about the possibility of receiving preexposure vaccination against rabies. Preexposure vaccination is suggested if:

- Your planned activity will bring you into contact with wild or domestic animals (for example, biologists, veterinarians, or agriculture specialists working with animals).

- You will be visiting remote areas where medical care is difficult to obtain or may be delayed (for example, hiking through remote villages where dogs are common).

- Your stay is longer than 1 month in an area where dog rabies is common (the longer you stay, the greater the chance of an encounter with an animal).

If I get preexposure vaccination before I travel, am I protected if I am bitten?

No. Preexposure prophylaxis is given for several reasons. First, although preexposure vaccination does not eliminate the need for additional therapy after a rabies exposure, it simplifies therapy by eliminating the need for human rabies immune globulin (HRIG) and decreasing the number of doses needed—a point of particular importance for persons at high risk of being exposed to rabies in areas where immunizing products may not be readily available. Second, it may protect persons whose postexposure therapy might be delayed. Finally, it may provide partial protection to persons with inapparent exposures to rabies.

Chapter 35

Raccoon Roundworm

Baylisascaris *(Bay-liss-ass-kuh-ris) Infection (Raccoon Roundworm) Infection*

What is Baylisascaris?

Baylisascaris is the scientific name of a type of intestinal round-worm that can infect a variety of carnivorous (meat-eating) animals. *Baylisascaris* procyonis is the name of the species found commonly in raccoons. When infective eggs of the roundworm are ingested by humans and other animals, *Baylisascaris* larvae hatch in the intestine and travel through the organs and muscles; this is called larva migrans syndrome. Infection rarely causes symptoms in raccoons.

How common is Baylisascaris *infection in raccoons?*

Fairly common. Infected raccoons have been found throughout the United States. The highest infection rates occur in the midwest, northeast, and west coast.

How common is Baylisascaris *infection in humans?*

Serious infection is rarely diagnosed; fewer than 30 cases have been reported. However, it is believed that some cases are incorrectly diagnosed as other infections or go undiagnosed.

"*Baylisascaris* Infection," Division of Parasitic Diseases, Centers for Disease Control and Prevention (CDC), reviewed January 4, 2002.

How is infection spread to humans?

Infected raccoons commonly shed millions of eggs in their feces, and the eggs usually develop to the infective stage in 2–4 weeks. The eggs are resistant to most environmental conditions and with adequate moisture, can survive for years. Infection is spread when infective eggs are accidentally ingested by a person or animal. People, especially young children, generally become infected from accidentally ingesting eggs from soil, water, hands, or other objects that have been contaminated with raccoon feces. The eggs must be ingested by a human or other animal to be able to hatch and release larvae. Animals may also become infected by eating a smaller animal that has been infected with *Baylisascaris*.

What are the signs and symptoms of Baylisascaris *infection?*

Signs and symptoms of infection depend on how many eggs are ingested and where in the body the larvae migrate (travel to). Once swallowed and inside the body, eggs hatch into larvae, which then cause disease when they migrate through the liver, brain, spinal cord, and other organs. Swallowing a few eggs may cause few or no symptoms. Ingesting large numbers of eggs may lead to serious symptoms. These symptoms may include nausea, tiredness, liver enlargement, lack of coordination, lack of attention to people and surroundings, loss of muscle control, coma, and blindness. Some cases have resulted in death. Signs and symptoms of infection may take a week or so after ingestion of eggs to develop.

Other animals (except raccoons) infected with *Baylisascaris* can develop similar symptoms, or may die as a result of infection.

What should I do if I think I have ingested Baylisascaris *eggs?*

See your health care provider immediately. Be sure to report that you have recently been in contact with raccoons.

How is infection diagnosed?

Infection is very difficult to diagnose and often is made by ruling out other infections that cause similar symptoms. Information on diagnosis and testing can be obtained through DPDx (a website of CDC's Division of Parasitic Diseases) at http://www.dpd.cdc.gov/dpdx/ or by calling the Parasitic Diseases Epidemiology Branch at 770-488-7760.

Who is at risk for infection?

Anyone who is exposed to environments where raccoons live is potentially at risk. Young children and developmentally disabled persons are at highest risk for infection because they spend time outdoors and they may put dirty fingers or objects into their mouths. Hunters, trappers, taxidermists, and wildlife rehabilitators may also be at increased risk if they handle raccoons or raccoon feces.

Is treatment available?

No effective, curative treatment is yet available. However, because early treatment might reduce serious damage caused by the infection, seek immediate medical attention for any person seen ingesting raccoon feces.

How can I prevent infection in myself, my children, or my neighbors?

- Avoid direct contact with raccoons, especially their feces. Do not keep, feed, or adopt raccoons as pets, Raccoons are wild animals.

- Discourage raccoons from living in and around your home or parks by removing access to food. Clear brush so raccoons are not likely to make a den on your property.

- Stay away from areas and materials that might be contaminated by raccoon feces. Raccoons typically defecate at the base of or in raised forks of trees, or on raised horizontal surfaces such as fallen logs, stumps, or large rocks. Raccoon feces also can be found on woodpiles, decks, rooftops, and in attics, garages, and haylofts. Feces usually are dark and tubular, have a pungent odor (usually worse than dog or cat feces), and often contain undigested seeds or other food items.

- To eliminate eggs, raccoon feces and material contaminated with raccoon feces should be removed carefully and burned, buried, or sent to a landfill. Care should be taken to avoid contaminating hands and clothes. Treat decks, patios, and other surfaces with boiling water or a propane flame-gun. (Exercise proper precautions) Prompt removal and destruction of raccoon feces will reduce risk for exposure and possible infection. Newly deposited eggs take at least 2–4 weeks to become infective.

• Contact your local animal control office for further assistance.

Chapter 36

Rickettsial Infections

Description

Several species of *Rickettsia* can cause illnesses in humans. These agents are usually not transmissible directly from person to person. Transmission occurs via an infected arthropod vector or through exposure to an infected animal reservoir host. In addition, transmission has been documented to occur via blood transfusion. Rickettsial agents that cause human disease are typically categorized not by disease manifestation but according to antigenic similarity. The clinical severity and duration of illnesses associated with different rickettsial infections vary considerably, even within a given antigenic group. Rickettsioses range in severity from diseases that are relatively mild (rickettsialpox and African tick-bite fever) to those that can be life-threatening (Rocky Mountain spotted fever and Oroya fever), and in duration from those that can be self-limiting (cat-scratch disease) to chronic (Q fever and Brill-Zinsser disease). Most patients with rickettsial infections recover with timely application of appropriate antibiotic therapy.

Travelers may be at risk for exposure to agents of rickettsial diseases if they engage in occupational or recreational activities that bring them into contact with habitats that support the vectors or animal reservoir species associated with these pathogens.

"Rickettsial Infections," Centers for Disease Control and Prevention (CDC), reviewed June 30, 2003.

Occurrence and Risk for Traveler

The geographic distribution and the risks for exposure to rickettsial agents are described below (by disease).

Epidemic Typhus and Trench Fever

Epidemic typhus and trench fever (caused by infection with *Rickettsia prowazekii and Bartonella quintana*, respectively) are transmitted from one person to another by the human body louse. Contemporary outbreaks of both diseases are rare in most developed countries and generally occur only in communities and populations in which body louse infestations are frequent (typically seen in refugee and prisoner populations, particularly during wars or famine). These diseases also occur sporadically in cooler mountainous regions of Africa, South America, Asia, and Mexico, especially during the colder months when louse-infested clothing is not laundered and person-to-person spread of lice is more frequent. Additional foci of trench fever among homeless populations in urban centers of industrialized countries have been recognized recently. Travelers who are not at risk of exposure to lice or to persons with lice are unlikely to acquire these illnesses. However, health-care workers who care for these patients may be at risk of acquiring louse-borne illnesses through inhalation or inoculation into the skin of infectious louse feces.

Murine Typhus

Murine typhus (caused by infection with *R. typhi*) occurs worldwide and is transmitted to humans by rat fleas. Flea-infested rats can be found throughout the year in humid tropical environments, but in temperate regions are most common during the warm summer months. Travelers who visit in rat-infested buildings and homes, especially in harbor or riverine environments, can be at risk for exposure to the agent of murine typhus.

Scrub Typhus

Mites ("chiggers") transmit *Orientia tsutsugamushi*, the agent of scrub typhus, to humans. These mites occur year round in a large area from the Indian subcontinent to Australia and in much of Asia, including Japan, China, Korea, and parts of Russia. Their prevalence, however, fluctuates with temperature and rainfall. Humans typically encounter the arthropod vector of scrub typhus in recently disturbed terrain (e.g., forest clearings).

Tick-Borne Rickettsioses

Tick-borne rickettsial diseases have a worldwide distribution, but are most apparent in temperate and subtropical regions. These diseases include Rocky Mountain spotted fever (caused by *R. rickettsii*), Mediterranean spotted fever (*R. conorii*), African tick-bite fever (*R. africae*), Queensland tick typhus (*R. australis*), and North Asian tick fever (*R. sibirica*), and ehrlichiosis (*Ehrlichia* spp., *Anaplasma phagocytophilum*, and *Neorickettsia sennetsu*). In general, peak transmission of tick-borne rickettsial pathogens occurs seasonally during spring and summer months. Travelers who participate in outdoor activities in grassy or wooded areas (e.g., trekking, camping, or going on safari) may be at risk for acquiring tick-borne illnesses, including those caused by *Rickettsia*, *Anaplasma*, and *Neorickettsia* species.

Rickettsialpox

Rickettsialpox is an urban, mite-vectored disease associated with *R. akari*-infected house mice. Outbreaks of this illness have occurred shortly after rodent extermination programs. *R. akari*-infected rodents have been found in urban centers in the former Soviet Union, South Africa, Korea, Croatia, and the United States.

Q Fever

Q fever occurs worldwide, most often in persons who have frequent contact with goat, sheep, and cattle carcasses (especially farmers, veterinarians, butchers, or meat packers). Travelers who visit farms or rural communities can be exposed to *Coxiella burnetii*, the agent of Q fever, through airborne transmission (via contaminated soil and dust), or possibly through consumption of unpasteurized milk products. Initially, these infections may result in only mild illnesses, but if untreated, infections may become chronic, particularly in persons with preexisting heart valve abnormalities or with prosthetic valves. Such persons can develop chronic and potentially fatal endocarditis.

Cat-Scratch Disease and Oroya Fever

Cat-scratch disease is contracted through scratches and bites from domestic cats infected with *Bartonella henselae*, and possibly from their fleas. Exposure can therefore occur wherever cats are found. Oroya fever can be transmitted by sandflies infected with *B. bacilliformis*. The agent of this disease is endemic in the Andean highlands.

Clinical Presentation

Clinical presentations of rickettsial illnesses vary, but early symptoms are generally nonspecific, involving fever, headache, and malaise. Rashes are often associated with rickettsioses, and an eschar (thick blackened scab) is seen in several spotted fever rickettsioses and in scrub typhus. Illnesses resulting from infection with rickettsial agents often go unrecognized or are attributed to other causes. Diagnosis of rickettsial diseases is based on two or more of the following: 1) clinical symptoms and an epidemiologic history compatible with a rickettsial disease, 2) the development of specific antibodies reactive with a given pathogen or antigenic group, 3) a positive polymerase chain reaction test result, or 4) isolation of a rickettsial agent. Ascertaining the place and the nature of potential exposures is particularly important for accurate diagnosis, as many rickettsial diseases have strong geographic links or are associated with exposure to specific animal reservoir species or arthropod vectors.

Prevention

With the exception of the louse-borne diseases described above, for which contact with infectious arthropod feces is the mode of transmission (via autoinoculation into a wound or inhalation), travelers and health-care providers are generally not at risk of becoming infected via exposure to an ill person. Infections result primarily from exposure to an infected vector or animal reservoir. Limiting these exposures remains the best means for reducing the risk for disease. Travelers should be advised that prevention is based on avoidance of vector-infested habitats, use of repellents and protective clothing, prompt detection and removal of arthropods on clothing and skin, and attention to hygiene. Disease management should focus on early detection and proper treatment to prevent severe complications of these illnesses.

Q fever and Bartonella group diseases may pose a special risk for persons with abnormal or prosthetic heart valves and persons who are immunocompromised. Special care should be taken by these groups of travelers to prevent potential exposures.

Treatment

Treatments for most rickettsial illnesses are similar and include administration of appropriate antibiotics (most often tetracyclines) and supportive care. Treatment should be initiated on the basis of clinical and epidemiologic clues, without waiting for laboratory confirmation. No commercially licensed vaccines are available in the United States, and vaccinations to prevent rickettsial infections are not required by any country as a condition for entry.

—Gregory Dasch, Mary Reynolds

Chapter 37

River Blindness

Description

Onchocerciasis—the world's second leading infectious cause of blindness—is present in 36 countries of Africa, the Arabian peninsula and the Americas. As a public health problem the disease is most closely associated with Africa, where it constitutes a serious obstacle to socio-economic development. Onchocerciasis is often called "river blindness" because of its most extreme manifestation and because the black fly vector abounds in fertile riverside areas, which frequently remain uninhabited for fear of infection.

Prevalence

- Out of some 120 million people world-wide who are at risk of onchocerciasis, 96% are in Africa.

- Of the 36 countries where the disease is endemic, 30 are in sub-Sahara Africa (plus Yemen) and six are in the Americas.

- A total of 18 million people are infected with the disease and have dermal microfilariae, of whom 99% are in Africa.

"Description," is excerpted from "Onchocerciasis (River Blindness)," World Health Organization, Fact Sheet No. 95, Revised February 2000, © 2000 World Health Organization, reprinted with permission; other sections are excerpted from "Onchocerciasis (River Blindness)," by Frank O. Richards, Jr., Centers for Disease Control and Prevention (CDC), Reviewed June 30, 2003.

- Of those infected with the disease, over 6.5 million suffer from severe itching or dermatitis and 270,000 are blind.

Characteristics

Onchocerciasis is caused by *Onchocerca volvulus*, a parasitic worm that lives for up to 14 years in the human body. Each adult female worm, thin but more than 1/2 metre in length, produces millions of microfilariae (microscopic larvae) that migrate throughout the body and give rise to a variety of symptoms: serious visual impairment, including blindness; rashes, lesions, intense itching and depigmentation of the skin; lymphadenitis, which results in hanging groins and elephantiasis of the genitals; and general debilitation. Onchocerciasis manifestations begin to occur in persons one to three years after the injection of infective larvae.

Microfilariae produced in one person are carried to another by the black fly, which in West Africa belongs to the *Simulium damnosum* species complex. The black fly lays its eggs in the water of fast-flowing rivers. Adults emerge after 8–12 days and live for up to four weeks, during which they can cover hundreds of kilometers in flight.

After mating, the female black fly seeks a bloodmeal and may ingest microfilariae if the meal is taken from a person infected with onchocerciasis. A few of these microfilariae may transform into infective larvae within the black fly, which are then injected into the person from whom the next meal is taken and subsequently develop into adult parasites, thus completing the life cycle of the parasite.

Occurrence

Onchocerciasis is endemic in more than 25 nations located in a broad band across the central part of Africa. Small endemic foci are also present in the Arabian Peninsula (Yemen) and in the Americas (Brazil, Colombia, Ecuador, Guatemala, southern Mexico, and Venezuela).

Risk for Travelers

Those traveling for short periods in onchocerciasis-endemic regions appear to be at low risk for acquiring this condition. However, those who visit or live in endemic regions for >3 months and live or work near black fly habitats are at greater risk for infection. Infections tend to occur in expatriate groups such as missionaries, field scientists, and Peace Corps volunteers.

Clinical Presentation

Infection with *O. volvulus* can result in dermatitis; subcutaneous nodules; lymphadenitis; and ocular lesions, which can progress to blindness. Symptoms may occur months to years after departure from endemic areas.

Prevention

No vaccine and no effective chemoprophylaxis are available. Protective measures include avoidance of black fly habitats and the use of personal protection measures against biting insects.

Treatment

Ivermectin is the drug of choice for onchocerciasis. Repeated oral doses are required for up to several years, because the drug kills the microfilaria but not the adult worm. Travelers should be advised to consult with a specialist in infectious diseases or tropical medicine.

Chapter 38

Rocky Mountain Spotted Fever

Introduction

Rocky Mountain spotted fever is the most severe and most frequently reported rickettsial illness in the United States. The disease is caused by *Rickettsia rickettsii*, a species of bacteria that is spread to humans by ixodid (hard) ticks. Initial signs and symptoms of the disease include sudden onset of fever, headache, and muscle pain, followed by development of rash. The disease can be difficult to diagnose in the early stages, and without prompt and appropriate treatment it can be fatal.

Rocky Mountain spotted fever was first recognized in 1896 in the Snake River Valley of Idaho and was originally called "black measles" because of the characteristic rash. It was a dreaded and frequently fatal disease that affected hundreds of people in this area. By the early 1900s, the recognized geographic distribution of this disease grew to encompass parts of the United States as far north as Washington and Montana and as far south as California, Arizona, and New Mexico.

The Organism

Rocky Mountain spotted fever is caused by *Rickettsia rickettsii*, a very small bacterium that must live inside the cells of its hosts. These bacteria range in size from 0.2 x 0.5 micrometers to 0.3 x 2.0 micrometers.

Viral and Rickettsial Zoonoses Branch, Division of Viral and Rickettsial Diseases, National Center for Infectious Diseases, Centers for Disease Control and Prevention (CDC), August 2000.

In humans, rickettsiae live and multiply primarily within cells that line small- to medium-sized blood vessels. Spotted fever group rickettsiae can grow in the nucleus or in the cytoplasm of the host cell. Once inside the host the rickettsiae multiply, resulting in damage and death of these cells. This causes blood to leak through tiny holes in vessel walls into adjacent tissues. This process causes the rash that is traditionally associated with Rocky Mountain spotted fever and causes damage to organs and tissues.

Epidemiology

Rocky Mountain spotted fever has been a reportable disease in the United States since the 1920s. In the last 50 years, approximately 250–200 cases of Rocky Mountain spotted fever have been reported annually, although it is likely that many more cases go unreported. CDC compiles the number of cases reported by the state health departments. To ensure standardization of reporting across the country, CDC advises that a consistent case definition be used by all states.

Seasonal Distribution of Rocky Mountain Spotted Fever

Over 90% of patients with Rocky Mountain spotted fever are infected during April through September. This period is the season for increased numbers of adult and nymphal *Dermacentor* ticks. A history of tick bite or exposure to tick-infested habitats is reported in approximately 60% of all cases of Rocky Mountain spotted fever.

Geography of Rocky Mountain Spotted Fever

Over half of Rocky Mountain spotted fever infections are reported from the south-Atlantic region of the United States (Delaware, Maryland, Washington D.C., Virginia, West Virginia, North Carolina, South Carolina, Georgia, and Florida). Infection also occurs in other parts of the United States, namely the Pacific region (Washington, Oregon, and California) and west south-central (Arkansas, Louisiana, Oklahoma, and Texas) region.

The states with the highest incidences of Rocky Mountain spotted fever are North Carolina and Oklahoma; these two states combined accounted for 35% of the total number of U.S. cases reported to CDC during 1993 through 1996. Although Rocky Mountain spotted fever was first identified in the Rocky Mountain states, less than 3% of the U.S. cases were reported from that area during the same interval (1993–1996).

Persons at Risk for Infection

The frequency of reported cases of Rocky Mountain spotted fever is highest among males, Caucasians, and children. Two-thirds of the Rocky Mountain spotted fever cases occur in children under the age of 15 years, with the peak age being 5 to 9 years old. Individuals with frequent exposure to dogs and who reside near wooded areas or areas with high grass may also be at increased risk of infection.

Worldwide

Infection with *Rickettsia rickettsii* has also been documented in Argentina, Brazil, Colombia, Costa Rica, Mexico, and Panama. Some synonyms for Rocky Mountain spotted fever in other countries include tick typhus, Tobia fever (Columbia), São Paulo fever and fiebre maculosa (Brazil), and fiebre manchada (Mexico). Closely related organisms cause other types of spotted fevers in other parts of the world.

Signs and Symptoms

Rocky Mountain spotted fever can be very difficult to diagnose in its early stages, even among experienced physicians who are familiar with the disease.

Patients infected with *R. rickettsii* generally visit a physician in the first week of their illness, following an incubation period of about 5–10 days after a tick bite. The early clinical presentation of Rocky Mountain spotted fever is nonspecific and may resemble a variety of other infectious and non-infectious diseases.

Initial symptoms may include:

- fever
- nausea
- vomiting

- severe headache
- muscle pain
- lack of appetite

Later signs and symptoms include:

- rash
- abdominal pain

- joint pain
- diarrhea

The classic triad of findings for this disease are fever, rash, and history of tick bite. However, this combination is often not identified when the patient initially presents for care.

The rash first appears 2–5 days after the onset of fever and is often not present or may be very subtle when the patient is initially seen by a physician. Younger patients usually develop the rash earlier than older patients. Most often it begins as small, flat, pink, non-itchy spots (macules) on the wrists, forearms, and ankles. These spots turn pale when pressure is applied and eventually become raised on the skin. The characteristic red, spotted (petechial) rash of Rocky Mountain spotted fever is usually not seen until the sixth day or later after onset of symptoms, and this type of rash occurs in only 35% to 60% of patients with Rocky Mountain spotted fever. The rash involves the palms or soles in as many as 50% to 80% of patients; however, this distribution may not occur until later in the course of the disease. As many as 10% to 15% of patients may never develop a rash.

Abnormal laboratory findings seen in patients with Rocky Mountain spotted fever may include thrombocytopenia, hyponatremia, or elevated liver enzyme levels.

Rocky Mountain spotted fever can be a very severe illness and patients often require hospitalization. Because *R. rickettsii* infects the cells lining blood vessels throughout the body, severe manifestations of this disease may involve the respiratory system, central nervous system, gastrointestinal system, or renal system. Host factors associated with severe or fatal Rocky Mountain spotted fever include advanced age, male sex, African-American race, chronic alcohol abuse, and glucose-6-phosphate dehydrogenase (G6PD) deficiency. Deficiency of G6PD is a sex-linked genetic condition affecting approximately 12% of the U.S. African-American male population; deficiency of this enzyme is associated with a high proportion of severe cases of Rocky Mountain spotted fever. This is a rare clinical course that is often fatal within 5 days of onset of illness.

Long-term health problems following acute Rocky Mountain spotted fever infection include partial paralysis of the lower extremities, gangrene requiring amputation of fingers, toes, or arms or legs, hearing loss, loss of bowel or bladder control, movement disorders, and language disorders. These complications are most frequent in persons recovering from severe, life-threatening disease, often following lengthy hospitalizations.

Treatment

Appropriate antibiotic treatment should be initiated *immediately* when there is a suspicion of Rocky Mountain spotted fever on the basis of clinical and epidemiologic findings. Treatment should **not** be delayed until laboratory confirmation is obtained.

If the patient is treated within the first 4–5 days of the disease, fever generally subsides within 24–72 hours after treatment with an appropriate antibiotic (usually a tetracycline). In fact, failure to respond to a tetracycline antibiotic argues against a diagnosis of RMSF. Severely ill patients may require longer periods before their fever resolves, especially if they have experienced damage to multiple organ systems. Preventive therapy in non-ill patients who have had recent tick bites is not recommended and may, in fact, only delay the onset of disease.

Doxycycline (100 mg every 12 hours for adults or 4 mg/kg body weight per day in two divided doses for children under 45 kg [100 lbs]) is the drug of choice for patients with Rocky Mountain spotted fever. Therapy is continued for at least 3 days after fever subsides and until there is unequivocal evidence of clinical improvement, generally for a minimum total course of 5 to 10 days. Severe or complicated disease may require longer treatment courses. Doxycycline is also the preferred drug for patients with ehrlichiosis, another tick-transmitted infection with signs and symptoms that may resemble Rocky Mountain spotted fever.

Tetracyclines are usually not the preferred drug for use in pregnant women because of risks associated with malformation of teeth and bones in unborn children. Chloramphenicol is an alternative drug that can be used to treat Rocky Mountain spotted fever; however, this drug may be associated with a wide range of side effects and may require careful monitoring of blood levels.

Prevention and Control

Limiting exposure to ticks is the most effective way to reduce the likelihood of Rocky Mountain spotted fever infection. In persons exposed to tick-infested habitats, prompt careful inspection and removal of crawling or attached ticks is an important method of preventing disease. It may take several hours of attachment before organisms are transmitted from the tick to the host. Currently, no licensed vaccine is available for Rocky Mountain spotted fever.

It is unreasonable to assume that a person can completely eliminate activities that may result in tick exposure. Therefore, prevention measures should be aimed at personal protection:

- Wear light-colored clothing to allow you to see ticks that are crawling on your clothing.

- Tuck your pants legs into your socks so that ticks cannot crawl up the inside of your pants legs.

- Apply repellants to discourage tick attachment. Repellents containing permethrin can be sprayed on boots and clothing, and will last for several days. Repellents containing DEET (n, n-diethyl-m-toluamide) can be applied to the skin, but will last only a few hours before reapplication is necessary. Use DEET with caution on children. Application of large amounts of DEET on children has been associated with adverse reactions.

- Conduct a body check upon return from potentially tick-infested areas by searching your entire body for ticks. Use a hand-held or full-length mirror to view all parts of your body. Remove any tick you find on your body.

- Parents should check their children for ticks, especially in the hair, when returning from potentially tick-infested areas. Additionally, ticks may be carried into the household on clothing and pets. Both should be examined carefully.

To remove attached ticks, use the following procedure:

1. Use fine-tipped tweezers or shield your fingers with a tissue, paper towel, or rubber gloves. When possible, persons should avoid removing ticks with bare hands.

2. Grasp the tick as close to the skin surface as possible and pull upward with steady, even pressure. Do not twist or jerk the tick; this may cause the mouthparts to break off and remain in the skin. (*If this happens, remove mouthparts with tweezers. Consult your health care provider if infection occurs.*)

3. Do not squeeze, crush, or puncture the body of the tick because its fluids (saliva, body fluids, gut contents) may contain infectious organisms.

4. After removing the tick, thoroughly disinfect the bite site and wash your hands with soap and water.

5. Save the tick for identification in case you become ill. This may help your doctor make an accurate diagnosis. Place the tick in a plastic bag and put it in your freezer. Write the date of the bite on a piece of paper with a pencil and place it in the bag.

Folklore Remedies Don't Work

Folklore remedies, such as the use of petroleum jelly or hot matches, do little to encourage a tick to detach from skin. In fact, they may make matters worse by irritating the tick and stimulating it to release additional saliva or regurgitate gut contents, increasing the chances of transmitting the pathogen. These methods of tick removal should be avoided. A number of tick removal devices have been marketed, but none are better than a plain set of fine tipped tweezers.

Tick Control

Strategies to reduce populations of vector ticks through area-wide application of acaricides (chemicals that will kill ticks and mites) and control of tick habitats (e.g., leaf litter and brush) have been effective in small-scale trials. New methods being developed include applying acaricides to rodents by using baited tubes, boxes, and feeding stations in areas where these pathogens are endemic. Biological control with fungi, parasitic nematodes, and parasitic wasps may play alternate roles in integrated tick control efforts. Community-based, integrated, tick-management strategies may prove to be an effective public health response to reduce the incidence of tick-borne infections. However, limiting exposure to ticks is currently the most effective method of prevention.

Chapter 39

Toxocariasis

What is toxocariasis?

Toxocariasis (TOX-o-kah-RYE-us-sis) is a zoonotic (animal to human) infection caused by the parasitic roundworms commonly found in the intestine of dogs (*Toxocara canis*) and cats (*T. cati*). In the United States, an estimated 10,000 cases of *Toxocara* infections occur yearly in humans.

What are the symptoms of toxocariasis?

There are two major forms of toxocariasis:

1. Ocular larva migrans (OLM): *Toxocara* infections can cause OLM, an eye disease that can cause blindness. OLM occurs when a microscopic worm enters the eye; it may cause inflammation and formation of a scar on the retina. Each year more than 700 people infected with *Toxocara* experience permanent partial loss of vision.

2. Visceral larva migrans (VLM): Heavier, or repeated *Toxocara* infections, while rare, can cause VLM, a disease that causes swelling of the body's organs or central nervous system.

"Toxocariasis," Division of Parasitic Diseases, Centers for Disease Control and Prevention (CDC), reviewed March 20, 2002. This information prepared in association with the American Association of Veterinary Parasitologists (AAVP).

Symptoms of VLM, which are caused by the movement of the worms through the body, include fever, coughing, asthma, or pneumonia.

How serious is infection with Toxocara?

In most cases, *Toxocara* infections are not serious, and many people, especially adults infected by a small number of larvae (immature worms), may not notice any symptoms. The most severe cases are rare, but are more likely to occur in young children, who often play in dirt, or eat dirt (pica) contaminated by dog or cat stool.

How is toxocariasis spread?

The most common *Toxocara* parasite of concern to humans is *T. canis*, which puppies usually contract from the mother before birth or from her milk. The larvae mature rapidly in the puppy's intestines; when the pup is 3 or 4 weeks old, they begin to produce large numbers of eggs that contaminate the environment through the animal's stool. The eggs soon develop into infective larvae.

How can I get toxocariasis?

You or your children can become infected after accidentally ingesting (swallowing) infective *Toxocara* eggs from larvae in soil or other contaminated surfaces.

What should I do if I think I have toxocariasis?

See your health care provider to discuss the possibility of infection and, if necessary, to be examined. A blood test is available for diagnosis.

What is the treatment for toxocariasis?

VLM is treated with antiparasitic drugs, usually in combination with anti-inflammatory medications. Treatment of OLM is more difficult and usually consists of measures to prevent progressive damage to the eye.

Who is at risk for toxocariasis?

Young children; owners of dogs and cats.

How can you prevent toxocariasis?

- Have your veterinarian treat your dogs and cats, especially young animals, regularly for worms.

- Wash your hands well with soap and water after playing with your pets and after outdoor activities, especially before you eat. Teach children to always wash their hands after playing with dogs and cats and after playing outdoors.

- Do not allow children to play in areas that are soiled with pet or other animal stool.

- Clean your pet's living area at least once a week. Feces should be either buried or bagged and disposed of in the trash.

- Teach children that it is dangerous to eat dirt or soil.

For More Information

1. Glickman LT, Schantz PM. Epidemiology and pathogenesis of zoonotic toxocariasis. *Epidemiol Rev* 1981;3:230-50.

2. Kazacos KR. Visceral and ocular larva migrans. *Semin Vet Med Surg (Small Anim)* 1991;6:227-35.

3. Schantz PM. *Toxocara* larva migrans now. *Am J Trop Med Hyg* 1989;41(3) Suppl:21-34.

Chapter 40

Toxoplasmosis

What is toxoplasmosis?

Toxoplasmosis is an infection caused by a single-celled parasite called *Toxoplasma gondii*. The parasite is found throughout the world. More than 60 million people in the United States probably carry the *Toxoplasma* parasite, but very few have symptoms because the immune system usually keeps the parasite from causing illness. However, pregnant women and those with compromised immune systems should be cautious because a *Toxoplasma* infection can cause serious problems.

How can I get toxoplasmosis?

- Through accidental ingestion of contaminated cat feces. This can occur if you accidentally touch your hands to your mouth after gardening, cleaning a cat's litter box, or touching anything that has come into contact with cat feces.

- Through ingestion of raw or partly cooked meat, especially pork, lamb, or venison, or by touching your hands to your mouth after handling undercooked meat.

- Through contamination of knives, utensils, cutting boards, and other foods that have had contact with raw meat.

"Toxoplasmosis," Division of Parasitic Diseases, Centers for Disease Control and Prevention (CDC), reviewed January 10, 2003.

- Through drinking water contaminated with *Toxoplasma*.

- Although extremely rare, by receiving an infected organ transplant or blood transfusion.

What are the symptoms of toxoplasmosis?

You may feel like you have the "flu," swollen lymph glands, or muscle aches and pains that last for a month or more. Rarely, a person with a "normal" immune system may develop eye damage from toxoplasmosis. However, most people who become infected with toxoplasmosis do not know it. Persons with weak immune systems, such as infants, those with HIV/AIDS, those taking certain types of chemotherapy, or persons who have recently received an organ transplant, may develop severe toxoplasmosis. This can cause damage to the brain or the eyes. Most infants who are infected while in the womb have no symptoms at birth but may develop symptoms later in life. Only a small percentage of infected newborns have serious eye or brain damage at birth.

Who is at risk for severe toxoplasmosis?

- Infants born to mothers who became infected with *Toxoplasma* for the first time during or just before pregnancy.

- Persons with severely weakened immune systems, such as persons with AIDS. This results from an acute *Toxoplasma* infection or an infection that occurred earlier in life that reactivates and causes damage to the brain, eyes, or other organs.

How do I know if I have toxoplasmosis?

See your health care provider who may order a blood sample to be taken. There are several different kinds of blood tests for toxoplasmosis. The results from the different tests can help your provider determine if you have *Toxoplasma* infection and if the infection is recent ("acute").

What should I do if I think I am at risk for severe toxoplasmosis?

- If you have a weakened immune system, have your blood tested for *Toxoplasma*. If your test is positive, your doctor can tell you if and when you need to take medicine to prevent the infection from reactivating. If your test is negative, it means you have never been infected and you need to take precautions to avoid infection. (See below.)

- If you are planning to become pregnant, your health care provider may test you for *Toxoplasma*. If the test is positive it means you have already been infected sometime in your life. There usually is little need to worry about passing the infection to your baby. If the test is negative, take necessary precautions to avoid infection (See below.)

- If you are already pregnant, you and your health care provider should discuss your risk for toxoplasmosis. Your health care provider may order a blood sample for testing.

How can I prevent toxoplasmosis?

There are several general sanitation and food safety steps you can take to reduce your chances of becoming infected.

- Wear gloves when you garden or do anything outdoors that involves handling soil. Cats, which may pass the parasite in their feces, often use gardens and sandboxes as litter boxes. Wash your hands well with soap and water after outdoor activities, especially before you eat or prepare any food.

- When preparing raw meat, wash any cutting boards, sinks, knives, and other utensils that might have touched the raw meat thoroughly with soap and hot water to avoid cross-contaminating other foods. Wash your hands well with soap and water after handling raw meat.

- Cook all meat thoroughly; that is, to an internal temperature of 160° F and until it is no longer pink in the center or until the juices become colorless. Do not taste meat before it is fully cooked.

Am I able to keep my cat?

Yes, but if you have a weakened immune system or are pregnant there are some steps to take to avoid being exposed to *Toxoplasma*.

- Help prevent your cat from becoming infected with *Toxoplasma*. Keep it indoors and feed it dry or canned cat food. A cat can become infected by eating infected prey or being fed raw or undercooked meat infected with the parasite.

- Do not bring a new cat into your house that might have spent time out of doors or might have been fed raw meat. Avoid stray cats and kittens and their adopted habitat. Your veterinarian can answer any other questions you may have regarding your cat and risk for toxoplasmosis.

- Have someone who is healthy and not pregnant change your cat's litter box daily. If this is not possible, wear gloves and clean the litter box daily (the parasite found in cat feces needs one or more days after being passed to become infectious.) Wash your hands well with soap and water afterwards.

Once infected with Toxoplasma *is my cat always able to spread the infection to me?*

No. Cats spread *Toxoplasma* in their feces for only a few weeks of their lives, usually after they are first infected with the parasite. Like humans, cats rarely have symptoms when first infected, so most people do not know if their cat has been infected with *Toxoplasma*. It is not helpful to have your cat or your cat's feces tested for *Toxoplasma*.

What is the treatment for toxoplasmosis?

Once a diagnosis of toxoplasmosis is confirmed, you and your health care provider can discuss whether treatment is necessary. In an otherwise healthy person who is not pregnant, treatment usually is not needed. Symptoms typically go away within a few weeks. For pregnant women or persons who have weakened immune systems, drugs are available to treat toxoplasmosis.

For More Information

- Centers for Disease Control and Prevention. CDC recommendations regarding selected conditions affecting women's health: preventing congenital toxoplasmosis. *MMWR* 2000;49(RR02):57–75.

- Centers for Disease Control and Prevention. 1999 USPHS/IDSA Guidelines for the prevention of opportunistic infections in persons infected with Human Immunodeficiency Virus. *MMWR* 1999;48(RR10):1–59.

- Centers for Disease Control and Prevention. Guidelines for the prevention of opportunistic infections among HIV-infected persons—2002. Recommendations of the U.S. Public Health Service and the Infectious Disease Society of America. *MMWR* 2002; 51(RR08): 1–52.

- Dubey JP. Toxoplasmosis (Zoonosis Update). *J Am Vet Med Assoc*. 1994 Dec. 1; 205(11): 1593–8.

- Frenkel JK. Fishback JL. Toxoplasmosis. *Hunter's Tropical Medicine and Emerging Diseases, 8th Ed.*, 2000. G. Thomas Strickland, Ed. W.B. Saunders and Company.

- Jones JL, Lopez A, Wilson M, Schulkin J, Gibbs R. Congenital toxoplasmosis: A review. *Obstet Gynecol Surv*. 2001 May;56(5): 296–305.

Chapter 41

Trypanosomiasis Diseases

Chagas Disease

What is Chagas disease?

Also called American trypanosomiasis (tri-PAN-o-SO-my-a-sis), Chagas (SHA-gus) disease is an infection caused by the parasite *Trypanosoma cruzi*. It is estimated that 16–18 million people are infected with Chagas disease; of those infected, 50,000 will die each year.

How is Chagas disease spread?

Reduviid bugs, or "kissing bugs" live in cracks and holes of substandard housing primarily found in South and Central America. Insects become infected after biting an animal or person who already has Chagas disease. Infection is spread to humans when an infected bug deposits feces on a person's skin, usually while the person is sleeping at night. The person often accidentally rubs the feces into the bite wound, an open cut, the eyes, or mouth. Animals can become infected the same way, and they can also contract the disease by eating an infected bug.

How can I become infected?

- By infective feces contacting your eyes, mouth, or open cuts.

"Chagas Disease," October 2002, and "West African Trypanosomiasis," August 1999, Division of Parasitic Diseases, Centers for Disease Control and Prevention (CDC).

- By infected mothers passing infection to their baby during pregnancy, at delivery, or while breastfeeding.

- By blood transfusion or organ transplant.

- By eating uncooked food contaminated with infective feces of "kissing bugs."

Is Chagas disease a serious illness?

Yes. Chagas disease primarily affects low income people living in rural areas. Many people get the infection during childhood. The early stage of infection (acute Chagas disease) usually is not severe, but sometimes it can cause death, particularly in infants. However, in about one-third of those who get the infection, chronic symptoms develop after 10–20 years. For these persons who develop chronic symptoms, the average life expectancy decreases by an average of 9 years.

What are the symptoms of Chagas disease?

There are three stages of infection with Chagas disease; each stage has different symptoms. Some persons may be infected and never develop symptoms.

Acute: Acute symptoms only occur in about 1% of cases. Most people infected do not seek medical attention. The most recognized symptom of acute Chagas infection is the Romaña's sign, or swelling of the eye on one side of the face, usually at the bite wound or where feces were rubbed into the eye. Other symptoms are usually not specific for Chagas infection. These symptoms may include fatigue, fever, enlarged liver or spleen, and swollen lymph glands. Sometimes, a rash, loss of appetite, diarrhea, and vomiting occur. In infants and in very young children with acute Chagas disease, swelling of the brain can develop in acute Chagas disease, and this can cause death. In general, symptoms last for 4–8 weeks and then they go away, even without treatment.

Indeterminate: Eight to 10 weeks after infection, the indeterminate stage begins. During this stage, people do not have symptoms.

Chronic: Ten to 20 years after infection, people may develop the most serious symptoms of Chagas disease. Cardiac problems, including an enlarged heart, altered heart rate or rhythm, heart failure, or cardiac arrest are symptoms of chronic disease. Chagas disease can also lead to enlargement of parts of the digestive tract, which result in severe constipation or problems with swallowing. In persons who are immune compromised, including persons with HIV/AIDS, Chagas disease can be severe. Not everyone will develop the chronic symptoms of Chagas disease.

How soon after infection will I have symptoms of Chagas disease?

Symptoms may occur within a few days to weeks. Most people do not have symptoms until the chronic stage of infection, 10–20 years after first being infected.

Can I take medication to prevent Chagas disease?

No. There is neither a vaccine nor recommended drug available to prevent Chagas disease.

What should I do if I think I have Chagas disease?

See your health care provider who will order blood tests to look for the parasite or for antibodies in your blood.

What is the treatment for Chagas disease?

Medication for Chagas disease is usually effective when given during the acute stage of infection. Once the disease has progressed to later stages, medication may be less effective. In the chronic stage, treatment involves managing symptoms associated with the disease.

Where can I contract Chagas disease?

Chagas disease is locally transmitted in Argentina, Belize, Bolivia, Brazil, Chile, Colombia, Costa Rica, Ecuador, El Salvador, French Guiana, Guatemala, Guyana, Honduras, Mexico, Nicaragua, Panama, Paraguay, Peru, Suriname, Uruguay, and Venezuela.

Who is at risk for Chagas disease?

Those people who sleep in poorly constructed houses found in the rural areas of the above-mentioned countries are at elevated risk of infection. Houses constructed from mud, adobe, or thatch present the greatest risk.

Travelers planning to stay in hotels, resorts, or other well-constructed housing facilities are NOT at high risk for contracting Chagas disease from reduviid bugs.

How can I prevent Chagas disease?

- Avoid sleeping in thatch, mud, or adobe houses.

- Use insecticides to kill insects and reduce the risk of transmission.

- Be aware that, in some countries, the blood supply may not always be screened for Chagas disease, and blood transfusions may carry a risk of infection.

For More Information

1. Hagar JM, Rahimtoola SH. Chagas' heart disease. *Curr Probl Cardiol* 1995;20:825–924.

2. Herwaldt BL, Grijalva MJ, Newsome AL, McGhee CR, Powell MR, Nemec DG, Steurer FJ, Eberhard ML. Use of polymerase chain reaction to diagnose the fifth reported US case of autochthonous transmission of *Trypanosoma cruzi*, in Tennessee, 1998. *J Infect Dis* 2000;181;395–399.

3. Herwaldt BL, Juranek DD. Laboratory-acquired malaria, leishmaniasis, trypanosomiasis, and toxoplasmosis. *Am J Trop Med Hyg* 1993;48:313–23.

4. Kirchoff LV. American trypanosomiasis (Chagas' disease). *Gastroenterol Clin North Am* 1996;25:517–532.

5. Kirchhoff LV. American trypanosomiasis (Chagas' disease)—a tropical disease now in the United States. *New Engl J Med* 1993;329:639–44.

West African Trypanosomiasis

What is African trypanosomiasis?

There are two types of African trypanosomiasis, also called sleeping sickness, named for the areas in Africa in which they are found. West African trypanosomiasis, also called Gambian sleeping sickness, is caused by a parasite called *Trypanosoma brucei gambiense* (tri-PAN-o-SO-ma brew-see-eye gam-be-ense). Worldwide, 20,000 new cases of both East and West African trypanosomiasis are reported each year. Few cases of West African trypanosomiasis have been reported in the United States.

How can I get West African trypanosomiasis?

- Through the bite of an infected tsetse fly, found only in Africa.

Rarely:

- If you are infected and pregnant, you may pass infection to your baby.
- Through blood transfusion or by organ transplant.

Is West African trypanosomiasis a serious illness?

Yes. If left untreated, death will occur.

What are the symptoms of West African trypanosomiasis?

A bite by the tsetse fly is often painful. Occasionally, 1–2 weeks after the tsetse fly bite, a red sore, also called a chancre (SHAN-ker) appears at the site of the infective bite. Several weeks to months later, other symptoms of sleeping sickness occur. These include fever, rash, swelling around the eye and hands, severe headaches, extreme fatigue, aching muscles and joints. You may develop swollen lymph nodes on the back of your neck called Winterbottom's sign. Weight loss occurs as the illness progresses. Personality changes, irritability, loss of concentration, progressive confusion, slurred speech, seizures, and difficulty in walking and talking occurs when infection has invaded the central nervous system. These symptoms become worse as illness progresses. Sleeping for long periods of the day and having insomnia at night is a common symptom. If left untreated, infection becomes worse and death will occur within several months to years after infection.

How soon after infection will I have symptoms of West African trypanosomiasis?

Symptoms occur within months to years after infection.

Can I take medication to prevent West African trypanosomiasis?

There is neither a vaccine nor recommended drug available to prevent West African trypanosomiasis.

What should I do if I think I have African trypanosomiasis?

See your health care provider who will order several tests to look for the parasite. Common tests include blood samples and a spinal tap. Your physician may also take a sample of fluid from swollen lymph nodes.

What is the treatment for West African trypanosomiasis?

Treatment should be started as soon as possible and is based on the infected person's symptoms and laboratory results. Medication for the treatment of West African trypanosomiasis is available. Hospitalization for treatment is necessary and periodic follow-up exams that include a spinal tap are required for 2 years.

Where can I contract West African trypanosomiasis?

West African trypanosomiasis can be contracted in parts of Western and Central Africa. The tsetse fly lives only in Africa; areas where infection is spread are largely determined by where the infected tsetse fly is found.

Who is at risk for contracting West African trypanosomiasis?

Tsetse flies can be found in Western and Central African forests, in areas of thick shrubbery and trees by rivers and waterholes. Risk of infection increases with the number of times a person is bitten by the tsetse fly. Therefore, tourists are not at great risk for contracting West African trypanosomiasis unless they are traveling and spending long periods of time in rural areas of Western and Central Africa.

How can I prevent African trypanosomiasis and other insect bites?

- Wear protective clothing, including long-sleeved shirts and pants. The tsetse fly can bite through thin fabrics, so clothing should be made of thick material.

- Wear khaki or olive colored clothing. The tsetse fly is attracted to bright colors and very dark colors.

- Use insect repellant. Though insect repellants have not proven effective in preventing tsetse fly bites, they are effective in preventing other insects from biting and causing illness.

- When sleeping, use bednets.

- Inspect vehicles for tsetse flies before entering.

- Don't ride in the back of jeeps, pickup trucks or other open vehicles. The tsetse fly is attracted to the dust that moving vehicles and wild animals create.

- Avoid bushes. The tsetse fly is less active during the hottest period of the day. It rests in bushes but will bite if disturbed.

For More Information

1. Bryan R, Waskin J, Richards F, et al. African trypanosomiasis in American travelers: a 20-year review. *Travel Medicine.* Steffen R, Lobel HO, Haworth J, Bradley DJ, eds. Berlin: Springer-Verlag, 1989:384–8.

2. McGovern TW, William W, Fitzpatrick JE, et al. Cutaneous manifestations of African trypanosomiasis. *Arch Dermatol* 1995;131:1178–82.

Chapter 42

Tularemia

Overview

Tularemia (also known as deerfly fever or rabbit fever) is an infectious disease caused by the bacterium *Francisella tularensis*. It is naturally found in small mammals such as rabbits, rodents, and hares, as well as the insects that feed on these animals. The bacteria can survive for weeks at low temperatures in water, moist soil, hay, straw, or decaying animal carcasses. Tularemia was first described by scientists in 1911, and its ability to infect whole populations was seen during outbreaks of waterborne disease in Europe and the Soviet Union in the 1930s and 1940s.

There are about 200 reported cases of human tularemia in the United States every year. Most occur in rural areas in the south-central and western states. Of these cases, less than 2 percent are fatal.

The Microbe

F. tularensis has two subspecies.

- Type A is common in North America and may be highly virulent in humans and animals.

- Type B probably causes all human tularemia in Europe and Asia.

"Tularemia," National Institute of Allergy and Infectious Diseases (NIAID), National Institutes of Health (NIH), February 2003.

Transmission

The most common ways people contract tularemia are

- Being bitten by flies or ticks carrying the disease
- Handling infected animal tissue or fluids
- Eating insufficiently cooked rabbit meat in which the bacteria were not destroyed by cooking

Tularemia also can be spread by

- Having direct contact with or ingesting bacteria-contaminated water, food, or soil
- Handling contaminated animal skins
- Inhaling infective aerosols

In Europe, there have been cases of the disease caused by inhaling airborne bacteria generated during farm work, such as moving infected hay. Laboratory workers also can become infected by inhaling bacteria while examining an open culture plate, for example.

There are no documented cases of human-to-human transmission.

Symptoms

Tularemia infection varies from a mild illness to acute sepsis (serious infection of the blood or other tissues) and rapid death. After exposure to the bacteria, a person will usually develop symptoms within 3 to 5 days, but they can take up to 21 days to appear. Symptoms include

- Sudden, abrupt onset of fever
- Chills
- Headaches
- Muscle aches
- Joint stiffness or pain
- Weakness

In most patients, progressive weakness leads to a dry cough and pneumonia. Tularemia-induced pneumonia can cause chest pain, bloody sputum, and trouble breathing. Depending on how a person was exposed to the bacteria, other symptoms may include

- A red spot on the skin that enlarges to an ulcer
- Ulcers in the mouth
- Swollen and painful lymph glands
- Swollen and painful eyes
- Sore throat

The inhalation form of tularemia begins 3 to 5 days after exposure. In some cases, pneumonia develops after several days or weeks. If left untreated, the disease could lead to respiratory failure.

Diagnosis

Health care workers can diagnosis tularemia by doing laboratory tests on blood or sputum.

Treatment

Antibiotics, such as doxycycline or ciprofloxacin, can effectively treat people with tularemia. A tularemia vaccine strain is being reviewed by the U.S. Food and Drug Administration, but its future availability is uncertain, mainly because of the length of time it takes for the vaccine to work (about 2 weeks).

The U.S. Department of Defense also has developed an experimental tularemia vaccine. To date, health officials have limited the use of this vaccine to laboratory and other high-risk workers.

How Common Is Tularemia?

Health experts believe that tularemia is underrecognized and underreported. There are approximately 200 reported cases in the United States each year. Most cases occur in rural areas from June through September (tick season) and generally infect hunters. From 1995 to 1997, approximately half of all U.S. tularemia cases were reported from Missouri, Oklahoma, Kansas, and Arkansas. Worldwide, the disease occurs in Eurasia-most commonly in northern and central Europe-and almost always in rural areas.

Research

The National Institute of Allergy and Infectious Diseases (NIAID) is part of the National Institutes of Health, an agency of the U.S.

Department of Health and Human Services. NIAID supports research on the diagnosis, prevention, and treatment of infections caused by microbes, including those that have the potential for use as biological weapons. The research program to address biodefense includes both short- and long-term studies targeted at designing, developing, evaluating, and approving specific tools (diagnostics, therapies, and vaccines) needed to defend against possible bioterrorist-caused disease outbreaks.

Institute research goals to diagnose, prevent, and treat tularemia include

- Developing quick and inexpensive ways to diagnose tularemia

- Developing antimicrobials and immunotherapies with novel mechanisms of action to treat tularemia

- Identifying new *F. tularensis* vaccine candidates that can prevent or modulate infection both before and after exposure

- Conducting clinical trials of vaccine candidates

More Information

National Institute of Allergy and Infectious Diseases
31 Center Drive, MSC 2520
Bethesda, MD 20892-2520
Website: http://www.niaid.nih.gov

National Library of Medicine
MEDLINEplus
8600 Rockville Pike
Bethesda, MD 20894
Phone: 1-800-338-7657
Website: http://www.nlm.nih.gov/medlineplus

U.S. Centers for Disease Control and Prevention
1600 Clifton Road
Atlanta, GA 30333
Phone: 1-888-232-3228
Website: http://www.bt.cdc.gov

Johns Hopkins University Center for Civilian Biodefense Studies
Website: http://www.hopkins-biodefense.org/pages/agents/agent
tularemia.html

Chapter 43

Viral Hemorrhagic Fevers

What are Viral Hemorrhagic Fevers?

Viral hemorrhagic fevers (VHFs) refer to a group of illnesses that are caused by several distinct families of viruses. In general, the term "viral hemorrhagic fever" is used to describe a severe multisystem syndrome (multisystem in that multiple organ systems in the body are affected). Characteristically, the overall vascular system is damaged, and the body's ability to regulate itself is impaired. These symptoms are often accompanied by hemorrhage (bleeding); however, the bleeding is itself rarely life-threatening. While some types of hemorrhagic fever viruses can cause relatively mild illnesses, many of these viruses cause severe, life-threatening disease.

How are hemorrhagic fever viruses grouped?

VHFs are caused by viruses of four distinct families: arenaviruses, filoviruses, bunyaviruses, and flaviviruses. Each of these families share a number of features:

This chapter contains excerpts from "Viral Hemorrhagic Fevers," January 2002, "Arenaviruses," January 2002," "Ebola Hemorrhagic Fever," August 2003, "Lassa Fever," April 2002, "Marburg Hemorrhagic Fever," April 2002, "Rift Valley Fever," May 2002, Centers for Disease Prevention and Control (CDC), Special Pathogens Branch, and "Dengue and Dengue Hemorrhagic Fever: Questions and Answers," February 2002, Centers for Disease Prevention and Control (CDC), Division of Vector-Borne Infectious Diseases.

- They are all RNA viruses, and all are covered, or enveloped, in a fatty (lipid) coating.

- Their survival is dependent on an animal or insect host, called the natural reservoir.

- The viruses are geographically restricted to the areas where their host species live.

- Humans are not the natural reservoir for any of these viruses. Humans are infected when they come into contact with infected hosts. However, with some viruses, after the accidental transmission from the host, humans can transmit the virus to one another.

- Human cases or outbreaks of hemorrhagic fevers caused by these viruses occur sporadically and irregularly. The occurrence of outbreaks cannot be easily predicted.

- With a few noteworthy exceptions, there is no cure or established drug treatment for VHFs.

In rare cases, other viral and bacterial infections can cause a hemorrhagic fever; scrub typhus is a good example.

How are hemorrhagic fever viruses transmitted?

Viruses causing hemorrhagic fever are initially transmitted to humans when the activities of infected reservoir hosts or vectors and humans overlap. The viruses carried in rodent reservoirs are transmitted when humans have contact with urine, fecal matter, saliva, or other body excretions from infected rodents. The viruses associated with arthropod vectors are spread most often when the vector mosquito or tick bites a human, or when a human crushes a tick. However, some of these vectors may spread virus to animals, livestock, for example. Humans then become infected when they care for or slaughter the animals.

Some viruses that cause hemorrhagic fever can spread from one person to another, once an initial person has become infected. Ebola, Marburg, Lassa and Crimean-Congo hemorrhagic fever viruses are examples. This type of secondary transmission of the virus can occur directly, through close contact with infected people or their body fluids. It can also occur indirectly, through contact with objects contaminated with infected body fluids. For example, contaminated syringes and needles have played an important role in spreading infection in outbreaks of Ebola hemorrhagic fever and Lassa fever.

What are the symptoms of viral hemorrhagic fever illnesses?

Specific signs and symptoms vary by the type of VHF, but initial signs and symptoms often include marked fever, fatigue, dizziness, muscle aches, loss of strength, and exhaustion. Patients with severe cases of VHF often show signs of bleeding under the skin, in internal organs, or from body orifices like the mouth, eyes, or ears. However, although they may bleed from many sites around the body, patients rarely die because of blood loss. Severely ill patient cases may also show shock, nervous system malfunction, coma, delirium, and seizures. Some types of VHF are associated with renal (kidney) failure.

Arenaviruses

What are the Arenaviridae?

The Arenaviridae are a family of viruses whose members are generally associated with rodent-transmitted disease in humans. Each virus usually is associated with a particular rodent host species in which it is maintained. Arenavirus infections are relatively common in humans in some areas of the world and can cause severe illnesses.

What viruses are included in the virus family?

The arenaviruses are divided into two groups: the New World or Tacaribe complex and the Old World or LCM [lymphocytic choriomeningitis virus]/Lassa complex. Viruses in these groups that cause illness in humans are listed below:

* Lassa virus: Lassa fever
* Junin virus: Argentine hemorrhagic fever
* Machupo virus: Bolivian hemorrhagic fever
* Guanarito virus: Venezuelan hemorrhagic fever
* Sabia virus: Brazilian hemorrhagic fever

What kinds of animal hosts do these viruses have?

These viruses are zoonotic, meaning that, in nature, they are found in animals. Each virus is associated with either one species or a few closely related rodents, which constitute the virus' natural reservoir. Tacaribe complex viruses are generally associated with the New World rats and mice (family Muridae, subfamily Sigmodontinae). The LCM/Lassa complex viruses are associated with the Old World rats and mice (family Muridae, subfamily Murinae). Taken together, these types of rodents are located across the greater proportion of the earth's land mass, including Europe, Asia, Africa, and the Americas. One notable exception is Tacaribe virus, found in Trinidad, which was isolated from a bat.

How are arenaviruses spread?

The rodent hosts of arenaviruses are chronically infected with the viruses; however, the viruses do not appear to cause obvious illness in them. Some Old World arenaviruses appear to be passed from mother rodents to their offspring during pregnancy, and thus remain in the rodent population generation after generation. Some New World arenaviruses are transmitted among adult rodents, likely via fighting and inflicting bites. Only a portion of the rodents in each host species is infected at any one time, and in many cases only in a limited portion of the host's geographical range. The viruses are shed into the environment in the urine or droppings of their infected hosts.

Human infection with arenaviruses is incidental to the natural cycle of the viruses and occurs when an individual comes into contact with the excretions or materials contaminated with the excretions of an infected rodent, such as ingestion of contaminated food, or by direct contact of abraded or broken skin with rodent excrement. Infection can also occur by inhalation of tiny particles soiled with rodent urine or saliva (aerosol transmission). The types of incidental contact depend on the habits of both humans and rodents. For example, where the infected rodent species prefers a field habitat, human infection is associated with agricultural work. In areas where the rodent species' habitat includes human homes or other buildings, infection occurs in domestic settings.

Some arenaviruses, such as Lassa and Machupo viruses, are associated with secondary person-to-person and nosocomial (health-care setting) transmission. This occurs when a person infected by exposure to the virus from the rodent host spreads the virus to other humans. This may occur in a variety of ways. Person-to-person transmission is associated with direct contact with the blood or other excretions, containing virus particles, of infected individuals. Airborne transmission has also been reported in connection with certain viruses. Contact with objects contaminated with these materials, such as medical equipment, is also associated with transmission. In these situations, use of protective clothing and disinfection procedures (together called barrier nursing) help prevent further spread of illness.

Dengue and Dengue Hemorrhagic Fever

What is dengue?

Dengue (pronounced den' gee) is a disease caused by any one of four closely related viruses (DEN-1, DEN-2, DEN-3, or DEN-4). The viruses are transmitted to humans by the bite of an infected mosquito. In the Western Hemisphere, the *Aedes aegypti* mosquito is the most important transmitter or vector of dengue viruses, although a 2001 outbreak in Hawaii was transmitted by *Aedes albopictus*. It is estimated that there are over 100 million cases of dengue worldwide each year.

What is dengue hemorrhagic fever (DHF)?

DHF is a more severe form of dengue. It can be fatal if unrecognized and not properly treated. DHF is caused by infection with the same viruses that cause dengue. With good medical management, mortality due to DHF can be less than 1%.

How are dengue and dengue hemorrhagic fever (DHF) spread?

Dengue is transmitted to people by the bite of an *Aedes* mosquito that is infected with a dengue virus. The mosquito becomes infected with dengue virus when it bites a person who has dengue or DHF and after about a week can transmit the virus while biting a healthy person. Dengue cannot be spread directly from person to person.

What are the symptoms of the disease?

The principal symptoms of dengue are high fever, severe headache, backache, joint pains, nausea and vomiting, eye pain, and rash. Generally, younger children have a milder illness than older children and adults.

Dengue hemorrhagic fever is characterized by a fever that lasts from 2 to 7 days, with general signs and symptoms that could occur with many other illnesses (e.g., nausea, vomiting, abdominal pain, and headache). This stage is followed by hemorrhagic manifestations, tendency to bruise easily or other types of skin hemorrhages, bleeding nose or gums, and possibly internal bleeding. The smallest blood vessels (capillaries) become excessively permeable ("leaky"), allowing the fluid component to escape from the blood vessels. This may lead to failure of the circulatory system and shock, followed by death, if circulatory failure is not corrected.

What is the treatment for dengue?

There is no specific medication for treatment of a dengue infection. Persons who think they have dengue should use analgesics (pain relievers) with acetaminophen and avoid those containing aspirin. They should also rest, drink plenty of fluids, and consult a physician.

Is there an effective treatment for dengue hemorrhagic fever (DHF)?

As with dengue, there is no specific medication for DHF. It can however be effectively treated by fluid replacement therapy if an early clinical diagnosis is made. Hospitalization is frequently required in order to adequately manage DHF. Physicians who suspect that a patient has DHF may want to consult the Dengue Branch at CDC, for more information.

Ebola Hemorrhagic Fever

What is Ebola hemorrhagic fever?

The disease is caused by infection with Ebola virus, named after a river in the Democratic Republic of the Congo (formerly Zaire) in Africa, where it was first recognized. The virus is one of two members of a family of RNA viruses called the Filoviridae. There are four identified subtypes of Ebola virus. Three of the four have caused disease in humans: Ebola-Zaire, Ebola-Sudan, and Ebola-Ivory Coast. The fourth, Ebola-Reston, has caused disease in nonhuman primates, but not in humans.

Where is Ebola virus found in nature?

The exact origin, locations, and natural habitat (known as the "natural reservoir") of Ebola virus remain unknown. However, on the basis of available evidence and the nature of similar viruses, researchers believe that the virus is zoonotic (animal-borne) and is normally maintained in an animal host that is native to the African continent. A similar host is probably associated with Ebola-Reston which was isolated from infected cynomolgus monkeys that were imported to the United States and Italy from the Philippines. The virus is not known to be native to other continents, such as North America.

Where do cases of Ebola hemorrhagic fever occur?

Confirmed cases of Ebola HF have been reported in the Democratic Republic of the Congo, Gabon, Sudan, the Ivory Coast, Uganda, and the Republic of the Congo. An individual with serologic evidence of infection but showing no apparent illness has been reported in Liberia, and a laboratory worker in England became ill as a result of an accidental needle-stick. No case of the disease in humans has ever been reported in the United States. Ebola-Reston virus caused severe illness and death in monkeys imported to research facilities in the United States and Italy from the Philippines; during these outbreaks, several research workers became infected with the virus, but did not become ill.

Ebola HF typically appears in sporadic outbreaks, usually spread within a health-care setting (a situation known as amplification). It is likely that sporadic, isolated cases occur as well, but go unrecognized.

How is Ebola virus spread?

Infections with Ebola virus are acute. There is no carrier state. Because the natural reservoir of the virus is unknown, the manner in which the virus first appears in a human at the start of an outbreak has not been determined. However, researchers have hypothesized that the first patient becomes infected through contact with an infected animal.

After the first case-patient in an outbreak setting is infected, the virus can be transmitted in several ways. People can be exposed to Ebola virus from direct contact with the blood and/or secretions of an infected person. Thus, the virus is often spread through families and friends because they come in close contact with such secretions when caring for infected persons. People can also be exposed to Ebola virus through contact with objects, such as needles, that have been contaminated with infected secretions.

Nosocomial transmission refers to the spread of a disease within a health-care setting, such as a clinic or hospital. It occurs frequently during Ebola HF outbreaks. It includes both types of transmission described above. In African health-care facilities, patients are often cared for without the use of a mask, gown, or gloves. Exposure to the virus has occurred when health care workers treated individuals with Ebola HF without wearing these types of protective clothing. In addition, when needles or syringes are used, they may not be of the disposable type, or may not have been sterilized, but only rinsed before reinsertion into multi-use vials of medicine. If needles or syringes become contaminated with virus and are then reused, numerous people can become infected.

Ebola-Reston appeared in a primate research facility in Virginia, where it may have been transmitted from monkey to monkey through the air. While all Ebola virus species have displayed the ability to be spread through airborne particles (aerosols) under research conditions, this type of spread has not been documented among humans in a real-world setting, such as a hospital or household.

What are the symptoms of Ebola hemorrhagic fever?

The incubation period for Ebola HF ranges from 2 to 21 days. The onset of illness is abrupt and is characterized by fever, headache, joint and muscle aches, sore throat, and weakness, followed by diarrhea, vomiting, and stomach pain. A rash, red eyes, hiccups and internal and external bleeding may be seen in some patients.

Researchers do not understand why some people are able to recover from Ebola HF and others are not. However, it is known that patients who die usually have not developed a significant immune response to the virus at the time of death.

How is Ebola hemorrhagic fever treated?

There is no standard treatment for Ebola HF. Patients receive supportive therapy. This consists of balancing the patient's fluids and electrolytes, maintaining their oxygen status and blood pressure, and treating them for any complicating infections.

Lassa Fever

What is Lassa fever?

Lassa fever is an acute viral illness that occurs in West Africa. The illness was discovered in 1969 when two missionary nurses died in Nigeria, West Africa. The cause of the illness was found to be Lassa virus, named after the town in Nigeria where the first cases originated. The virus, a member of the virus family Arenaviridae, is a single-stranded RNA virus and is zoonotic, or animal-borne.

In areas of Africa where the disease is endemic (that is, constantly present), Lassa fever is a significant cause of morbidity and mortality. While Lassa fever is mild or has no observable symptoms in about 80% of people infected with the virus, the remaining 20% have a severe multisystem disease. Lassa fever is also associated with occasional epidemics, during which the case-fatality rate can reach 50%.

Where is Lassa fever found?

Lassa fever is an endemic disease in portions of West Africa. It is recognized in Guinea, Liberia, Sierra Leone, as well as Nigeria. However, because the rodent species which carry the virus are found throughout West Africa, the actual geographic range of the disease may extend to other countries in the region.

How many people become infected?

The number of Lassa virus infections per year in West Africa is estimated at 100,000 to 300,000, with approximately 5,000 deaths. Unfortunately, such estimates are crude, because surveillance for cases of the disease is not uniformly performed. In some areas of Sierra Leone and Liberia, it is known that 10%–16% of people admitted to hospitals have Lassa fever, which indicates the serious impact of the disease on the population of this region.

How do humans get Lassa fever?

There are a number of ways in which the virus may be transmitted, or spread, to humans. The Mastomys rodents shed the virus in urine and droppings. Therefore, the virus can be transmitted through direct contact with these materials, through touching objects or eating food contaminated with these materials, or through cuts or sores. Because Mastomys rodents often live in and around homes and scavenge on human food remains or poorly stored food, transmission of this sort is common. Contact with the virus also may occur when a person inhales tiny particles in the air contaminated with rodent excretions. This is called aerosol or airborne transmission. Finally, because Mastomys rodents are sometimes consumed as a food source, infection may occur via direct contact when they are caught and prepared for food.

Lassa fever may also spread through person-to-person contact. This type of transmission occurs when a person comes into contact with virus in the blood, tissue, secretions, or excretions of an individual infected with the Lassa virus. The virus cannot be spread through casual contact (including skin-to-skin contact without exchange of body fluids). Person-to-person transmission is common in both village and health care settings, where, along with the above-mentioned modes of transmission, the virus also may be spread in contaminated medical equipment, such as reused needles (this is called nosocomial transmission).

What are the symptoms of Lassa fever?

Signs and symptoms of Lassa fever typically occur 1–3 weeks after the patient comes into contact with the virus. These include fever, retrosternal pain (pain behind the chest wall), sore throat, back pain, cough, abdominal pain, vomiting, diarrhea, conjunctivitis, facial swelling, proteinuria (protein in the urine), and mucosal bleeding. Neurological problems have also been described, including hearing loss, tremors, and encephalitis. Because the symptoms of Lassa fever are so varied and nonspecific, clinical diagnosis is often difficult.

Are there complications after recovery?

The most common complication of Lassa fever is deafness. Various degrees of deafness occur in approximately one-third of cases, and in many cases hearing loss is permanent. As far as is known, severity of the disease does not affect this complication: deafness may develop in mild as well as in severe cases. Spontaneous abortion is another serious complication.

What proportion of people die from the illness?

Approximately 15%–20% of patients hospitalized for Lassa fever die from the illness. However, overall only about 1% of infections with Lassa virus result in death. The death rates are particularly high for women in the third trimester of pregnancy, and for fetuses, about 95% of which die in the uterus of infected pregnant mothers.

How is Lassa fever treated?

Ribavirin, an antiviral drug, has been used with success in Lassa fever patients. It has been shown to be most effective when given early in the course of the illness. Patients should also receive supportive care consisting of maintenance of appropriate fluid and electrolyte balance, oxygenation and blood pressure, as well as treatment of any other complicating infections.

Marburg Hemorrhagic Fever

What is Marburg hemorrhagic fever?

Marburg hemorrhagic fever is a rare, severe type of hemorrhagic fever which affects both humans and non-human primates. Caused by a genetically unique zoonotic (that is, animal-borne) RNA virus of the filovirus family, its recognition led to the creation of this virus family. The four species of Ebola virus are the only other known members of the filovirus family.

Where is Marburg virus found?

Recorded cases of the disease are rare, and have appeared in only a few locations. Marburg virus is indigenous to Africa. While the geographic area to which it is native is unknown, this area appears to include at least parts of Uganda and Western Kenya, and perhaps Zimbabwe. As with Ebola virus, the actual animal host for Marburg virus also remains a mystery. Both of the men infected in 1980 in western Kenya had traveled extensively, including making a visit to a cave, in that region. The cave was investigated by placing sentinels animals inside to see if they would become infected, and by taking samples from numerous animals and arthropods trapped during the investigation. The investigation yielded no virus: The sentinel animals remained healthy and no virus isolations from the samples obtained have been reported.

How do humans get Marburg hemorrhagic fever?

Just how the animal host first transmits Marburg virus to humans is unknown. However, as with some other viruses which cause viral hemorrhagic fever, humans who become ill with Marburg hemorrhagic fever may spread the virus to other people. This may happen in several ways. Persons who have handled infected monkeys and have come in direct contact with their fluids or cell cultures, have become infected. Spread of the virus between humans has occurred in a setting of close contact, often in a hospital. Droplets of body fluids, or direct contact with persons, equipment, or other objects contaminated with infectious blood or tissues are all highly suspect as sources of disease.

What are the symptoms of the disease?

After an incubation period of 5–10 days, the onset of the disease is sudden and is marked by fever, chills, headache, and myalgia.

341

Around the fifth day after the onset of symptoms, a maculopapular rash, most prominent on the trunk (chest, back, stomach), may occur. Nausea, vomiting, chest pain, a sore throat, abdominal pain, and diarrhea then may appear. Symptoms become increasingly severe and may include jaundice, inflammation of the pancreas, severe weight loss, delirium, shock, liver failure, massive hemorrhaging, and multiorgan dysfunction.

Because many of the signs and symptoms of Marburg hemorrhagic fever are similar to those of other infectious diseases, such as malaria or typhoid fever, diagnosis of the disease can be difficult, especially if only a single case is involved.

Antigen-capture enzyme-linked immunosorbent assay (ELISA) testing, IgM-capture ELISA, polymerase chain reaction (PCR), and virus isolation can be used to confirm a case of Marburg hemorrhagic fever within a few days of the onset of symptoms. The IgG-capture ELISA is appropriate for testing persons later in the course of disease or after recovery. The disease is readily diagnosed by immunohistochemistry, virus isolation, or PCR of blood or tissue specimens from deceased patients.

Are there complications after recovery?

Recovery from Marburg hemorrhagic fever may be prolonged and accompanied by orchitis, recurrent hepatitis, transverse myelitis or uveitis. Other possible complications include inflammation of the testis, spinal cord, eye, parotid gland, or by prolonged hepatitis.

Is the disease ever fatal?

Yes. The case-fatality rate for Marburg hemorrhagic fever is between 23–25%.

How is Marburg hemorrhagic fever treated?

A specific treatment for this disease is unknown. However, supportive hospital therapy should be utilized. This includes balancing the patient's fluids and electrolytes, maintaining their oxygen status and blood pressure, replacing lost blood and clotting factors and treating them for any complicating infections.

Sometimes treatment also has used transfusion of fresh-frozen plasma and other preparations to replace the blood proteins important in clotting. One controversial treatment is the use of heparin (which blocks clotting) to prevent the consumption of clotting factors. Some researchers believe the consumption of clotting factors is part of the disease process.

Rift Valley Fever

What is Rift Valley fever?

Rift Valley fever (RVF) is an acute, fever-causing viral disease that affects domestic animals (such as cattle, buffalo, sheep, goats, and camels) and humans. RVF is most commonly associated with mosquito-borne epidemics during years of unusually heavy rainfall.

The disease is caused by the RVF virus, a member of the genus *Phlebovirus* in the family Bunyaviridae. The disease was first reported among livestock by veterinary officers in Kenya in the early 1900s.

Where is the disease found?

RVF is generally found in regions of eastern and southern Africa where sheep and cattle are raised, but the virus also exists in most countries of sub-Saharan Africa and in Madagascar. In September 2000, a RVF outbreak was reported in Saudi Arabia and subsequently Yemen. These cases represent the first Rift Valley fever cases identified outside Africa.

How do humans get RVF?

Humans can get RVF as a result of bites from mosquitoes and possibly other bloodsucking insects that serve as vectors. Humans can also get the disease if they are exposed to either the blood or other body fluids of infected animals. This exposure can result from the slaughtering or handling of infected animals or by touching contaminated meat during the preparation of food. Infection through aerosol transmission of RVF virus has resulted from contact with laboratory specimens containing the virus.

What are the symptoms of RVF?

RVF virus can cause several different disease syndromes. People with RVF typically have either no symptoms or a mild illness associated with fever and liver abnormalities. However, in some patients the illness can progress to hemorrhagic fever (which can lead to shock or hemorrhage), encephalitis (inflammation of the brain, which can lead to headaches, coma, or seizures), or ocular disease (diseases affecting the eye). Patients who become ill usually experience fever, generalized weakness, back pain, dizziness, and extreme weight loss at the onset of the illness. Typically, patients recover within two days to one week after onset of illness.

Are there complications after recovery?

The most common complication associated with RVF is inflammation of the retina (a structure connecting the nerves of the eye to the brain). As a result, approximately 1%–10% of affected patients may have some permanent vision loss.

Is the disease ever fatal?

Approximately 1% of humans that become infected with RVF die of the disease. Case-fatality proportions are significantly higher for infected animals. The most severe impact is observed in pregnant livestock infected with RVF, which results in abortion of virtually 100% of fetuses.

How is RVF treated?

There is no established course of treatment for patients infected with RVF virus. However, studies in monkeys and other animals have shown promise for ribavirin, an antiviral drug, for future use in humans. Additional studies suggest that interferon, immune modulators, and convalescent-phase plasma may also help in the treatment of patients with RVF.

Chapter 44

West Nile Virus

Overview

West Nile virus belongs to a group of disease-causing viruses known as flaviviruses, which are spread by insects, usually mosquitoes. Other flaviviruses include yellow fever virus, Japanese encephalitis virus, dengue virus, and Saint Louis encephalitis virus. West Nile virus is the most familiar flavivirus and represents an emerging infectious disease in the United States.

Most human infections are mild, causing fever, headache, and body aches, often accompanied by a skin rash and swollen lymph glands. If the virus crosses the blood-brain barrier, however, it can cause life-threatening encephalitis (inflammation of the brain) or meningitis (inflammation of the lining of the brain and spinal cord). Recent cases have indicated that West Nile virus can be transmitted by transfusion or transplantation. In addition, it appears that West Nile virus can also be transmitted from mother to child before birth and through breast milk.

The first step in the transmission cycle of West Nile virus occurs when a mosquito bites an infected bird. Although the virus primarily cycles between mosquitoes and birds, infected female mosquitoes can transmit West Nile virus to humans and other incidental "hosts" when they bite and take a blood meal. Crows are commonly associated with the virus because they are highly susceptible to infection. Scientists have identified at least 75 other infected bird species as well.

"NIAID Research on West Nile Virus," National Institute of Allergy and Infectious Diseases (NIAID), National Institutes of health (NIH), June 2003.

345

West Nile virus was first isolated in Uganda in 1937. Today it is most commonly found in Africa, West Asia, Europe, and the Middle East. In 1999, it emerged in the Western Hemisphere for the first time in the New York City area. Although health officials hoped the virus would not survive the first winter, in early spring 2000 it re-emerged in birds and mosquitoes and spread to other parts of the eastern United States.

Between 1999 and 2001, West Nile virus caused 18 deaths and sickened 131 other people. By the summer of 2002, the virus had quickly spread west and south. For 2002, state health departments reported 4,156 cases of West Nile virus in people, resulting in 284 deaths. (See www.cdc.gov/od/oc/media/wncount.htm for the Centers for Disease Control and Prevention [CDC] Web page about the current number of reported human cases of West Nile virus infections in the United States.) Researchers continue to monitor and test birds and mosquitoes throughout the United States for evidence of the virus (see www.nationalatlas.gov/virusmap.html for the latest information).

There are no drugs to treat the virus and no vaccines available to prevent infection. Because West Nile virus is now established in the United States, scientists and health experts at the National Institute of Allergy and Infectious Diseases (NIAID), along with public health officials, have enhanced research. This effort is part of NIAID's comprehensive emerging infectious disease program, which supports research on bacterial, viral, and other types of disease-causing microbes.

NIAID Research

Research is underway to develop a vaccine, antiviral medicines, and new diagnostic tests for West Nile virus. Additionally, basic research is providing new clues about the virus itself, the disease in humans and animals, and how the virus is maintained in the environment. This knowledge is essential to develop strategies to prevent, treat, and eventually control this disease.

These areas of research include the following.

Basic Research on the Virus, on the Disease in Humans, and on Its Maintenance in Nature

NIAID supports basic research to better understand factors associated with the animal or human hosts, the microbe, and the environment that influence disease emergence. For example, basic research is helping scientists determine which flavivirus proteins contribute to the virus' ability to cause disease. Researchers are investigating how protective immune responses are elicited within the central nervous system during acute flavivirus encephalitis.

Factors influencing the pattern of emergence and distribution of West Nile include those associated with the virus itself, the agent's hosts and vectors, and the environment in which agent and host interact. The specific factors contributing to emergence of West Nile, however, are poorly understood. Nonetheless, knowledge of these principles is essential in planning strategies to prevent, treat, and control this disease. The overall objective of this basic research is to develop the knowledge and public health tools needed for the United States to combat West Nile virus.

NIAID also supports researchers investigating how West Nile virus disseminates throughout the environment. An International Centers for Infectious Disease Research program is supporting research in Mexico to study whether migrating bird populations carry the virus from its presumed point of entrance into the Western Hemisphere (New York City) to points in Central and South America. The emergence of West Nile virus in these new areas, which harbor abundant mosquito populations, could set up conditions for a potentially severe epidemic. Researchers are examining wild birds and chickens in the Yucatan Peninsula for evidence of exposure to West Nile virus.

Researchers are also examining the ecology and persistence of mosquito-borne encephalitis viruses and the effect of genetic variation on the virus' spread and virulence. They are looking at how birds might be year-round reservoirs for the viruses that cause encephalomyelitis and St. Louis encephalitis. They are also comparing the genetics of St. Louis encephalitis viruses from throughout California and different parts of the United States to determine the rate at which the virus is changing, and whether birds carry it between discrete geographic areas.

NIAID also supports research to better understand the insects and ticks that transmit flaviviruses. Such an understanding will allow improved monitoring and surveillance, and enable developing and preliminary testing strategies to control carriers of the virus.

Lastly, NIAID-supported basic research is important for maintaining the national and international scientific expertise required to respond to future health threats.

Research to Prevent and Control Spread of the Disease

For several years, NIAID has supported research to develop a vaccine against West Nile. In 1999, NIAID funded a fast-track project to develop a candidate West Nile virus vaccine with Acambis, a biotechnology company with vaccine development laboratories in Boston.

Since then, scientists have developed a prototype vaccine that has shown promise in animal tests. Scientists construct the vaccine by using vaccine licensed for preventing yellow fever (caused by another flavivirus) as the backbone.

For the West Nile vaccine, researchers substituted the surface protein of West Nile virus for the deleted yellow fever virus protein. They are also applying this method of creating so-called chimeric flavivirus vaccines to make vaccines for dengue and for Japanese encephalitis virus. The Acambis vaccine has undergone preclinical evaluations in hamsters, mice, monkeys, and horses with encouraging results. The company is moving forward toward Phase I human trials and is expected to soon file an investigational new drug (IND) application with the U.S. Food and Drug Administration. Trials are anticipated to begin in 2003.

NIAID intramural scientists, who pioneered the concept of creating chimeric flavivirus vaccines in 1992, also have developed a West Nile vaccine candidate which they have tested in monkeys with promising results. This experimental vaccine, using a dengue virus as a backbone to carry West Nile virus genes, will be tested in Phase I human trials beginning in late 2003.

The NIAID Vaccine Research Center (VRC) has started to develop a candidate vaccine for West Nile virus. The VRC's proposed candidates are DNA constructs that express West Nile virus proteins. Vectors have been constructed using West Nile virus genes modified to increase protein expression. Preclinical studies are now underway. Further preclinical evaluation and viral challenge studies will be performed in the near future. The VRC plans to produce clinical grade plasmid DNA for future Phase I trials in hopes of identifying a protective vaccine against the virus.

Last year, NIAID-supported researchers developed a hamster model of West Nile virus, which closely mimics human disease. This animal model has proved useful in evaluating strategies for preventing the complications associated with this emerging infectious disease. Using this animal model, researchers were able to determine that prior infection with other related viruses provides complete or partial immunity to West Nile virus.

Research to Treat the Disease

Drugs may be effective against West Nile virus because the infection is typically not chronic and antiviral drugs have been identified to be effective in the laboratory against other flaviviruses. NIH has funded investigators to establish a system to screen chemical compounds for possible antiviral activity against West Nile virus. Any promising antiviral drug candidates will be tested in the hamster model. This resource allows scientists to evaluate a drug's safety and efficacy before moving on to possible human trials. Other research projects are investigating emerging diseases and developing candidate drugs to fight West Nile virus. More than 550 drugs have been screened, and about 3 percent have shown promise for additional testing in animals. Immunotherapeutics (treatments that supply protective antibodies donated from other patients that have recovered from West Nile) are also being explored.

Research to Improve Rapid Diagnosis

Research is also underway to allow for more rapid detection of West Nile in samples from humans, other animals, or mosquitoes. This research occurs mainly at small biotechnology companies attempting to develop new, commercially available diagnostic tests.

Research Resources

NIAID maintains the World Reference Center for Arboviruses at the University of Texas Medical Branch at Galveston. The Center has reference anti-West Nile virus sera and seed lots of various strains of the virus. This international program involves characterizing viruses transmitted to people and domestic animals by mosquitoes and other arthropods and researching the epidemiology of arboviruses of the United States and overseas. During the last 3 years, these reagents were provided on request to investigators in the United States and Canada.

NIAID has recently expanded its West Nile and related viruses research portfolio. This includes establishing two Emerging Viral Diseases Research Centers in New York and Texas, with collaborating laboratories in Colorado, Massachusetts, and elsewhere. These centers include a focus on West Nile and related viruses. NIAID has also funded a project entitled "Development of Novel Antiviral Agents Against West Nile Virus" under the Partnerships for Development of Novel Therapeutic and Vector-Control Strategies. In addition, many of the programs that have been recently developed and expanded for biodefense are available for other emerging infectious diseases, including West Nile.

Chapter 45

Yellow Fever

Yellow fever is a viral disease that has caused large epidemics in Africa and the Americas. It can be recognized from historic texts stretching back 400 years. Infection causes a wide spectrum of disease, from mild symptoms to severe illness and death. The "yellow" in the name is explained by the jaundice that affects some patients. Although an effective vaccine has been available for 60 years, the number of people infected over the last two decades has increased and yellow fever is now a serious public health issue again.

Cause

The disease is caused by the yellow fever virus, which belongs to the flavivirus group. In Africa there are two distinct genetic types (called topotypes) associated with East and West Africa. South America has two different types, but since 1974 only one has been identified as the cause of disease outbreaks.

Symptoms

The virus remains silent in the body during an incubation period of three to six days. There are then two disease phases. While some infections have no symptoms whatsoever, the first, "acute", phase is

---

"Yellow Fever," Fact Sheet No. 100, revised December 2001, © 2002 World Health Organization (WHO).

normally characterized by fever, muscle pain (with prominent back-ache), headache, shivers, loss of appetite, nausea and/or vomiting. Often, the high fever is paradoxically associated with a slow pulse. After three to four days most patients improve and their symptoms disappear.

However, 15% enter a "toxic phase" within 24 hours. Fever reappears and several body systems are affected. The patient rapidly develops jaundice and complains of abdominal pain with vomiting. Bleeding can occur from the mouth, nose, eyes and/or stomach. Once this happens, blood appears in the vomit and feces. Kidney function deteriorates; this can range from abnormal protein levels in the urine (albuminuria) to complete kidney failure with no urine production (anuria). Half of the patients in the "toxic phase" die within 10–14 days. The remainder recover without significant organ damage.

Yellow fever is difficult to recognize, especially during the early stages. It can easily be confused with malaria, typhoid, rickettsial diseases, hemorrhagic viral fevers (e.g., Lassa), arboviral infections (e.g., dengue), leptospirosis, viral hepatitis and poisoning (e.g., carbon tetrachloride). A laboratory analysis is required to confirm a suspect case. Blood tests (serology assays) can detect yellow fever antibodies that are produced in response to the infection. Several other techniques are used to identify the virus itself in blood specimens or liver tissue collected after death. These tests require highly trained laboratory staff using specialized equipment and materials.

Regions Affected

The virus is constantly present with low levels of infection (i.e., endemic) in some tropical areas of Africa and the Americas. This viral presence can amplify into regular epidemics. Until the start of this century, yellow fever outbreaks also occurred in Europe, the Caribbean islands and Central and North America. Even though the virus is not felt to be present in these areas now, they must still be considered at risk for yellow fever epidemics.

Thirty-three countries, with a combined population of 508 million, are at risk in Africa. These lie within a band from 15°N to 10°S of the equator. In the Americas, yellow fever is endemic in nine South American countries and in several Caribbean islands. Bolivia, Brazil, Colombia, Ecuador and Peru are considered at greatest risk.

There are 200,000 estimated cases of yellow fever (with 30,000 deaths) per year. However, due to underreporting, only a small percentage of these cases are identified. Small numbers of imported cases also occur in countries free of yellow fever. Although yellow fever has never been reported from Asia, this region is at risk because the appropriate primates and mosquitoes are present.

Transmission

Humans and monkeys are the principal animals to be infected. The virus is carried from one animal to another (horizontal transmission) by a biting mosquito (the vector). The mosquito can also pass the virus via infected eggs to its offspring (vertical transmission). The eggs produced are resistant to drying and lie dormant through dry conditions, hatching when the rainy season begins. Therefore, the mosquito is the true reservoir of the virus, ensuring transmission from one year to the next.

Several different species of the *Aedes* and *Haemagogus* (S. America only) mosquitoes transmit the yellow fever virus. These mosquitoes are either domestic (i.e. they breed around houses), wild (they breed in the jungle) or semi-domestic types (they display a mixture of habits). Any region populated with these mosquitoes can potentially harbor the disease. Control programs successfully eradicated mosquito habitats in the past, especially in South America. However, these programs have lapsed over the last 30 years and mosquito populations have increased. This favors epidemics of yellow fever.

Infection of Humans

There are three types of transmission cycle for yellow fever: sylvatic, intermediate and urban. All three cycles exist in Africa, but in South America, only sylvatic and urban yellow fever occur.

- Sylvatic (or jungle) yellow fever: In tropical rainforests, yellow fever occurs in monkeys that are infected by wild mosquitoes. The infected monkeys can then pass the virus onto other mosquitoes that feed on them. These infected wild mosquitoes bite humans entering the forest resulting in sporadic cases of yellow fever. The majority of cases are young men working in the forest (logging, etc.). On occasion, the virus spreads beyond the affected individual.

- Intermediate yellow fever: In humid or semi-humid savannahs of Africa, small-scale epidemics occur. These behave differently from urban epidemics; many separate villages in an area suffer cases simultaneously, but fewer people die from infection. Semi-domestic mosquitoes infect both monkey and human hosts. This area is often called the "zone of emergence", where increased contact between man and infected mosquito leads to disease. This is the most common type of outbreak seen in recent decades in Africa. It can shift to a more severe urban-type epidemic if the infection is carried into a suitable environment (with the presence of domestic mosquitoes and unvaccinated humans).

- Urban yellow fever: Large epidemics can occur when migrants introduce the virus into areas with high human population density. Domestic mosquitoes (of one species, *Aedes aegypti*) carry the virus from person to person; no monkeys are involved in transmission. These outbreaks tend to spread outwards from one source to cover a wide area.

Treatment

There is no specific treatment for yellow fever. Dehydration and fever can be corrected with oral rehydration salts and paracetamol. Any superimposed bacterial infection should be treated with an appropriate antibiotic. Intensive supportive care may improve the outcome for seriously ill patients, but is rarely available in poorer, developing countries.

Prevention

Vaccination is the single most important measure for preventing yellow fever. In populations where vaccination coverage is low, vigilant surveillance is critical for prompt recognition and rapid control of outbreaks. Mosquito control measures can be used to prevent virus transmission until vaccination has taken effect.

Vaccination

Yellow fever vaccine is safe and highly effective. The protective effect (immunity) occurs within one week in 95% of people vaccinated. A single dose of vaccine provides protection for 10 years and probably for life. Over 300 million doses have been given and serious side effects are extremely rare. However, recently a few serious adverse outcomes, including deaths, have been reported in Brazil, Australia and the United States. Scientists are investigating the cause of these adverse events, and monitoring to ensure detection of any similar incidents.

The risk to life from yellow fever is far greater than the risk from the vaccine, so those who may be exposed to yellow fever should be protected by immunization. If there is no risk of exposure, for example, if a person will not be visiting an endemic area, there is no necessity to receive the vaccine. Since most of the other known side effects have occurred in children less than six months old, vaccine is not administered to this age group. The vaccine should only be given to pregnant women during vaccination campaigns in the midst of an epidemic.

Vaccination can be part of a routine preventive immunization program or can be done in mass "catch-up" campaigns to increase vaccination coverage in areas where it is low. The World Health Organization (WHO) strongly recommends routine childhood vaccination. The vaccine can be administered at age nine months, at the same time as the measles vaccine. Eighteen African nations have agreed to incorporate yellow fever vaccine into their routine national vaccination programs. This is more cost effective and prevents more cases (and deaths) than when emergency vaccination campaigns are performed to control an epidemic.

Past experience shows the success of this strategy. Between 1939 and 1952 yellow fever cases almost vanished from French West Africa after intensive vaccination campaigns. Similarly, Gambia instituted mass routine vaccination after its 1979/1980 epidemic and later incorporated yellow fever vaccine into its childhood immunization program. Gambia reported 85% vaccine coverage in 2000. No cases have been reported since 1980, yet the virus remains present in the environment.

To prevent an epidemic in a country, at least 80% of the population must have immunity to yellow fever. This can only be achieved through the effective incorporation of yellow fever into childhood immunization programs and the implementation of mass catch-up campaigns. The latter is the only way to ensure that coverage of all susceptible age groups is achieved and will prevent outbreaks from spreading. Very few countries in Africa have achieved this level to date.

Vaccination is highly recommended for travelers to high-risk areas. A vaccination certificate is required for entry to many countries, particularly for travelers arriving in Asia from Africa or South America. Fatal cases in unvaccinated tourists have been reported.

Surveillance

Because vaccination coverage in many areas is not optimal, prompt detection of yellow fever cases and rapid response (emergency vaccination campaigns) are essential for controlling disease outbreaks. Improvement in yellow fever surveillance is needed as evidenced by the gross underreporting of cases (estimates as to the true number of cases vary widely and have put the underreporting factor between three- and 250-fold). A surveillance system must be sensitive enough to detect and appropriately investigate suspect cases. This is facilitated by a standardized definition of possible yellow fever cases, that is "acute fever followed by jaundice within two weeks of onset of symptoms, or with bleeding symptoms or with death within three weeks of onset." Suspect cases are reported to health authorities on a standardized case investigation form.

Ready access to laboratory testing is essential for confirming cases of yellow fever, as many other diseases have similar symptoms. WHO has recently recommended that every at-risk country have at least one national laboratory where basic yellow fever blood tests can be performed. Training programs are being conducted and test materials are provided by WHO.

Given the likelihood that other cases have occurred (but have not been detected), one confirmed case of yellow fever is considered to be an outbreak. An investigation team should subsequently explore and define the outbreak. This produces data for analysis, which guides the epidemic control committee in preparing the appropriate outbreak response (e.g., emergency vaccination programs, mosquito control activities). This committee should also plan for the long term by implementing or strengthening routine childhood yellow fever vaccination.

Mosquito Control

In general, eliminating potential mosquito breeding sites is an important and effective means for controlling mosquito-transmitted diseases. For prevention and control of yellow fever, priority is placed on vaccination programs. For example, mosquito control programs against wild mosquitoes in forested areas are not practical or cost-effective for preventing sylvatic infections. Spraying to kill adult mosquitoes during epidemics may have value by interrupting virus transmission. This "buys time" for immunity to develop after an emergency vaccination campaign.

In Summary

Over the last 20 years the number of yellow fever epidemics has risen and more countries are reporting cases. Mosquito numbers and habitats are increasing. In both Africa and the Americas, there is a large susceptible, unvaccinated population. Changes in the world's environment, such as deforestation and urbanization, have increased contact with the mosquito/virus. Widespread international travel could play a role in spreading the disease. The priorities are vaccination of exposed populations, improved surveillance and epidemic preparedness.

In March 1998, WHO held a technical consensus meeting in Geneva to identify obstacles to yellow fever prevention and control. Priorities identified included: prevention through routine immunization and preventive mass immunization campaigns; detection, reporting and investigation of suspect cases; laboratory support; outbreak response; vaccine supply; and furthering research. Guidelines for investigation and control of yellow fever outbreaks, and a background document reviewing topics of importance discussed at this meeting have been published, and are available on the WHO web site at: http://www.who .int/emc-documents/yellow_fever/whoepigen9809c.html

Part Four

Environmental Contamination and Microbe Overgrowth

Chapter 46

Acanthamoeba *Infection*

What is an Acanthamoeba *infection?*

Acanthamoeba are microscopic ameba commonly found in the environment. Several species of *Acanthamoeba* have been found to infect humans, *A. culbertsoni, A. polyphaga, A. castellanii, A. healyi, (A. astronyxis), A. hatchetti, A. rhysodes*, and possibly others.

Where are Acanthamoeba *found?*

Acanthamoeba spp. (spp. means several species) are found worldwide. Most commonly, *Acanthamoeba* are found in the soil and dust, in fresh water sources such as lakes, rivers, and hot springs and in hot tubs. *Acanthamoeba* may also be found in brackish water and in sea water. Amebas can also be found in Heating, Venting, and Air Conditioner units (HVAC), humidifiers, dialysis units, and contact lens paraphernalia.

Acanthamoeba have been found in the nose and throat of healthy people as well as those with compromised immune systems.

How does infection with Acanthamoeba *occur?*

Acanthamoeba can enter the skin through a cut, wound, or through the nostrils. Once inside the body, amebas can travel to the lungs and through the bloodstream to other parts of the body, especially the central nervous system (brain and spinal cord).

"*Acanthamoeba* Infection," Division of Parasitic Diseases, Centers for Disease Control and Prevention (CDC), reviewed March 2001.

Through improper storage, handling, and disinfection of contact lenses, *Acanthamoeba* can enter the eye and cause a serious infection.

What are the signs and symptoms of Acanthamoeba infection?

There are several ways *Acanthamoeba* spp. can affect the body.

Each year, many people are infected with *Acanthamoeba*. Eye infections result from contact lens cases becoming contaminated after improper cleaning and handling. Risk of *Acanthamoeba* infection is higher for people who make their own contact lens cleaning solution. *Acanthamoeba* enter the eye via contact lenses or through a corneal cut or sore. Infection or a corneal ulcer results.

In addition, *Acanthamoeba* spp. can cause skin lesions and/or a systemic (whole body) infection. *Acanthamoeba* spp. cause a serious, most often deadly infection called granulomatous amebic encephalitis (GAE). Once infected, a person may suffer with headaches, stiff neck, nausea and vomiting, tiredness, confusion, lack of attention to people and surroundings, loss of balance and bodily control, seizures, and hallucinations. Signs and symptoms progresses over several weeks; death generally occurs.

Who is at risk for infection with Acanthamoeba?

Infections caused by *Acanthamoeba* spp. occur more frequently in people with compromised immune systems or those who are chronically ill.

Is there treatment for infection with Acanthamoeba?

Yes. Eye and skin infections are generally treatable. Although most cases of brain (CNS) infection with *Acanthamoeba* have been fatal, a few however, have recovered from the infection with proper treatment. *Acanthamoeba* infections of the brain (CNS) are almost always fatal.

Can infection be spread from person to person?

No cases have ever been reported.

How can I prevent an infection with Acanthamoeba?

Eye infections may be prevented by using commercially prepared contact lens cleaning solution rather than making and using home-made solutions. There is little that can be done to prevent skin and body infection.

For More Information

1. Centers for Disease Control. *Acanthamoeba* keratitis associated with contact lenses—United States. *MMWR* 1986:35: 405–8.

2. Centers for Disease Control. *Acanthamoeba* keratitis associated with soft contact lens wearers—United States. *MMWR* 1987; 36:397–8, 403–4.

3. Ma P, Visvesvara GS, Martinez AJ, Theodore FH, Daggett PM, Sawyer TK. Naegleria and *Acanthamoeba* infections: Review. *Rev Infect Dis* 1990; 12:490–513.

4. Visvesvara GS, Stehr-Green JK. Epidemiology of free-living ameba infections. *J Protozool* 1990; 37:25S–33S.

5. Martinez AJ, Visvesvara GS. Free-living, amphizoic and opportunistic amebas. *Brain Pathol* 1997; 7:583–598.

Chapter 47

Anthrax

What is anthrax?

Anthrax is an acute infectious disease caused by the spore-forming bacterium *Bacillus anthracis*. Anthrax most commonly occurs in wild and domestic lower vertebrates (cattle, sheep, goats, camels, antelopes, and other herbivores), but it can also occur in humans when they are exposed to infected animals or tissue from infected animals.

How common is anthrax and who can get it?

Anthrax is most common in agricultural regions where it occurs in animals. These include South and Central America, Southern and Eastern Europe, Asia, Africa, the Caribbean, and the Middle East. When anthrax affects humans, it is usually due to an occupational exposure to infected animals or their products. Workers who are exposed to dead animals and animal products from other countries where anthrax is more common may become infected with *B. anthracis* (industrial anthrax). Anthrax in wild livestock has occurred in the United States.

How is anthrax transmitted?

Anthrax infection can occur in three forms: cutaneous (skin), inhalation, and gastrointestinal. *B. anthracis* spores can live in the soil for many years, and humans can become infected with anthrax by

"Anthrax," Division of Bacterial and Mycotic Diseases, Centers for Disease Control and Prevention (CDC), reviewed May 2, 2003.

handling products from infected animals or by inhaling anthrax spores from contaminated animal products. Anthrax can also be spread by eating undercooked meat from infected animals. It is rare to find infected animals in the United States.

What are the symptoms of anthrax?

Symptoms of disease vary depending on how the disease was contracted, but symptoms usually occur within 7 days.

Cutaneous: Most (about 95%) anthrax infections occur when the bacterium enters a cut or abrasion on the skin, such as when handling contaminated wool, hides, leather, or hair products (especially goat hair) of infected animals. Skin infection begins as a raised itchy bump that resembles an insect bite but within 1–2 days develops into a vesicle and then a painless ulcer, usually 1–3 cm in diameter, with a characteristic black necrotic (dying) area in the center. Lymph glands in the adjacent area may swell. About 20% of untreated cases of cutaneous anthrax will result in death. Deaths are rare with appropriate antimicrobial therapy.

Inhalation: Initial symptoms may resemble a common cold. After several days, the symptoms may progress to severe breathing problems and shock. Inhalation anthrax is usually fatal.

Intestinal: The intestinal disease form of anthrax may follow the consumption of contaminated meat and is characterized by an acute inflammation of the intestinal tract. Initial signs of nausea, loss of appetite, vomiting, and fever are followed by abdominal pain, vomiting of blood, and severe diarrhea. Intestinal anthrax results in death in 25% to 60% of cases.

Where is anthrax usually found?

Anthrax can be found globally. It is more common in developing countries or countries without veterinary public health programs. Certain regions of the world (South and Central America, Southern and Eastern Europe, Asia, Africa, the Caribbean, and the Middle East) report more anthrax in animals than others.

Can anthrax be spread from person-to-person?

Direct person-to-person spread of anthrax is extremely unlikely to occur. Communicability is not a concern in managing or visiting with patients with inhalational anthrax.

Is there a way to prevent infection?

In countries where anthrax is common and vaccination levels of animal herds are low, humans should avoid contact with livestock and animal products and avoid eating meat that has not been properly slaughtered and cooked. Also, an anthrax vaccine has been licensed for use in humans. The vaccine is reported to be 93% effective in protecting against anthrax.

What is the anthrax vaccine?

The anthrax vaccine is manufactured and distributed by BioPort Corporation, Lansing, Michigan. The vaccine is a cell-free filtrate vaccine, which means it contains no dead or live bacteria in the preparation. The final product contains no more than 2.4 mg of aluminum hydroxide as adjuvant. Anthrax vaccines intended for animals should not be used in humans.

Who should get vaccinated against anthrax?

The Advisory Committee on Immunization Practices has recommended anthrax vaccination for the following groups:

- Persons who work directly with the organism in the laboratory

- Persons who work with imported animal hides or furs in areas where standards are insufficient to prevent exposure to anthrax spores.

- Persons who handle potentially infected animal products in high-incidence areas. (Incidence is low in the United States, but veterinarians who travel to work in other countries where incidence is higher should consider being vaccinated.)

- Military personnel deployed to areas with high risk for exposure to the organism (as when it is used as a biological warfare weapon).

The anthrax Vaccine Immunization Program in the U.S. Army Surgeon General's Office can be reached at 1-877-GETVACC (1-877-438-8222). http://www.anthrax.osd.mil

Pregnant women should be vaccinated only if absolutely necessary.

What is the protocol for anthrax vaccination?

The immunization consists of three subcutaneous injections given 2 weeks apart followed by three additional subcutaneous injections given at 6, 12, and 18 months. Annual booster injections of the vaccine are recommended thereafter.

Are there adverse reactions to the anthrax vaccine?

Mild local reactions occur in 30% of recipients and consist of slight tenderness and redness at the injection site. Severe local reactions are infrequent and consist of extensive swelling of the forearm in addition to the local reaction. Systemic reactions occur in fewer than 0.2% of recipients.

How is anthrax diagnosed?

Anthrax is diagnosed by isolating *B. anthracis* from the blood, skin lesions, or respiratory secretions or by measuring specific antibodies in the blood of persons with suspected cases.

Is there a treatment for anthrax?

Doctors can prescribe effective antibiotics. To be effective, treatment should be initiated early. If left untreated, the disease can be fatal.

Where can I get more information about the recent Department of Defense decision to require men and women in the Armed Services to be vaccinated against anthrax?

The Department of Defense recommends that servicemen and women contact their chain of command on questions about the vaccine and its distribution. The anthrax Vaccine Immunization Program in the U.S. Army Surgeon General's Office can be reached at 1-877-GETVACC (1-877-438-8222). http://www.anthrax.osd.mil

Chapter 48

Ascaris *Infection*

What is an Ascaris *infection?*

An ascarid is a worm that lives in the small intestine. Infection with ascarids is called ascariasis (ass-kuh-rye-uh-sis). Adult female worms can grow over 12 inches in length, adult males are smaller.

How common is ascariasis?

Ascariasis is the most common human worm infection. Infection occurs worldwide and is most common in tropical and subtropical areas where sanitation and hygiene are poor. Children are infected more often than adults. In the United States, infection is rare, but most common in rural areas of the southeast.

What are the signs and symptoms of an Ascaris *infection?*

Most people have no symptoms. A person may be infected with only a few worms—or dozens. Symptoms usually occur in people who have large numbers of worms. If you are heavily infected, you may have abdominal pain. Sometimes, while the immature worms migrate through the lungs, you may cough and have difficulty breathing. If you have a very heavy worm infection, your intestines may become blocked.

"*Ascaris* Infection," Division of Parasitic Diseases, Centers for Disease Control and Prevention (CDC), reviewed August 15, 1999. Reviewed and revised by David A. Cooke, M.D., on January 26, 2004.

How is an Ascaris *infection spread?*

Ascarid eggs are found in the soil. Infection occurs when a person accidentally ingests (swallows) infective ascarid eggs. Once in the stomach, larvae (immature worms) hatch from the eggs. The larvae are carried through the lungs then to the throat where they are then swallowed. Once swallowed, they reach the intestines and develop into adult worms. Adult female worms lay eggs that are then passed in feces; this cycle will take between 2–3 months.

Pigs can be infected with ascarids. Occasionally, a pig ascarid infection can be spread to humans; this occurs when infective eggs, found in the soil and manure, are ingested. Infection is more likely if pig feces is used as fertilizer in the garden; crops then become contaminated with ascarid eggs.

How can I get ascariasis?

You or your children can become infected after touching your mouth with your hands contaminated with eggs from soil or other contaminated surfaces.

What should I do if I think I have ascariasis?

See your health care provider.

How is diagnosis of Ascaris *made?*

Your health care provider will ask you to provide stool samples for testing. Some people notice infection when a worm is passed in stool or is coughed up. These worms may resemble earthworms. If this happens, bring in the worm specimen to your health care provider for diagnosis. There is no blood test used to diagnose an ascarid infection. Worms are sometimes visible on x-rays or CAT scans of the abdomen.

What is the treatment for ascariasis?

In the United States, *Ascaris* infections are generally treated for 1–3 days with medication prescribed by your health care provider. The drugs are effective and appear to have few side-effects. Your health care provider will likely request additional stool exams 1 to 2 weeks after therapy; if the infection is still present, treatment will be repeated.

I am pregnant and have just been diagnosed with ascariasis. Can I be treated?

Infection with ascarid worms is generally light and is not considered an emergency. Unless your infection is heavy, and your health may be at risk, treatment is generally postponed until after delivery of the baby.

How can I prevent infection with ascarids?

- Avoid contacting soil that may be contaminated with human feces.

- Do not defecate outdoors.

- Dispose of diapers properly.

- Wash hands with soap and water before handling food.

- When traveling to countries where sanitation and hygiene are poor, avoid water or food that may be contaminated.

- Wash, peel or cook all raw vegetables and fruits before eating.

Should I be concerned about spreading infection to the rest of my household?

No. Infection is not spread from person to person.

For More Information

Sarinas PS, Chitkara RK. Ascariasis and hookworm. *Semin Respir Infect* 1997 Jun;12(2):130–7

Chapter 49

Aspergillosis

Definition

Aspergillosis is an infection, a growth, or an allergic response caused by the *Aspergillus* fungus.

Causes, Incidence, and Risk Factors

Aspergillosis is caused by a fungus (*Aspergillus*), which is commonly found growing on dead leaves, stored grain, compost piles, or in other decaying vegetation.

It causes illness in three ways: as an allergic reaction in people with asthma (Pulmonary aspergillosis—allergic bronchopulmonary type); as a colonization and growth in an old healed lung cavity from previous disease (such as tuberculosis or lung abscess) where it produces a fungus ball called aspergilloma; and as an invasive infection with pneumonia that is spread to other parts of the body by the bloodstream (Pulmonary aspergillosis—invasive type).

The invasive infection can affect the eye, causing blindness, and any other organ of the body, but especially the heart, lungs, brain, and kidneys. The third form occurs almost exclusively in people who are immunosuppressed because of cancer, AIDS, leukemia, organ transplants, high doses of corticosteroid drugs, chemotherapy, or other diseases that reduce the number of normal white blood cells.

Symptoms

Symptoms of allergic aspergillosis:

- Fever
- Malaise
- Cough
- Coughing up blood or brownish mucous plugs
- Wheezing
- Weight loss
- Recurrent episodes of lung obstruction

Symptoms of invasive infection:

- Fever
- Chills
- Headaches
- Cough
- Shortness of breath
- Chest pain
- Increased sputum production, which may be bloody
- Bone pain
- Blood in the urine
- Decreased urine output
- Weight loss
- Symptoms involving specific organs
    - Brain: meningitis
    - Eye: blindness or visual impairment
    - Sinuses: sinusitis
    - Heart: endocarditis

Signs and Tests

- Abnormal chest x-ray or CT scan

- Sputum stain and culture showing *Aspergillus*
- Tissue biopsy (see bronchoscopy with transtracheal biopsy) for aspergillosis
- *Aspergillus* antigen skin test
- Aspergillosis precipitin antibody
- Elevated serum total IgE (immunoglobulin)
- Peripheral eosinophilia with allergic disease

Treatment

The goal of treatment is to control symptomatic infection. A fungus ball usually does not require treatment unless bleeding into the lung tissue is associated with the infection, then surgical excision is required.

Invasive aspergillosis is treated with several weeks of intravenous amphotericin B, an antifungal medication. Itraconazole can also be used.

Endocarditis caused by *Aspergillus* is treated by surgical removal of the infected heart valves and long-term amphotericin B therapy.

Allergic aspergillosis is treated with oral prednisone. Some people may benefit from allergy desensitization. Antifungal agents do not help people with allergic aspergillosis.

Expectations (prognosis)

Gradual improvement is seen in patients with allergic aspergillosis. Invasive aspergillosis may resist drug treatment and progress to death. The underlying disease and immune status of a person with invasive aspergillosis will also affect the overall prognosis.

Complications

- Amphotericin B can cause kidney impairment and severely unpleasant side effects.
- Invasive lung disease can cause massive bleeding from the lung.

Calling Your Health Care Provider

Call the health care provider if symptoms suggest this disease; if urine output becomes decreased while receiving antifungal medication; or if fever, chills, headache or other worsening symptoms develop.

Prevention

Be cautious in the use of drugs that suppress the immune system. Prevention of AIDS prevents opportunistic diseases, including aspergillosis, that are associated with a damaged or incompetent immune system.

Chapter 50

Candidiasis

Genital Candidiasis (Vulvovaginal Candidiasis (VVC), vaginal yeast infections)

What is genital candidiasis/VVC?

Candidiasis, also known as a "yeast infection" or VVC, is a common fungal infection that occurs when there is overgrowth of the fungus called *Candida*. *Candida* is always present in the body in small amounts. However, when an imbalance occurs, such as when the normal acidity of the vagina changes or when hormonal balance changes, *Candida* can multiply. When that happens, symptoms of candidiasis appear.

What are the symptoms of genital candidiasis/VVC?

Women with VVC usually experience genital itching or burning, with or without a "cottage cheese-like" vaginal discharge. Males with genital candidiasis may experience an itchy rash on the penis.

How common is genital candidiasis/VVC, and who can get it?

Nearly 75% of all adult women have had at least one genital "yeast infection" in their lifetime. On rare occasions, men may also experience genital candidiasis. VVC occurs more frequently and more severely

"Genital Candidiasis," "Invasive Candidiasis," "Oropharyngeal Candidiasis," Division of Bacterial and Mycotic Diseases, Centers for Disease Control and Prevention (CDC), reviewed April 6, 2000.

in people with weakened immune systems. There are some other conditions that may put a woman at risk for genital candidiasis:

- Pregnancy
- Diabetes mellitus
- Use of broad-spectrum antibiotics
- Use of corticosteroid medications

How is genital candidiasis/VVC transmitted?

Most cases of *Candida* infection are caused by the person's own *Candida* organisms. *Candida* yeasts usually live in the mouth, gastrointestinal tract, and vagina without causing symptoms. Symptoms develop only when *Candida* becomes overgrown in these sites. Rarely, *Candida* can be passed from person to person, such as through sexual intercourse.

How is genital candidiasis/VVC diagnosed?

The symptoms of genital candidiasis are similar to those of many other genital infections. Making a diagnosis usually requires laboratory testing of a genital swab taken from the affected area by a physician.

How is genital candidiasis/VVC treated?

Antifungal drugs which are taken orally, applied directly to the affected area, or used vaginally are the drugs of choice for vaginal yeast infections. Although these drugs usually work to cure the infection (80%–90% success rate), infections that do not respond to treatment are becoming more common, especially in HIV-infected women receiving long-term antifungal therapy. Prolonged and frequent use of these treatments can lessen their effectiveness.

What is the difference between the 3-day treatments and the 7-day treatments for genital candidiasis/VVC?

The only difference between these is the length of treatment. Three-day and 7-day treatments may both be effective.

Are over-the-counter (OTC) treatments for genital candidiasis/VVC safe to use?

Over-the-counter treatments for VVC are becoming more available. As a result more women are diagnosing themselves with VVC and using one of a family of drugs called "azoles" for therapy. However, misdiagnosis is common, and studies have shown that as many as two-thirds of all OTC drugs sold to treat VVC were used by women without the disease. Using these drugs when they are not needed may lead to a resistant infection. Resistant infections are very difficult to treat with the currently available medications for VVC.

Can Candida *infections become resistant to treatment?*

Overuse of these antifungal medications can increase the chance that they will eventually not work (the fungus develops resistance to medications). Therefore, it is important to be sure of the diagnosis before treating with over-the-counter or other antifungal medications.

What will happen if a person does not seek treatment for genital candidiasis/VVC?

Symptoms, which may be very uncomfortable, may persist. There is a chance that the infection may be passed between sex partners.

How can someone tell the difference between genital candidiasis/VVC and a urinary tract infection?

Because VVC and urinary tract infections share similar symptoms, such as a burning sensation when urinating, it is important to see a doctor and obtain laboratory testing to determine the cause of the symptoms and to treat effectively.

Invasive Candidiasis (infections in the bloodstream and organs)

What is invasive candidiasis?

Invasive candidiasis is a fungal infection that occurs when *Candida* species enter the blood, causing bloodstream infection and then spreading throughout the body.

How common is invasive candidiasis and who can get it?

One form of invasive candidiasis, candidemia, is the fourth most common bloodstream infection among hospitalized patients in the United States. A survey conducted at CDC found that candidemia occurs in 8 of every 100,000 persons per year. Persons at high risk for candidemia include low-birth-weight babies, surgical patients, and those whose immune systems are deficient.

What are the symptoms of invasive candidiasis?

The symptoms of invasive candidiasis are not specific. Fever and chills that do not improve after antibiotic therapy are the most common symptoms. If the infection spreads to deep organs such as kidneys, liver, bones, muscles, joints, spleen, or eyes, additional specific symptoms may develop, which vary depending on the site of infection. If the infection does not respond to treatment, the patient's organs may fail and cause death.

How is invasive candidiasis transmitted?

Invasive candidiasis may result when a person's own *Candida* organisms, normally found in the digestive tract, enter the bloodstream. On rare occasions, it can also occur when medical equipment or devices become contaminated with *Candida*. In either case, the infection may spread throughout the body.

How is invasive candidiasis diagnosed?

Invasive candidiasis is usually diagnosed by either culture of blood or tissue or by examining samples of infected tissue under the microscope.

How is invasive candidiasis treated?

Invasive candidiasis is usually treated with Amphotericin B given intravenously (IV) (in the vein) or with azole drugs taken by mouth or IV.

Oropharyngeal Candidiasis (OPC, thrush)

What is OPC?

Candidiasis of the mouth and throat, also known as a "thrush" or oropharyngeal candidiasis (OPC), is a fungal infection that occurs when there is overgrowth of fungus called *Candida*. *Candida* is normally found on skin or mucous membranes. However, if the environment inside the mouth or throat becomes imbalanced, *Candida* can multiply. When this happens, symptoms of thrush appear.

How common is OPC and who can get it?

OPC can affect normal newborns, but it occurs more frequently and more severely in people with weakened immune systems, particularly in persons with AIDS.

What are the symptoms of OPC?

People with OPC infection usually have painless, white patches in the mouth. Symptoms of OPC in the esophagus may include pain and difficulty swallowing.

How do I get OPC?

Most cases of OPC are caused by the person's own *Candida* organisms which normally live in the mouth or digestive tract. A person has symptoms when overgrowth of *Candida* organisms occurs.

How is OPC diagnosed?

OPC is diagnosed in two ways. A doctor may take a swab or sample of infected tissue and look at it under a microscope. If there is evidence of *Candida* infection, the sample will be cultured to confirm the diagnosis.

How is OPC treated?

Prescription treatments such as, Oral fluconazole, clotrimazole troches, or nystatin suspension usually provide effective treatment for OPC.

What will happen if a person does not seek treatment for a OPC?

Symptoms, which may be uncomfortable, may persist. In rare cases, invasive candidiasis may occur.

Can Candida-causing OPC become resistant to treatment?

Overuse of antifungal medications can increase the chance that they will eventually not work (the fungus develops resistance to medications). Therefore, it is important to be sure of the diagnosis from before treating with over-the-counter or other antifungal medications.

Chapter 51

Cryptococcosis

Definition

A rare fungal infection caused by inhaling the fungus, *Cryptococcus neoformans*.

Causes, Incidence, and Risk Factors

Cryptococcus neoformans, the fungus that causes this disease, is ordinarily found in soil. Once inhaled, infection with cryptococcosis may heal on its own, remain localized in the lungs, or spread throughout the body (disseminate).

Most cases occur in people whose resistance to infection is lowered (such as by HIV infection, high doses of corticosteroid medications, cancer chemotherapy, or Hodgkin's disease).

In people with normal immune systems, the pulmonary (lung) form may have no symptoms. However, in people with impaired immune systems, the cryptococcus organism may spread to the brain.

The onset of neurological symptoms is gradual. The majority of people with this condition have meningoencephalitis (swelling and irritation of the brain and spinal cord) at the time of diagnosis.

Cryptococcus is one of the most common life-threatening fungal infections in AIDS patients.

"Cryptococcosis," © 2002, A.D.A.M., Inc., reprinted with permission, updated August 14, 2002. Updated by: Donna R. Cooper, MD, MPH. Department of Medicine, Massachusetts General Hospital, Boston, MA. Review provided by VeriMed Healthcare Network.

Symptoms

- Chest pain
- Dry cough
- Headache
- Nausea
- Confusion
- Blurred vision or double vision (diplopia)
- Fatigue
- Fever
- Unusual and excessive sweating at night
- Glands, swollen without nearby areas appearing infected (e.g., red, painful, swollen)
- Prolonged bleeding, bruising easily
- Skin rash may be present
  - Skin rash or lesion; pinpoint red spots (petechiae)
  - Bleeding into the skin
  - Bruises (ecchymoses)
- Unintentional weight loss
- Appetite loss
- Abdominal fullness prematurely after meals
- Abdominal pain
- Abdomen swollen
- Weakness
- Bone pain or tenderness of the breastbone (sternum)
- Numbness and tingling
  - Nerve pain or pain along the path of a specific nerve
  - Pain along a nerve root (major pathway from the spinal cord)

Note: In individuals with normal immune systems there may be no symptoms.

Signs and Tests

- Sputum culture and stain
- Lung biopsy

- Bronchoscopy
- CSF culture and stain
- Chest x-ray

Treatment

Some infections require no treatment. However, medical observation should continue for a year to detect any progression of the disease. If pulmonary lesions are present or the disease spreads, antifungal medications are prescribed, and treatment with these agents may be prolonged.

Medications include:

- Amphotericin B
- Flucytosine
- Fluconazole

Expectations (prognosis)

Central nervous system involvement often has a fatal outcome, or leads to permanent damage.

Complications

- Relapse of infection
- Meningitis
- Permanent brain or nerve damage
- Side effects of medications (such as Amphotericin B) can be severe

Calling Your Health Care Provider

Call your health care provider if symptoms develop that are suggestive of cryptococcosis, particularly if you have an impaired immune system.

Prevention

Minimize doses of corticosteroid medications. Safer sex practices reduce the risk of acquiring HIV and the subsequent opportunistic infections associated with a weakened immune system.

Chapter 52

Histoplasmosis

Frequently asked Questions

What is histoplasmosis?

Histoplasmosis is a disease caused by the fungus *Histoplasma capsulatum*. Its symptoms vary greatly, but the disease primarily affect the lungs. Occasionally, other organs are affected. This form of the disease is called disseminated histoplasmosis, and it can be fatal if untreated.

Can anyone get histoplasmosis?

Yes. Positive histoplasmin skin tests occur in as many as 80% of the people living in areas where *H. capsulatum* is common, such as the eastern and central United States. Infants, young children, and older persons, in particular those with chronic lung disease are at increased risk for severe disease. Disseminated disease is more frequently seen in people with cancer or AIDS.

How is someone infected with H. capsulatum?

H. capsulatum grows in soil and material contaminated with bat or bird droppings. Spores become airborne when contaminated soil

"Histoplasmosis: Frequently asked Questions," Division of Bacterial and Mycotic Diseases, National Center for Infectious Diseases, Centers for Disease Control and Prevention (CDC), reviewed March 7, 2003, and "Histoplasmosis," National Eye Institute, National Institutes of Health (NIH), October 2002.

is disturbed. Breathing the spores causes infection. The disease is not transmitted from an infected person to someone else.

What are the symptoms of histoplasmosis?

Most infected persons have no apparent ill effects. The acute respiratory disease is characterized by respiratory symptoms, a general ill feeling, fever, chest pains, and a dry or nonproductive cough. Distinct patterns may be seen on a chest x-ray. Chronic lung disease resembles tuberculosis and can worsen over months or years. The disseminated form is fatal unless treated.

When do symptoms start?

If symptoms occur, they will start within 3 to 17 days after exposure; the average is 10 days.

Is histoplasmosis treatable?

Yes. Antifungal medications are used to treat severe cases of acute histoplasmosis and all cases of chronic and disseminated disease. Mild disease usually resolves without treatment. Past infection results in partial protection against ill effects if reinfected.

Where is H. capsulatum *found?*

H. capsulatum is found throughout the world and is endemic in certain areas of the United States. The fungus has been found in poultry house litter, caves, areas harboring bats, and in bird roosts.

What can be done to prevent histoplasmosis?

It is not practical to test or decontaminate most sites that may be contaminated with *H. capsulatum*, but the following precautions can be taken to reduce a person's risk of exposure:

- Avoid areas that may harbor the fungus, e.g., accumulations of bird or bat droppings.

- Before starting a job or activity having a risk for exposure to *H. capsulatum*, consult the NIOSH/NCID Document "Histoplasmosis: Protecting Workers at Risk." This document contains information on work practices and personal protective equipment that will reduce the risk of infection. A copy can also be obtained by requesting publication No. 97-146 from:

National Institute for Occupational Safety and Health
Publications Dissemination
4676 Columbia Parkway
Mail Stop C-13
Cincinnati, OH 45226-1998
Phone: 1-800-356-4674

Ocular Histoplasmosis Syndrome (OHS)

What is OHS?

Histoplasmosis, even mild cases, can later cause a serious eye disease called ocular histoplasmosis syndrome (OHS), a leading cause of vision loss in Americans ages 20 to 40.

How does histoplasmosis cause ocular histoplasmosis syndrome?

Scientists believe that *Histoplasma capsulatum* (histo) spores spread from the lungs to the eye, lodging in the choroid, a layer of blood vessels that provides blood and nutrients to the retina. The retina is the light-sensitive layer of tissue that lines the back of the eye. Scientists have not yet been able to detect any trace of the histo fungus in the eyes of patients with ocular histoplasmosis syndrome. Nevertheless, there is good reason to suspect the histo organism as the cause of OHS.

How does OHS develop?

OHS develops when fragile, abnormal blood vessels grow underneath the retina. These abnormal blood vessels form a lesion known as choroidal neovascularization (CNV). If left untreated, the CNV lesion can turn into scar tissue and replace the normal retinal tissue in the macula. The macula is the central part of the retina that provides the sharp, central vision that allows us to read a newspaper or drive a car. When this scar tissue forms, visual messages from the retina to the brain are affected, and vision loss results.

Vision is also impaired when these abnormal blood vessels leak fluid and blood into the macula. If these abnormal blood vessels grow toward the center of the macula, they may affect a tiny depression called the fovea. The fovea is the region of the retina with the highest concentration of special retinal nerve cells, called cones, that produce sharp, daytime vision. Damage to the fovea and the cones can severely impair, and even destroy, this straight-ahead vision. Early treatment of OHS is essential; if the abnormal blood vessels have affected the fovea, controlling the disease will be more difficult. Since OHS rarely affects side, or peripheral vision, the disease does not cause total blindness.

What are the symptoms of OHS?

OHS usually has no symptoms in its early stages; the initial OHS infection usually subsides without the need for treatment. This is true for other histo infections; in fact, often the only evidence that the inflammation ever occurred are tiny scars called "histo spots," which remain at the infection sites. Histo spots do not generally affect vision, but for reasons that are still not well understood, they can result in complications years—sometimes even decades—after the original eye infection. Histo spots have been associated with the growth of the abnormal blood vessels underneath the retina.

In later stages, OHS symptoms may appear if the abnormal blood vessels cause changes in vision. For example, straight lines may appear crooked or wavy, or a blind spot may appear in the field of vision. Because these symptoms indicate that OHS has already progressed enough to affect vision, anyone who has been exposed to histoplasmosis and perceives even slight changes in vision should consult an eye care professional.

Who is at risk for OHS?

Although only a tiny fraction of the people infected with the histo fungus ever develops OHS, any person who has had histoplasmosis should be alert for any changes in vision similar to those described above. Studies have shown the OHS patients usually test positive for previous exposure to histoplasmosis.

In the United States, the highest incidence of histoplasmosis occurs in a region often referred to as the "Histo Belt," where up to 90 percent of the adult population has been infected by histoplasmosis. This region includes all of Arkansas, Kentucky, Missouri, Tennessee, and West Virginia as well as large portions of Alabama, Illinois, Indiana, Iowa, Kansas, Louisiana, Maryland, Mississippi, Nebraska, Ohio, Oklahoma, Texas, and Virginia. Since most cases of histoplasmosis are undiagnosed, anyone who has ever lived in an area known to have a high rate of histoplasmosis should consider having their eyes examined for histo spots.

How is OHS diagnosed?

An eye care professional will usually diagnose OHS if a careful eye examination reveals two conditions: (1) The presence of histo spots, which indicate previous exposure to the histo fungus spores; and (2) Swelling of the retina, which signals the growth of new, abnormal blood vessels. To confirm the diagnosis, a dilated eye examination must be performed. This means that the pupils are enlarged temporarily with special drops, allowing the eye care professional to better examine the retina.

If fluid, blood, or abnormal blood vessels are present, an eye care professional may want to perform a diagnostic procedure called fluorescein angiography. In this procedure, a dye, injected into the patient's arm, travels to the blood vessels of the retina. The dye allows a better view of the CNV lesion, and photographs can document the location and extent to which it has spread. Particular attention is paid to how close the abnormal blood vessels are to the fovea.

How is OHS treated?

The only proven treatment for OHS is a form of laser surgery called photocoagulation. A small, powerful beam of light destroys the fragile, abnormal blood vessels, as well as a small amount of the overlying retinal tissue. Although the destruction of retinal tissue during the procedure can itself cause some loss of vision, this is done in the hope of protecting the fovea and preserving the finely-tuned vision it provides.

How effective is laser surgery?

Controlled clinical trials, sponsored by the National Eye Institute, have shown that photocoagulation can reduce future vision loss from OHS by more than half. The treatment is most effective when:

- The CNV has not grown into the center of the fovea, where it can affect vision.

- The eye care professional is able to identify and destroy the entire area of CNV.

Does laser surgery restore lost vision?

Laser photocoagulation usually does not restore lost vision. However, it does reduce the chance of further CNV growth and any resulting vision loss.

Does laser surgery cure OHS?

No. OHS cannot be cured. Once contracted, OHS remains a threat to a person's sight for their lifetime.

People with OHS who experience one bout of abnormal blood vessel growth may have recurrent CNV. Each recurrence can damage vision and may require additional laser therapy. It is crucial to detect and treat OHS as early as possible before it causes significant visual impairment.

Is there a simple way to check for signs of OHS damage to the macula?

Yes. A person can check for signs of damage to the macula by looking at a printed pattern called an Amsler grid. If the macula has been damaged, the vertical and horizontal lines of the grid may appear curved, or a blank spot may seem to appear.

Many eye care professionals advise patients who have received treatment for OHS, as well as those with histo spots, to check their vision daily with the Amsler grid one eye at a time. Patients with OHS in one eye are likely to develop it in the other.

What help is available for people who have already lost significant vision from OHS?

Scientists and engineers have developed many useful devices to help people with severe visual impairment in both eyes. These devices, called low vision aids, use special lenses or electronics to create enlarged visual images. An eye care professional can suggest sources that provide information on counseling, training, and special services for people with low vision. Many organizations for people who are blind also serve those with low vision.

What research is being conducted on the ocular histoplasmosis syndrome?

The National Eye Institute (NEI) supports research aimed at learning more about the relationship between histoplasmosis and OHS and how to treat OHS effectively. One such multicenter clinical study is called the Submacular Surgery Trials (SST). This clinical study is examining whether CNV in the fovea, which cannot be treated by laser photocoagulation, can be successfully removed through traditional surgery. Patients with OHS who would like to receive more information about the Submacular Surgery Trials should call the SST Chairman's Office toll-free at 1-888-554-0412. Information on the Submacular Surgery Trials is also available on the NEI web site at http://www.nei .nih.gov/neitrials/index.htm.

Where can I obtain information on histoplasmosis of the lungs and other parts of the body?

Information on systemic histoplasmosis can be obtained from:

The National Institute of Allergy and Infectious Diseases (NIAID)
The National Institutes of Health
Building 31, Room 7A50
31 Center Drive, MSC 2520
Bethesda, MD, 20892-2520
Phone: 301-496-5717
Website: http://www.niaid.nih.gov

Chapter 53

Hookworm

What is hookworm infection?

Hookworms are small parasitic worms (adult stage is approximately 1 centimeter long) which can infect the small intestines. There are two major species of hookworms for which humans are the usual host, and three species that primarily infect dogs and cats that can also cause infection in humans.

Who gets hookworm infection?

Hookworm is estimated to affect one-fourth of the world's population. It is widely found in tropical and subtropical countries such as Asia (particularly Southeast Asia), East Africa, the South Pacific, and South America. It is also found occasionally in the southeastern United States. Hookworm infection occurs where sanitary disposal of human waste is not available and where the temperature and other environmental conditions favor the development of infective larvae.

How is hookworm spread?

Hookworm is not spread directly from one person to another. It is transmitted when the microscopic hookworm eggs in human or animal feces (stool) are deposited on the ground, hatch, and develop into tiny larvae. People become infected when the larvae penetrate the

---

"Hookworm Infection," Wisconsin Department of Health and Family Services, revised July 2, 2001.

skin, usually of the foot. The larvae eventually migrate to the small intestine where they attach to the intestinal wall, mature into adult hookworms and produce eggs in 6–7 weeks. Without treatment the infection may persist for several years.

What are the symptoms of hookworm?

When the larvae penetrate the skin, they produce a characteristic skin rash termed "ground itch." Abdominal pain, diarrhea, and weight loss may occur when the worms attach to the intestinal wall. If the infection is light, few or no symptoms may occur. If the infection is heavy, iron deficiency and anemia may develop. Prolonged heavy infections can retard mental and physical development.

How soon after exposure do symptoms appear?

Although "ground itch" may occur immediately, other symptoms may develop from a few weeks to many months after exposure, depending on the intensity of the infection and the iron intake of the person infected.

How is hookworm diagnosed?

Infection is confirmed in a medical laboratory by finding the microscopic hookworm eggs in the feces (stool).

What is the treatment for hookworm infection?

Doctors treat hookworm infections with an antiparasitic drug. The currently available drugs result in a very high rate of cure. If the infected person is also anemic, this should be corrected with iron therapy. It is recommended that a stool specimen be submitted for testing two weeks after therapy has been completed. If there is still evidence of infection, retreatment is recommended.

How can hookworm be prevented?

Hookworm can be prevented by improving general sanitary conditions, especially installing sanitary disposal systems for feces. Nightsoil (soil containing human feces) and sewage effluent are dangerous to use as fertilizer. Shoes should be worn when walking in areas where hookworm disease is common. Persons immigrating from endemic to non-endemic areas, such as refugees from Southeast Asia, should be examined and treated if infected.

Chapter 54

Legionnaires' Disease and Pontiac Fever

Legionellosis is an infection caused by the bacterium *Legionella pneumophila*. The disease has two distinct forms:

- Legionnaires' disease, the more severe form of infection which includes pneumonia, and

- Pontiac fever, a milder illness.

Legionnaires' disease acquired its name in 1976 when an outbreak of pneumonia occurred among persons attending a convention of the American Legion in Philadelphia. Later, the bacterium causing the illness was named *Legionella*.

How common is legionellosis in the United States?

An estimated 8,000 to 18,000 people get Legionnaires' disease in the United States each year. Some people can be infected with the *Legionella* bacterium and have mild symptoms or no illness at all.

Outbreaks of Legionnaires' disease receive significant media attention. However, this disease usually occurs as a single, isolated case not associated with any recognized outbreak. When outbreaks do occur, they are usually recognized in the summer and early fall, but cases

---

"Legionellosis: Legionnaire's Disease (LD) and Pontiac Fever," Division of Bacterial and Mycotic Diseases, Centers for Disease Control and Prevention (CDC), reviewed June 20, 2001.

may occur year-round. About 5% to 30% of people who have Legionnaires' disease die.

What are the usual symptoms of legionellosis?

Patients with Legionnaires' disease usually have fever, chills, and a cough, which may be dry or may produce sputum. Some patients also have muscle aches, headache, tiredness, loss of appetite, and, occasionally, diarrhea. Laboratory tests may show that these patients' kidneys are not functioning properly. Chest x-rays often show pneumonia. It is difficult to distinguish Legionnaires' disease from other types of pneumonia by symptoms alone; other tests are required for diagnosis.

Persons with Pontiac fever experience fever and muscle aches and do not have pneumonia. They generally recover in 2 to 5 days without treatment.

The time between the patient's exposure to the bacterium and the onset of illness for Legionnaires' disease is 2 to 10 days; for Pontiac fever, it is shorter, generally a few hours to 2 days.

How is legionellosis diagnosed?

The diagnosis of legionellosis requires special tests not routinely performed on persons with fever or pneumonia. Therefore, a physician must consider the possibility of legionellosis in order to obtain the right tests.

Several types of tests are available. The most useful tests detect the bacteria in sputum, find *Legionella* antigens in urine samples, or compare antibody levels to *Legionella* in two blood samples obtained 3 to 6 weeks apart.

Who gets legionellosis?

People of any age may get Legionnaires' disease, but the illness most often affects middle-aged and older persons, particularly those who smoke cigarettes or have chronic lung disease. Also at increased risk are persons whose immune system is suppressed by diseases such as cancer, kidney failure requiring dialysis, diabetes, or AIDS. Those that take drugs that suppress the immune system are also at higher risk.

Pontiac fever most commonly occurs in persons who are otherwise healthy.

What is the treatment for legionellosis?

Erythromycin is the antibiotic currently recommended for treating persons with Legionnaires' disease. In severe cases, a second drug, rifampin, may be used in addition. Other drugs are available for patients unable to tolerate erythromycin.

Pontiac fever requires no specific treatment.

How is legionellosis spread?

Outbreaks of legionellosis have occurred after persons have breathed mists that come from a water source (e.g., air conditioning cooling towers, whirlpool spas, showers) contaminated with *Legionella* bacteria. Persons may be exposed to these mists in homes, workplaces, hospitals, or public places. Legionellosis is not passed from person to person, and there is no evidence of persons becoming infected from auto air conditioners or household window air-conditioning units.

Where is the Legionella bacterium found?

Legionella organisms can be found in many types of water systems. However, the bacteria reproduce to high numbers in warm, stagnant water (90°–105° F), such as that found in certain plumbing systems and hot water tanks, cooling towers and evaporative condensers of large air-conditioning systems, and whirlpool spas. Cases of legionellosis have been identified throughout the United States and in several foreign countries. It is believed to occur worldwide.

What is being done to prevent legionellosis?

Improved design and maintenance of cooling towers and plumbing systems to limit the growth and spread of *Legionella* organisms are the foundations of legionellosis prevention.

During outbreaks, CDC and health department investigators seek to identify the source of disease transmission and recommend appropriate prevention and control measures, such as decontamination of the water source. Current research will likely identify additional prevention strategies.

Chapter 55

Schistosomiasis

What is schistosomiasis?

Schistosomiasis, also known as bilharzia (bill-HAR-zi-a), is a disease caused by parasitic worms. Infection with *Schistosoma mansoni*, *S. haematobium*, and *S. japonicum* causes illness in humans. Although schistosomiasis is not found in the United States, 200 million people are infected worldwide.

How can I get schistosomiasis?

Infection occurs when your skin comes in contact with contaminated fresh water in which certain types of snails that carry schistosomes are living.

Fresh water becomes contaminated by *Schistosoma* eggs when infected people urinate or defecate in the water. The eggs hatch, and if certain types of snails are present in the water, the parasites grow and develop inside the snails. The parasite leaves the snail and enters the water where it can survive for about 48 hours. *Schistosoma* parasites can penetrate the skin of persons who are wading, swimming, bathing, or washing in contaminated water. Within several weeks, worms grow inside the blood vessels of the body and produce eggs. Some of these eggs travel to the bladder or intestines and are passed into the urine or stool.

"Schistosomiasis," Division of Parasitic Diseases, Centers for Disease Control and Prevention (CDC), reviewed August 15, 1999. Reviewed by David A. Cooke, M.D. on January 26, 2004.

What are the symptoms of schistosomiasis?

Within days after becoming infected, you may develop a rash or itchy skin. Fever, chills, cough, and muscle aches can begin within 1–2 months of infection. Most people have no symptoms at this early phase of infection.

Eggs travel to the liver or pass into the intestine or bladder. Rarely, eggs are found in the brain or spinal cord and can cause seizures, paralysis, or spinal cord inflammation. For people who are repeatedly infected for many years, the parasite can damage the liver, intestines, lungs, and bladder.

Symptoms of schistosomiasis are caused by the body's reaction to the eggs produced by worms, not by the worms themselves.

What should I do if I think I have schistosomiasis?

See your health care provider. If you have traveled to countries where schistosomiasis is found and had contact with fresh water, describe in detail where and for how long you traveled. Explain that you may have been exposed to contaminated water.

How is schistosomiasis diagnosed?

Your health care provider may ask you to provide stool or urine samples to see if you have the parasite. A blood test has been developed and is available at CDC (Centers for Disease Control and Prevention). For accurate results, you must wait 6–8 weeks after your last exposure to contaminated water before the blood sample is taken.

What is the treatment for schistosomiasis?

Safe and effective drugs are available for the treatment of schistosomiasis. You will be given pills to take for 1–2 days.

Am I at risk?

If you live in or travel to areas where schistosomiasis occurs and your skin comes in contact with fresh water from canals, rivers, streams, or lakes, you are at risk of getting schistosomiasis.

In what areas of the world does schistosomiasis occur?

- Africa: southern Africa, sub-Saharan Africa, Lake Malawi, the Nile River valley in Egypt

- South America: including Brazil, Suriname, Venezuela

- Caribbean: Antigua, Dominican Republic, Guadeloupe, Martinique, Montserrat, Saint Lucia (risk is low)

- The Middle East: Iran, Iraq, Saudi Arabia, Syrian Arab Republic, Yemen

- Southern China

- Southeast Asia: Philippines, Laos, Cambodia, Japan, central Indonesia, Mekong delta.

How can I prevent schistosomiasis?

- Avoid swimming or wading in fresh water when you are in countries in which schistosomiasis occurs. Swimming in the ocean and in chlorinated swimming pools is generally thought to be safe.

- Drink safe water. Because there is no way to make sure that water coming directly from canals, lakes, rivers, streams or springs is safe, you should either boil water for 1 minute or filter water before drinking it. Boiling water for at least 1 minute will kill any harmful parasites, bacteria, or viruses present. Iodine treatment alone will not guarantee that water is safe and free of all parasites.

- Bath water should be heated for 5 minutes at 150° F. Water held in a storage tank for at least 48 hours should be safe for showering.

- Vigorous towel drying after an accidental, very brief water exposure may help to prevent the *Schistosoma* parasite from penetrating the skin. You should not rely on vigorous towel drying to prevent schistosomiasis.

For More Information

1.   Centers for Disease Control and Prevention. Schistosomiasis in Peace Corps volunteers—Malawi, *MMWR* 1993;42:565-70.

2.   Cetron MS, Chitsulo L, Sullivan JJ, et al. Schistosomiasis in Lake Malawi. *Lancet* 1996;348:1274-8.

3.   Jordan P. *Schistosomiasis. The St. Lucia Project. New York*: Cambridge University Press, 1985.

4. Jordan P, Webbe G, Sturrock RF, eds. *Human schistosomiasis*. Wallingford: CAB International, 1993.

5. Rollinson D. Simpson AJG, eds. *The biology of schistosomes from genes to latrines*. London: Academic Press, 1987.

6. Tsang VCW, Wilkins PP. Immunodiagnosis of schistosomiasis. Screen with FAST-ELISA and confirm with immunoblot. *Clin Lab Med* 1991;11:1029-39.

7. World Health Organization. *The control of schistosomiasis: Second report of the WHO Expert Committee. WHO Technical Report Series 830*. Geneva: WHO, 1993.

Chapter 56

Sepsis

Alternative Names

Systemic inflammatory response syndrome (SIRS)

Definition

Sepsis is a severe illness caused by overwhelming infection of the bloodstream by toxin-producing bacteria.

Causes, Incidence, and Risk Factors

Sepsis occurs in 2 of every 100 hospital admissions. It is caused by bacterial infection that can originate anywhere in the body. Common sites include the following:

- The kidneys (upper urinary tract infection)
- The liver or the gall bladder
- The bowel (usually seen with peritonitis)
- The skin (cellulitis)
- The lungs (bacterial pneumonia)

"Sepsis," © 2002, A.D.A.M., Inc., reprinted with permission, updated August 7, 2002. Updated by: Camille Kotton, M.D., Infectious Diseases Division, Massachusetts General Hospital and Brigham and Women's Hospital, Boston, MA. Review provided by VeriMed Healthcare Network.

Meningitis may also be accompanied by sepsis. In children, sepsis may accompany infection of the bone (osteomyelitis). In hospitalized patients, common sites of infection include intravenous lines, surgical wounds, surgical drains, and sites of skin breakdown known as decubitus ulcers or bedsores.

The infection is often confirmed by a positive blood culture, though blood cultures may be negative in individuals who have been receiving antibiotics. In sepsis, blood pressure drops, resulting in shock. Major organs and systems, including the kidneys, liver, lungs, and central nervous system, stop functioning normally.

A change in mental status and hyperventilation may be the earliest signs of impending sepsis.

Sepsis is often life-threatening, especially in people with a weakened immune system or other medical illnesses.

Symptoms

- Fever or hypothermia (low body temperature)
- Hyperventilation
- Chills
- Shaking
- Warm skin
- Skin rash
- Rapid heart beat (tachycardia)
- Confusion or delirium
- Decreased urine output

Signs and Tests

- White blood cell count that is low or high
- Platelet count that is low
- Blood culture that is positive for bacteria
- Blood gases that reveal acidosis
- Kidney function tests that are abnormal (early in the course of disease)

This disease may also alter the results of the following tests:

- Peripheral smear may demonstrate a low platelet count and destruction of red blood cells.

- Fibrin degradation products are often elevated, a condition that may be associated with a tendency to bleed.

- Blood differential—with immature white blood cells seen

Treatment

Septic patients usually require monitoring in an intensive care unit (ICU). "Broad spectrum" intravenous antibiotic therapy should be initiated as soon as sepsis is suspected.

The number of antibiotics administered may be decreased when the results of blood cultures become available and the causative organism is identified. The source of the infection should be discovered, if possible, which may mean further diagnostic testing. Sources such as infected intravenous lines or surgical drains should be removed, and sources such as abscesses should be surgically drained.

Supportive therapy with oxygen, intravenous fluids, and medications that increase blood pressure may be required for a good outcome. Dialysis may be necessary in the event of kidney failure, and mechanical ventilation is often required if respiratory failure occurs.

Expectations (Prognosis)

The death rate can be as high as 60% for people with underlying medical problems. Mortality is less (but still significant) in individuals without other medical problems.

Complications

- Septic shock
- Impaired blood flow to vital organs (brain, heart, kidneys)
- Disseminated intravascular coagulation

Calling Your Health Care Provider

Go to the emergency room or call the local emergency number (such as 911) if you suspect sepsis.

Prevention

Many cases are not preventable. Awareness of risk may allow earlier detection.

Chapter 57

Staph Infections

The Centers for Disease Control and Prevention (CDC) has received inquiries about infections with antibiotic-resistant *Staphylococcus aureus* (including methicillin-resistant *S. aureus* [MRSA]) among persons who have no apparent contact with the healthcare system. This chapter addresses some of the most frequently asked questions.

What is **Staphylococcus aureus?**

Staphylococcus aureus, often simply referred to simply as "staph," are bacteria commonly found on the skin and in the noses of healthy people. Occasionally, staph can cause infection; staph bacteria are one of the most common causes of skin infections in the United States. Most of these infections are minor (such as pimples, boils, and other skin conditions) and most can be treated without antimicrobial agents (also known as antibiotics or antibacterial agents). However, staph bacteria can also cause serious and sometimes fatal infections (such as bloodstream infections, surgical wound infections, and pneumonia). In the past, most serious staph bacterial infections were treated with a type of antimicrobial agent related to penicillin. Over the past 50 years, treatment of these infections has become more difficult because staph bacteria have become resistant to various antimicrobial agents, including

"MRSA, Methicillin Resistant *Staphylococcus aureus*," reviewed March 7, 2003, and "VISA/VRSA, Vancomycin-Intermediate/Resistant *Staphylococcus aureus*," reviewed April 1, 2003, Division of Healthcare Quality Promotion, Centers for Disease Control and Prevention (CDC).

the commonly used penicillin-related antibiotics. These resistant bacteria are called methicillin-resistant *Staphylococcus aureus*, or MRSA.

Where are staph and MRSA found?

Staph bacteria and MRSA can be found on the skin and in the nose of some people without causing illness.

What is the difference between colonization and infection?

Colonization occurs when the staph bacteria are present on or in the body without causing illness. Approximately 25 to 30% of the population is colonized in the nose with staph bacteria at a given time.[2]

Infection occurs when the staph bacteria cause disease in the person. People also may be colonized or infected with MRSA, the staph bacteria that are resistant to many antibiotics.

Who gets MRSA?

Staph bacteria can cause different kinds of illness, including skin infections, bone infections, pneumonia, severe life-threatening bloodstream infections, and others. Since MRSA is a staph bacterium, it can cause the same kinds of infection as staph in general; however, MRSA occurs more commonly among persons in hospitals and healthcare facilities.

MRSA infection usually develops in hospitalized patients who are elderly or very sick or who have an open wound (such as a bedsore) or a tube going into their body (such as a urinary catheter or intravenous [IV] catheter). MRSA infections acquired in hospitals and healthcare settings can be severe. In addition, certain factors can put some patients at higher risk for MRSA including prolonged hospital stay, receiving broad-spectrum antibiotics, being hospitalized in an intensive care or burn unit, spending time close to other patients with MRSA, having recent surgery, or carrying MRSA in the nose without developing illness. [3–6]

MRSA causes illness in persons outside of hospitals and healthcare facilities as well. Cases of MRSA diseases in the community have been associated with recent antibiotic use, sharing contaminated items, having active skin diseases, and living in crowded settings. Clusters of skin infections caused by MRSA have been described among injecting drug-users,[7,8] aboriginals in Canada,[9] New Zealand[10] or Australia,[11,12] Native Americans in the United States,[13] incarcerated persons,[14] players of close-contact sports,[15,16] and other populations.[17–23] Community-associated MRSA infections are typically skin infections, but also can cause severe illness as in the cases of four children who died from community-associated MRSA.[24] Most of the transmission in these settings appeared to be from people with active MRSA skin infections.

How common is staph and MRSA?

Staph bacteria are one of the most common causes of skin infection in the United States, and are a common cause of pneumonia and bloodstream infections. Staph and MRSA infections are not routinely reported to public health authorities, so a precise number is not known. According to some estimates, as many as 100,000 persons are hospitalized each year with MRSA infections, although only a small proportion of these persons have disease onset occurring in the community. Approximately 25 to 30% of the population is colonized in the nose with staph bacteria at a given time.[2] The number who are colonized with MRSA at any one time is not known. CDC is currently collaborating with state and local health departments to improve surveillance for MRSA. Active, population-based surveillance in selected regions of the United States is ongoing and will help characterize the scope and risk factors for MRSA in the community.

Are staph and MRSA infections treatable?

Yes. Most staph bacteria and MRSA are susceptible to several antibiotics. Furthermore, most staph skin infections can be treated without antibiotics by draining the sore. However, if antibiotics are prescribed, patients should complete the full course and call their doctors if the infection does not get better. Patients who are only colonized with staph bacteria or MRSA usually do not need treatment.

How are staph and MRSA spread?

Staph bacteria and MRSA can spread among people having close contact with infected people. MRSA is almost always spread by direct physical contact, and not through the air. Spread may also occur through indirect contact by touching objects (i.e., towels, sheets, wound dressings, clothes, workout areas, sports equipment) contaminated by the infected skin of a person with MRSA or staph bacteria.

How can I prevent staph or MRSA infections?

Practice good hygiene

1. Keep your hands clean by washing thoroughly with soap and water

2. Keep cuts and abrasions clean and covered with a proper dressing (e.g., bandage) until healed

3. Avoid contact with other people's wounds or material contaminated from wounds.

What should I do if I think I have a Staph or MRSA infection?

See your healthcare provider.

What is CDC doing to address MRSA in the community?

CDC is concerned about MRSA in communities and is working with multiple partners on prevention strategies.

- CDC is working with 4 states in a project to define the spectrum of disease, determine populations affected, and develop studies to define who is at particular risk for infection.

- CDC is working with state health departments to assist in the development of surveillance systems for tracking MRSA in the community.

- CDC is using the National Health and Nutritional Evaluation Survey (NHANES) to estimate the number of individuals in the United States who carry staph bacteria in their nose.

- CDC works with laboratories across the country to improve the detection of MRSA through training personnel and use of appropriate testing methods.

- CDC provides technical expertise to hospitals and state and local health departments on infection control in healthcare settings, including control of MRSA.

- CDC laboratories are working to characterize the unique features of MRSA strains from the community.

What are VISA and VRSA?

VISA and VRSA are specific types of antimicrobial-resistant staph bacteria. While most staph bacteria are susceptible to the antimicrobial agent vancomycin some have developed resistance. VISA and VRSA cannot be successfully treated with vancomycin because these organisms are no longer susceptible to vancomycin. However, to date, all VISA and VRSA isolates have been susceptible to other Food and Drug Administration (FDA) approved drugs.

How do VISA and VRSA get their names?

Staph bacteria are classified as VISA or VRSA based on laboratory tests. Laboratories perform tests to determine if staph bacteria are resistant to antimicrobial agents that might be used for treatment of infections. For vancomycin and other antimicrobial agents, laboratories determine how much of the agent it requires to inhibit the growth of the organism in a test tube. The result of the test is usually expressed as a minimum inhibitory concentration (MIC) or the minimum amount of antimicrobial agent that inhibits bacterial growth in the test tube. Therefore, staph bacteria are classified as VISA if the MIC for vancomycin is 8–16 µg/ml, and classified as VRSA if the vancomycin MIC is >32 µg/ml.

How common are VISA and VRSA infections?

VISA and VRSA infections are rare. Only eight cases of infection caused by VISA (Michigan 1997, New Jersey 1997, New York 1998, Illinois 1999, Minnesota 2000, Nevada 2000, Maryland 2000, and Ohio 2001) and two cases of infection caused by VRSA (Michigan 2002 and Pennsylvania 2002) have been reported in the United States.

Who gets VISA and VRSA infections?

Persons that developed VISA and VRSA infections had several underlying health conditions (such as diabetes and kidney disease), previous infections with methicillin-resistant *Staphylococcus aureus* (MRSA), tubes going into their bodies (such as intravenous [IV] catheters), recent hospitalizations, and recent exposure to vancomycin and other antimicrobial agents.

What should I do if I think I have a Staph, MRSA, VISA, or VRSA infection?

See your healthcare provider.

Are VISA and VRSA infections treatable?

Yes. To date, all VISA and VRSA isolates have been susceptible to several Food and Drug Administration (FDA) approved drugs.

413

How can the spread of VISA and VRSA be prevented?

Use of appropriate infection control practices (such as wearing gloves before and after contact with infectious body substances and adherence to hand hygiene) by healthcare personnel can reduce the spread of VISA and VRSA.

Because VISA and VRSA are only part of the larger problem of antimicrobial resistance in healthcare settings, CDC has started a Campaign to Prevent Antimicrobial Resistance. The campaign centers around four strategies that clinicians can use to prevent antimicrobial resistance: prevent infections; diagnose and treat infections effectively; use antimicrobials wisely; and prevent transmission. A series of evidence-based steps are described that can reduce the development and spread of resistant organisms such as VISA and VRSA.

What should I do if a family member or close friend has VISA or VRSA?

VISA and VRSA are types of antibiotic-resistant staph bacteria. Therefore, as with all staph bacteria, spread occurs among people having close physical contact with infected patients or contaminated material like bandages. Therefore, persons having close physical contact with infected patients while they are outside of the healthcare setting should: (1) keep their hands clean by washing thoroughly with soap and water, (2) avoid contact with other people's wounds or material contaminated from wounds. If you visit a friend or family member who is infected with VISA or VRSA while they are hospitalized, follow the hospital's recommended precautions.

What is CDC doing to address VISA and VRSA?

CDC has established several programs to promote appropriate use of antimicrobial agents because inappropriate antibiotic use is a major cause of antimicrobial resistance. One program that focuses on patients in healthcare facilities is the Campaign to Prevent Antimicrobial Resistance. The campaign centers around four strategies that clinicians can use to prevent antimicrobial resistance: prevent infections; diagnose and treat infections effectively; use antimicrobials wisely; and prevent transmission of infections. A series of evidence-based steps are described that can reduce the development and spread of resistant organisms, such as VISA and VRSA. CDC also has published guidance to prevent the spread of vancomycin resistance in healthcare settings.

In addition to providing guidance for clinicians and infection control personnel, CDC is also working with state and local health agencies, healthcare facilities, and clinical microbiology laboratories to ensure that laboratories are using proper methods to detect VISA and VRSA (S.E.A.R.C.H.). Recently CDC developed a training tool for laboratorians to enhance their understanding and improve their proficiency in performing antimicrobial susceptibility testing (M.A.S.T.E.R.). Accurate antimicrobial susceptibility test results not only help physicians choose the best therapy for their patients, but guide infection control efforts to the most serious infections.

References

1. Lowry FD. *Staphylococcus aureus* infections. *New England Journal of Medicine*. 1998;339:520-32.

2. Kluytmans J, Van Belkum A, Verbrugh H. Nasal carriage of *Staphylococcus aureus*: epidemiology, underlying mechanisms, and associated risks. *Clin Microbiol Rev*. 1997;10:505-20.

3. Boyce JM. Methicillin-resistant *Staphylococcus aureus*. Detection, epidemiology, and control measures. *Infect Dis Clinics of North Am*. 1989;3:901-13.

4. Herwaldt LA. Control of methicillin-resistant *Staphylococcus aureus* in the hospital setting. *Am J Medicine*. 1999;106:11S-18S; discussion 48S-52S.

5. Asensio A, Guerrero A, Quereda C, Lizan M, Martinez-Ferrer M. Colonization and infection with methicillin-resistant *Staphylococcus aureus*: associated factors and eradication. *Infec Control Hosp Epidemiol*. 1996;17:20-8.

6. Mulligan ME, Murray-Leisure KA, Ribner BD, et al. Methicillin-resistant *Staphylococcus aureus*: a consensus review of the microbiology, pathogenesis, and epidemiology with implications for prevention and management. *Am J Medicine*. 1993;94:313-28.

7. Saravolatz LD, Markowitz N, Arking L, Pohloh D, Fisher E. Methicillin-resistant *Staphylococcus aureus*. Epidemiologic observations during a community-acquired outbreak. *Annals of Internal Medicine*. 1982;96:11-16.

8. CDC. Community-acquired methicillin-resistant *Staphylococcus aureus* infections—Michigan. *MMWR*. 1981;30:185-7.

9. Embil J, Ramotar K, Romance L, et al. Methicillin-resistant *Staphylococcus aureus* in tertiary care institutions on the Canadian prairies 1990-1992. *Infection Control and Hospital Epidemiology* 1994; 15:646-51.

10. Rings T, Findlay R, Lang S. Ethnicity and methicillin-resistant *S. aureus* in South Auckland. *New Zealand Medical Journal* 1998; 111:151.

11. Maguire GP, Arthur AD, Boustead PJ, Dwyer B, Currie BJ. Emerging epidemic of community-acquired methicillin-resistant *Staphylococcus aureus* infection in the Northern Territory. *Medical Journal of Australia* 1996; 1996; 164:721-3.

12. Collignon P, Gosbell I, Vickery A, Nimmo G, Stylianopoulos T, Gottlieb T. Community-acquired methicillin-resistant *Staphylococcus aureus* in Australia. Australian Group on Antimicrobial Resistance. *Lancet* 1998; 352:145-6.

13. Groos A, Naimi T, Wolset D, Smith-Johnson K, Moore K, Cheek J. *Emergence of community-acquired methicillin-resistant Staphylococcus aureus in a rural American Indian community (Abstract 1230), 39th Annual Interscience Conference on Antimicrobial Agents and Chemotherapy*, San Francisco, CA, 1999.

14. Methicillin-resistant *Staphylococcus aureus* skin or soft tissue infections in a state prison—Mississippi, 2000. *MMWR* 2001 Oct. 26. 50 (42); 919-922.

15. Lindenmayer JM, Schoenfeld S, O'Grady R, Carney JK. Methicillin-resistant *Staphylococcus aureus* in a high school wrestling team and the surrounding community. *Archives of Internal Medicine* 1998; 158:895-9.

16. Stacey AR, Endersby KE, Chan PC, Marples RR. An outbreak of methicillin-resistant *Staphylococcus aureus* infection in a rugby football team. *British Journal of Sports Medicine* 1998; 332: 153-4.

17. Kallen AJ, Driscoll TJ, Thornton S, Olson PE, Wallace MR. Increase in community-acquired methicillin-resistant *Staphylococcus aureus* at a Naval Medical Center. *Infection Control and Hospital Epidemiology 2000*; 21: 223-6

18. Hussain FM, Boyle-Vavra S, Bethel CD, Daum RS. Current trends in community-acquired methicillin-resistant *Staphylococcus aureus* at a tertiary care pediatric facility. *Pediatric Infectious Disease Journal* 2000; 19: 1163-6.

19. Feder HM, Jr. Methicillin-resistant *Staphylococcus aureus* infections in 2 pediatric outpatients. *Archives of Family Medicine 2000*; 1163-6.

20. Goetz A, Posey K, Fleming J, et al. Methicillin-resistant *Staphylococcus aureus* in the community: a hospital-based study. *Infection Control and Hospital Epidemiology* 1999; 20: 689-91.

21. Frank AL, Marcinak JK, Mangat PD, Schreckenberger PC. Community-acquired and clindamycin-susceptible methicillin-resistant *Staphylococcus aureus* in children. *Pediatric Infectious Disease Journal* 1999; 18:993-1000.

22. Price MF, McBride ME, Wolf JE, Jr., Prevalence of methicillin-resistant *Staphylococcus aureus* in a dermatology outpatient population. *Southern Medical Journal* 1998: 91:369-71.

23. Herold BC, Immergluck LC, Maranan MC, et al. Community-acquired methicillin-resistant *Staphylococcus aureus* in children with no identified predisposing risk. *JAMA* 1998; 279:593-8.

24. From the Centers for Disease Control and Prevention. Four pediatric deaths from community-acquired methicillin-resistant *Staphylococcus aureus*—Minnesota and North Dakota, 1997-1999. *JAMA* 1999; 282: 1123-5.

Chapter 58

Swimmer's Itch

What is swimmer's itch?

Swimmer's itch, also called cercarial dermatitis (SIR-care-ee-uhl DER-muh-TIGHT-iss), is a skin rash caused by an allergic reaction to infection with certain parasites of birds and mammals. These microscopic parasites are released from infected snails to swim in fresh and salt water, such as lakes, ponds, and oceans used for swimming and wading. Infection is found throughout the world. Swimmer's itch generally occurs during summer months.

What are the signs and symptoms of swimmer's itch?

Within minutes to days after swimming in contaminated water, you may experience tingling, burning, or itching of the skin. Small reddish pimples appear within 12 hours. Pimples may develop into small blisters. Itching may last up to a week or more, but will gradually go away.

Because swimmer's itch is caused by an allergic reaction to infection, the more often you swim or wade in contaminated water, the more likely you are to develop more serious symptoms. The greater the number of exposures to contaminated water, the more intense and immediate symptoms of swimmer's itch will be.

Be aware that there are other causes of rash that may occur after swimming in fresh and salt water.

"Cercarial Dermatitis," Division of Parasitic Diseases, Centers for Disease Control and Prevention, reviewed March 2002.

419

Do I need to see my health care provider for treatment?

No. Most cases do not require medical attention.
If you have a rash, you may try the following for relief:

- corticosteroid cream
- cool compresses
- bath with baking soda
- baking soda paste to the rash
- anti-itch lotion
- calamine lotion
- colloidal oatmeal baths, such as Aveeno®

Try not to scratch. Scratching may cause the rash to become infected. If itching is severe, your health care provider may prescribe lotion or creams to lessen your symptoms.

How does water become infested with the parasite?

The adult parasite lives in the blood of infected animals such as ducks, geese, gulls, swans, as well as certain aquatic mammals such as muskrats and beavers. The parasites produce eggs that are passed in the feces of infected birds or mammals.

If the eggs land in the water, the water becomes contaminated. Eggs hatch, releasing small, free-swimming larvae. These larvae swim in the water in search of a certain species of aquatic snail.

If the larvae find one of these snails, they infect the snail and undergo further development. Infected snails release a different type of larvae (cercariae, hence the name cercarial dermatitis) into the water. This larval form then searches for a suitable host (bird, muskrat) so they can start the life cycle over again. Although humans are not a suitable host, the larvae burrow into the skin of swimmers, which may cause an allergic reaction/rash. The larvae cannot develop inside a human and they soon die.

Can swimmer's itch be spread from person-to-person?

No.

Who is at risk for swimmer's itch?

Anyone who swims or wades in infested water may be at risk. Larvae are more likely to be swimming along shallow water by the shoreline.

Children are most often affected because they swim, wade, and play in the shallow water more than adults. Also, they do not towel dry themselves when leaving the water.

Once an outbreak of swimmer's itch has occurred in water, will the water always be unsafe?

No. Many factors must be present for swimmer's itch to become a problem in water. Since these factors change (sometimes within a swim season), swimmer's itch will not always be a problem. However, there is no way to know how long water may be unsafe. Larvae are generally infective for 24 hours once they are released from the snail. However, an infected snail will continue to produce cercariae throughout the remainder of its life. For future snails to become infected, migratory birds or mammals in the area must also be infected so the life cycle can continue.

What can be done to reduce the risk of swimmer's itch?

- Avoid swimming in areas where swimmer's itch is a known problem or where signs have been posted warning of unsafe water.

- Avoid swimming near or wading in marshy areas where snails are commonly found.

- Towel dry or shower immediately after leaving the water.

- Encourage health officials to post signs on shorelines where swimmer's itch is a current problem.

- Do not attract birds by feeding them to areas where people are swimming.

For further information on protecting yourself from recreational water illnesses, please visit http://www.healthyswimming.org.

Is my swimming pool safe to swim in?

Yes. As long as your swimming pool is well-maintained and chlorinated, there is no risk of swimmer's itch.

Chapter 59

Tetanus

Facts about Tetanus for Children

Signs and Symptoms

Tetanus is the result of an infection that affects the muscles and nerves. It is usually due to a contaminated wound. Tetanus often begins with muscle spasms in the jaw (also called trismus or lockjaw), together with difficulty in swallowing, and stiffness or pain in muscles of the neck, shoulder, or back. Spasms soon spread to muscles of the abdomen, upper arms, and thighs.

Neonatal tetanus causes these same symptoms in newborns. Neonatal tetanus occurs after a baby is delivered in unsanitary conditions, especially if the umbilical cord cut is contaminated. Prior to immunizations, neonatal tetanus was a common cause of newborn death. Because of improved surgical techniques and because of maternal antibodies passed to the baby in the womb, newborn tetanus is now rare in developed countries.

"Facts about Tetanus for Children" is from "Tetanus," text provided by KidsHealth, one of the largest resources online for medically reviewed health information written for parents, kids, and teens. For more articles like this one, visit www.KidsHealth.org, or www.TeensHealth.org. © 2003 The Nemours Center for Children's Health, and "Facts about Tetanus for Adults" is reprinted with permission from the National Foundation for Infectious Diseases - National Coalition on Adult Immunization. © 2003. For additional information visit the National Foundation for Infectious Diseases website at www.nfid.org. or http://www.nfid.org/ncai.

Description

Tetanus is caused by a type of soil bacteria called *Clostridium tetani*, which produces a toxin (poison) called tetanospasmin. Tetanospasmin attaches to nerves around the wound area and is carried inside the nerves to the brain or spinal cord. There it interferes with the normal activity of nerves, especially nerves that send messages to the muscles.

In the United States, most cases of tetanus follow a cut or puncture injury. Sometimes the injury itself is so small that it was never seen by a doctor, and the tetanus bacteria grew unobserved in the wound. Other types of wounds that commonly lead to tetanus are: burns, frostbite, abortion, and drug abuse (especially "skin popping").

Many developing countries have no effective prevention and immunization program against tetanus, so the disease is much more common there than in the United States

Duration

Tetanus, although rare, is a serious illness. However, when the infection is diagnosed and treated early, recovery is possible. Recovery usually takes at least 4 to 6 weeks.

In infants, neonatal tetanus is almost always fatal.

Contagiousness

Tetanus is not contagious.

Incubation

The incubation period for tetanus is 3 to 14 days, with most symptoms beginning around day seven. In neonatal tetanus, symptoms start within the first 2 weeks of life.

Prevention

In children, tetanus can be prevented through immunizations given by your child's doctor as part of the DPT series of injections. After childhood, a tetanus booster is recommended every 10 years. Some doctors schedule a tetanus booster whenever an adult reaches a "5" age—for example, at age 25, 35, 45, etc.

Neonatal tetanus can be prevented by making sure that all pregnant women have proper immunization before delivery and by delivering all newborns in sanitary conditions.

When to Call Your Child's Doctor

If you are not sure whether your child has been immunized against tetanus, call your child's doctor's office. If your child has not received tetanus immunizations, call the doctor as soon as possible to schedule an office visit.

If it's been more than 10 years since either you or your child have had a tetanus booster, schedule an office visit with your doctors to bring your immunizations up to date.

If you are pregnant, discuss your immunization record with your obstetrician before your due date.

Professional Treatment

Children and adults with tetanus infections are treated in a hospital, usually in an intensive care unit. They receive antibiotics to kill tetanus bacteria and antitoxin to neutralize the toxin. They also receive medicines to control muscle spasms and medicines to stop the abnormal nerve activity that would otherwise cause disturbances in heartbeat, blood pressure, and body temperature.

Home Treatment

Anyone with a tetanus infection needs to be treated in a hospital. Hospitals have medicine and equipment to support recovering patients.

If you or your child have not been immunized against tetanus, arrange for immunization as soon as possible. Although it's always important to clean a child's wounds, remember that cleaning a wound will not substitute for immunization.

Facts about Tetanus for Adults

What is tetanus?

Tetanus, commonly called lockjaw, is a bacterial disease that affects the nervous system. It is contracted through a cut or wound that becomes contaminated with tetanus bacteria. The bacteria can get in through even a tiny pinprick or scratch, but deep puncture wounds or cuts like those made by nails or knives are especially susceptible to infection with tetanus. Tetanus bacteria are present worldwide and are commonly found in soil, dust and manure. Infection with tetanus causes severe muscle spasms, leading to "locking" of the jaw so the patient cannot open his/her mouth or swallow, and may even lead to death by suffocation. Tetanus is not transmitted from person to person.

Prevention

Vaccination is the best way to protect against tetanus. Due to widespread immunization, tetanus is now a rare disease in the U.S. A combination shot, called the Td vaccine, protects against both tetanus and diphtheria. A Td booster shot is recommended every 10 years. Adults who have never received immunization against tetanus should start with a 3-dose primary series given over 7–12 months.

Symptoms

Common first signs of tetanus are a headache and muscular stiffness in the jaw (lockjaw) followed by stiffness of the neck, difficulty in swallowing, rigidity of abdominal muscles, spasms, sweating and fever.

Symptoms usually begin 8 days after the infection, but may range in onset from 3 days to 3 weeks.

Who should get Td vaccine?

- All adults who have not had a Td booster shot in the last 10 years.
- Adults who have recovered from tetanus (lockjaw) disease.
- Adults who have never received immunization against tetanus.
- All adolescents and adults who deferred their regular booster during 2001–2002 because of shortages of the vaccine—the supply problems have been resolved.

Vaccine Safety

Tetanus vaccine and the combination Td vaccine are very safe and effective. When side effects do occur, they usually include soreness, redness or swelling at the injection site and a slight fever. As with any medicine, there are very small risks that serious problems, such as an allergic reaction or neurologic condition, could occur after getting a vaccine. However, the potential risks associated with tetanus disease are much greater than the potential risks associated with the tetanus vaccine. You cannot get tetanus from the vaccine.

Facts

- Tetanus can be prevented with a safe and effective vaccine.

- You cannot get tetanus from the vaccine.

- Tetanus is caused by a toxin produced by a type of bacteria found worldwide in soil, dust and manure.

- Tetanus is not transmitted from one person to another.

- Almost all reported cases of tetanus occur in persons who have either never been vaccinated, or those who completed a primary series but have not had a booster vaccination in the past 10 years.

- Approximately 11% of reported cases of tetanus are fatal. In the U.S., where 50 or fewer cases of tetanus occur each year, deaths are more likely to occur in persons 60 years of age and older.

- People with tetanus may have to spend several weeks in the hospital under intensive care.

- For adults, a tetanus-diphtheria (Td) shot every 10 years ensures protection against these two diseases.

- Recovery from tetanus illness may not result in immunity. Another infection could occur unless immunization is provided soon after the person's condition has stabilized.

Chapter 60

Urinary Tract Infections

Urinary tract infections are a serious health problem affecting millions of people each year.

Infections of the urinary tract are common—only respiratory infections occur more often. In 1997, urinary tract infections (UTIs) accounted for about 8.3 million doctor visits.* Women are especially prone to UTIs for reasons that are poorly understood. One woman in five develops a UTI during her lifetime. UTIs in men are not so common, but they can be very serious when they do occur.

The urinary system consists of the kidneys, ureters, bladder, and urethra. The key elements in the system are the kidneys, a pair of purplish-brown organs located below the ribs toward the middle of the back. The kidneys remove liquid waste from the blood in the form of urine, keep a stable balance of salts and other substances in the blood, and produce a hormone that aids the formation of red blood cells. Narrow tubes called ureters carry urine from the kidneys to the bladder, a triangle-shaped chamber in the lower abdomen. Urine is stored in the bladder and emptied through the urethra.

The average adult passes about a quart and a half of urine each day. The amount of urine varies, depending on the fluids and foods a person consumes. The volume formed at night is about half that formed in the daytime.

"Urinary Tract Infections in Adults," National Kidney and Urologic Diseases Information Clearinghouse (NKUDIC), National Institute of Diabetes and Digestive and Kidney Diseases (NIDDK), July 2002.

What Are the Causes of UTI?

Normal urine is sterile. It contains fluids, salts, and waste products, but it is free of bacteria, viruses, and fungi. An infection occurs when microorganisms, usually bacteria from the digestive tract, cling to the opening of the urethra and begin to multiply. Most infections arise from one type of bacteria, *Escherichia coli* (*E. coli*), which normally lives in the colon.

In most cases, bacteria first begin growing in the urethra. An infection limited to the urethra is called urethritis. From there bacteria often move on to the bladder, causing a bladder infection (cystitis). If the infection is not treated promptly, bacteria may then go up the ureters to infect the kidneys (pyelonephritis).

Microorganisms called *Chlamydia* and *Mycoplasma* may also cause UTIs in both men and women, but these infections tend to remain limited to the urethra and reproductive system. Unlike *E. coli*, *Chlamydia* and *Mycoplasma* may be sexually transmitted, and infections require treatment of both partners.

The urinary system is structured in a way that helps ward off infection. The ureters and bladder normally prevent urine from backing up toward the kidneys, and the flow of urine from the bladder helps wash bacteria out of the body. In men, the prostate gland produces secretions that slow bacterial growth. In both sexes, immune defenses also prevent infection. Despite these safeguards, though, infections still occur.

Who Is at Risk?

Some people are more prone to getting a UTI than others. Any abnormality of the urinary tract that obstructs the flow of urine (a kidney stone, for example) sets the stage for an infection. An enlarged prostate gland also can slow the flow of urine, thus raising the risk of infection.

A common source of infection is catheters, or tubes, placed in the bladder. A person who cannot void or who is unconscious or critically ill often needs a catheter that stays in place for a long time. Some people, especially the elderly or those with nervous system disorders who lose bladder control, may need a catheter for life. Bacteria on the catheter can infect the bladder, so hospital staff take special care to keep the catheter sterile and remove it as soon as possible.

People with diabetes have a higher risk of a UTI because of changes in the immune system. Any disorder that suppresses the immune system raises the risk of a urinary infection.

UTIs may occur in infants who are born with abnormalities of the urinary tract, which sometimes need to be corrected with surgery. UTIs are rarely seen in boys and young men. In women, though, the rate of UTIs gradually increases with age. Scientists are not sure why women have more urinary infections than men. One factor may be that a woman's urethra is short, allowing bacteria quick access to the bladder. Also, a woman's urethral opening is near sources of bacteria from the anus and vagina. For many women, sexual intercourse seems to trigger an infection, although the reasons for this linkage are unclear.

According to several studies, women who use a diaphragm are more likely to develop a UTI than women who use other forms of birth control. Recently, researchers found that women whose partners use a condom with spermicidal foam also tend to have growth of E. coli bacteria in the vagina.

Recurrent Infections

Many women suffer from frequent UTIs. Nearly 20 percent of women who have a UTI will have another, and 30 percent of those will have yet another. Of the last group, 80 percent will have recurrences.

Usually, the latest infection stems from a strain or type of bacteria that is different from the infection before it, indicating a separate infection. (Even when several UTIs in a row are due to E. coli, slight differences in the bacteria indicate distinct infections.)

Research funded by the National Institutes of Health (NIH) suggests that one factor behind recurrent UTIs may be the ability of bacteria to attach to cells lining the urinary tract. A recent NIH-funded study has also shown that women with recurrent UTIs tend to have certain blood types. Some scientists speculate that women with these blood types are more prone to UTIs because the cells lining the vagina and urethra may allow bacteria to attach more easily. Further research will show whether this association is sound and proves useful in identifying women at high risk for UTIs.

Infections in Pregnancy

Pregnant women seem no more prone to UTIs than other women. However, when a UTI does occur, it is more likely to travel to the kidneys. According to some reports, about 2 to 4 percent of pregnant women develop a urinary infection. Scientists think that hormonal

431

changes and shifts in the position of the urinary tract during pregnancy make it easier for bacteria to travel up the ureters to the kidneys. For this reason, many doctors recommend periodic testing of urine.

What Are the Symptoms of UTI?

Not everyone with a UTI has symptoms, but most people get at least some. These may include a frequent urge to urinate and a painful, burning feeling in the area of the bladder or urethra during urination. It is not unusual to feel bad all over—tired, shaky, washed out—and to feel pain even when not urinating. Often, women feel an uncomfortable pressure above the pubic bone, and some men experience a fullness in the rectum. It is common for a person with a urinary infection to complain that, despite the urge to urinate, only a small amount of urine is passed. The urine itself may look milky or cloudy, even reddish if blood is present. A fever may mean that the infection has reached the kidneys. Other symptoms of a kidney infection include pain in the back or side below the ribs, nausea, or vomiting.

In children, symptoms of a urinary infection may be overlooked or attributed to another disorder. A UTI should be considered when a child or infant seems irritable, is not eating normally, has an unexplained fever that does not go away, has incontinence or loose bowels, or is not thriving. The child should be seen by a doctor if there are any questions about these symptoms, especially if there is a change in the child's urinary pattern.

How Is UTI Diagnosed?

To find out whether you have a UTI, your doctor will test a sample of urine for pus and bacteria. You will be asked to give a "clean catch" urine sample by washing the genital area and collecting a "midstream" sample of urine in a sterile container. (This method of collecting urine helps prevent bacteria around the genital area from getting into the sample and confusing the test results.) Usually, the sample is sent to a laboratory, although some doctors' offices are equipped to do the testing.

In the urinalysis test, the urine is examined for white and red blood cells and bacteria. Then the bacteria are grown in a culture and tested against different antibiotics to see which drug best destroys the bacteria. This last step is called a sensitivity test.

Some microbes, like Chlamydia and Mycoplasma, can be detected only with special bacterial cultures. A doctor suspects one of these infections when a person has symptoms of a UTI and pus in the urine, but a standard culture fails to grow any bacteria.

When an infection does not clear up with treatment and is traced to the same strain of bacteria, the doctor will order a test that makes images of the urinary tract. One of these tests is an intravenous pyelogram (IVP), which gives x-ray images of the bladder, kidneys, and ureters. An opaque dye visible on x-ray film is injected into a vein, and a series of x-rays is taken. The film shows an outline of the urinary tract, revealing even small changes in the structure of the tract.

If you have recurrent infections, your doctor also may recommend an ultrasound exam, which gives pictures from the echo patterns of sound waves bounced back from internal organs. Another useful test is cystoscopy. A cystoscope is an instrument made of a hollow tube with several lenses and a light source, which allows the doctor to see inside the bladder from the urethra.

How Is UTI Treated?

UTIs are treated with antibacterial drugs. The choice of drug and length of treatment depend on the patient's history and the urine tests that identify the offending bacteria. The sensitivity test is especially useful in helping the doctor select the most effective drug. The drugs most often used to treat routine, uncomplicated UTIs are trimethoprim (Trimpex), trimethoprim/sulfamethoxazole (Bactrim, Septra, Cotrim), amoxicillin (Amoxil, Trimox, Wymox), nitrofurantoin (Macrodantin, Furadantin), and ampicillin. A class of drugs called quinolones includes four drugs approved in recent years for treating UTI. These drugs include ofloxacin (Floxin), norfloxacin (Noroxin), ciprofloxacin (Cipro), and trovafloxacin (Trovan).

Often, a UTI can be cured with 1 or 2 days of treatment if the infection is not complicated by an obstruction or nervous system disorder. Still, many doctors ask their patients to take antibiotics for a week or two to ensure that the infection has been cured. Single-dose treatment is not recommended for some groups of patients, for example, those who have delayed treatment or have signs of a kidney infection, patients with diabetes or structural abnormalities, or men who have prostate infections. Longer treatment is also needed by patients with infections caused by *Mycoplasma* or *Chlamydia*, which are usually treated with tetracycline, trimethoprim/sulfamethoxazole (TMP/SMZ), or doxycycline. A followup urinalysis helps to confirm that the urinary tract is infection-free. It is important to take the full course of treatment because symptoms may disappear before the infection is fully cleared.

Severely ill patients with kidney infections may be hospitalized until they can take fluids and needed drugs on their own. Kidney infections generally require several weeks of antibiotic treatment. Researchers at the University of Washington found that 2-week therapy with TMP/SMZ was as effective as 6 weeks of treatment with the same drug in women with kidney infections that did not involve an obstruction or nervous system disorder. In such cases, kidney infections rarely lead to kidney damage or kidney failure unless they go untreated.

Various drugs are available to relieve the pain of a UTI. A heating pad may also help. Most doctors suggest that drinking plenty of water helps cleanse the urinary tract of bacteria. For the time being, it is best to avoid coffee, alcohol, and spicy foods. (And one of the best things a smoker can do for his or her bladder is to quit smoking. Smoking is the major known cause of bladder cancer.)

Recurrent Infections in Women

Women who have had three UTIs are likely to continue having them. Four out of five such women get another within 18 months of the last UTI. Many women have them even more often. A woman who has frequent recurrences (three or more a year) should ask her doctor about one of the following treatment options:

- Take low doses of an antibiotic such as TMP/SMZ or nitrofurantoin daily for 6 months or longer. (If taken at bedtime, the drug remains in the bladder longer and may be more effective.) NIH-supported research at the University of Washington has shown this therapy to be effective without causing serious side effects.

- Take a single dose of an antibiotic after sexual intercourse.

- Take a short course (1 or 2 days) of antibiotics when symptoms appear.

Dipsticks that change color when an infection is present are now available without prescription. The strips detect nitrite, which is formed when bacteria change nitrate in the urine to nitrite. The test can detect about 90 percent of UTIs when used with the first morning urine specimen and may be useful for women who have recurrent infections.

Doctors suggest some additional steps that a woman can take on her own to avoid an infection:

- Drink plenty of water every day.

- Urinate when you feel the need; don't resist the urge to urinate.
- Wipe from front to back to prevent bacteria around the anus from entering the vagina or urethra.
- Take showers instead of tub baths.
- Cleanse the genital area before sexual intercourse.
- Avoid using feminine hygiene sprays and scented douches, which may irritate the urethra.
- Some doctors suggest drinking cranberry juice.

Infections in Pregnancy

A pregnant woman who develops a UTI should be treated promptly to avoid premature delivery of her baby and other risks such as high blood pressure. Some antibiotics are not safe to take during pregnancy. In selecting the best treatments, doctors consider various factors such as the drug's effectiveness, the stage of pregnancy, the mother's health, and potential effects on the fetus.

Complicated Infections

Curing infections that stem from a urinary obstruction or nervous system disorder depends on finding and correcting the underlying problem, sometimes with surgery. If the root cause goes untreated, this group of patients is at risk of kidney damage. Also, such infections tend to arise from a wider range of bacteria, and sometimes from more than one type of bacteria at a time.

Infections in Men

UTIs in men usually stem from an obstruction—for example, a urinary stone or enlarged prostate—or from a medical procedure involving a catheter. The first step is to identify the infecting organism and the drugs to which it is sensitive. Usually, doctors recommend lengthier therapy in men than in women, in part to prevent infections of the prostate gland.

Prostate infections (chronic bacterial prostatitis) are harder to cure because antibiotics are unable to penetrate infected prostate tissue effectively. For this reason, men with prostatitis often need long-term treatment with a carefully selected antibiotic. UTIs in older men are frequently associated with acute bacterial prostatitis, which can be fatal if not treated immediately.

Is There a Vaccine to Prevent Recurrent UTIs?

In the future, scientists may develop a vaccine that can prevent UTIs from coming back. Researchers in different studies have found that children and women who tend to get UTIs repeatedly are likely to lack proteins called immunoglobulins, which fight infection. Children and women who do not get UTIs are more likely to have normal levels of immunoglobulins in their genital and urinary tracts.

Early tests indicate that a vaccine helps patients build up their own natural infection-fighting powers. The dead bacteria in the vaccine do not spread like an infection; instead, they prompt the body to produce antibodies that can later fight against live organisms. Researchers are testing injection and oral vaccines to see which works best. Another method being considered for women is to apply the vaccine directly as a suppository in the vagina.

Suggestions for Additional Reading

The following materials can be found in medical libraries, many college and university libraries, and through inter-library loan in most public libraries. Internet addresses are given for materials available on the World Wide Web.

Answers to Your Questions About Urinary Tract Infections. A patient information booklet prepared by the Bladder Health Council, American Foundation for Urologic Disease, 1128 North Charles Street, Baltimore, MD 21201. Phone: (410) 468-1800; fax: (410) 468-1808.

Blumberg, Emily A., and Abrutyn, Elias. (1997). Methods for the reduction of urinary tract infection. *Current Opinion in Urology*, 7, 47-51.

Gillenwater, Jay A., et al. (Eds.). (1996). *Adult and pediatric urology*. (3rd ed.). St. Louis: Mosby-Year Book.

Kunin, Calvin M. (1997). *Urinary tract infections: Detection, prevention, and management*. (5th ed.). Baltimore: Williams & Wilkins.

Uehling, David T., et al. (1995). Vaginal mucosal immunization in recurrent UTIs. *Infections in Urology* 8(2):57-61.

Urinary Tract Infections in Children. A patient education fact sheet prepared by the National Institute of Diabetes and Digestive and Kidney Diseases, NIH, 2000.

Walsh, Patrick C., et al. (Eds.). (1997). *Campbell's urology.* (Vol. 1, 7th ed.). Philadelphia: W. B. Saunders.

Additional Resources

More information is available from

American Foundation for Urologic Disease
1128 North Charles Street
Baltimore, MD 21201
Phone: 1-800-242-2383 or (410) 727-2908
E-mail: admin@afud.org
Website: http://www.afud.org

The Prostatitis Foundation
1063 30th Street, Box 8
Smithshire, IL 61478
Phone: 1-888-891-4200
Fax: (309) 325-7184
E-mail: mailto:Mcaoston@aol.com
Website: http://www.prostatitis.org

The U.S. Government does not endorse or favor any specific commercial product or company. Trade, proprietary, or company names appearing in this document are used only because they are considered necessary in the context of the information provided. If a product is not mentioned, this does not mean or imply that the product is unsatisfactory.

National Kidney and Urologic Diseases Information Clearinghouse
3 Information Way
Bethesda, MD 20892-3580
E-mail: http://kidney.niddk.nih.gov/about/contact.htm

The National Kidney and Urologic Diseases Information Clearinghouse (NKUDIC) is a service of the National Institute of Diabetes and Digestive and Kidney Diseases (NIDDK). The NIDDK is part of the National Institutes of Health under the U.S. Department of Health and Human Services. Established in 1987, the clearinghouse provides information about diseases of the kidneys and urologic system to people with kidney and urologic disorders and to their families, health care professionals, and the public. NKUDIC answers inquiries, develops and distributes publications, and works closely with professional and patient organizations and Government agencies to coordinate resources about kidney and urologic diseases.

Publications produced by the clearinghouse are carefully reviewed by both NIDDK scientists and outside experts.

Note

Ambulatory Care Visits to Physician Offices, Hospital Outpatient Departments, and Emergency Departments: United States, 1997. Atlanta, GA: National Center for Health Statistics, Centers for Disease Control and Prevention, U.S. Dept. of Health and Human Services; November 1999. Vital and Health Statistics. Series 13, No. 143.

Part Five

The Threat of Bioterrorism

Chapter 61

Be Informed Regarding Biological Threats

Biological Threats

Overview

A biological attack is the deliberate release of germs or other biological substances that can make you sick. Many agents must be inhaled, enter through a cut in the skin, or be eaten to make you sick. Some biological agents, such as anthrax, do not cause contagious diseases. Others, like the smallpox virus, can result in diseases you can catch from other people.

If There Is a Biological Threat

Unlike an explosion, a biological attack may or may not be immediately obvious. While it is possible that you will see signs of a biological attack, as was sometimes the case with the anthrax mailings, it is perhaps more likely that local health care workers will report a pattern of unusual illness or there will be a wave of sick people seeking emergency medical attention. You will probably learn of the danger through an emergency radio or TV broadcast, or some other signal used in your community. You might get a telephone call or emergency response workers may come to your door.

"Biological Threat," U.S. Department of Homeland Security, 2003, "Public Health Emergency Preparedness and Response: Other FAQs," Centers for Disease Control and Prevention (CDC), October 2001, and "Biothreats—Are Claims to Treat Really Just a Trick?," Federal Trade Commission (FTC), February 2002.

In the event of a biological attack, public health officials may not immediately be able to provide information on what you should do. It will take time to determine exactly what the illness is, how it should be treated, and who is in danger. However, you should watch TV, listen to the radio, or check the Internet for official news including the following:

- Are you in the group or area authorities consider in danger?
- What are the signs and symptoms of the disease?
- Are medications or vaccines being distributed?
- Where?
- Who should get them?
- Where should you seek emergency medical care if you become sick?

Protect Yourself

If you become aware of an unusual and suspicious release of an unknown substance nearby, it doesn't hurt to protect yourself. Quickly get away. Cover your mouth and nose with layers of fabric that can filter the air but still allow breathing. Examples include two to three layers of cotton such as a t-shirt, handkerchief, or towel. Otherwise, several layers of tissue or paper towels may help. Wash with soap and water and contact authorities.

Symptoms and Hygiene

At the time of a declared biological emergency, if a family member becomes sick, it is important to be suspicious. Do not automatically assume, however, that you should go to a hospital emergency room or that any illness is the result of the biological attack. Symptoms of many common illnesses may overlap. Use common sense, practice good hygiene and cleanliness to avoid spreading germs, and seek medical advice.

Frequently Asked Questions: Preparedness and Response

What should I do to be prepared?

We continue to hear stories of the public buying gas masks and hoarding medicine in anticipation of a possible bioterrorist or chemical attack. We do not recommend either. As Secretary Thompson said recently, people should not be scared into thinking they need a gas mask. In the event of a public health emergency, local and state health departments will inform the public about the actions individuals need to take.

Does every city have an adequate emergency response system, especially one geared for a bioterrorist attack? How quickly can it be implemented?

The emergency response system varies from community to community on the basis of each community's investment in its public health infrastructure. Some components of these emergency systems can be implemented very quickly, while others may take longer.

Are hospitals prepared to handle a sudden surge in demand for health care?

The preparedness level in hospitals depends on the biological agent used in an attack. Because a sudden surge in demand could overwhelm an individual hospital's resources, hospitals collaborate with other hospitals in their area in order to respond to a bioterrorist attack on a citywide or regional basis. Hospitals are required to maintain disaster response plans and to practice applying them as part of their accreditation process. Many components of such plans are useful in responding to bioterrorism. Specific plans for bioterrorism have been added to the latest accreditation requirements of the Joint Commission on Accreditation of Healthcare Organizations. In an emergency, local medical care capacity will be supplemented with federal resources.

Are health department labs equipped/capable of doing testing?

CDC, the Association of Public Health Laboratories, and other officials are working together to ensure that all state health departments are capable of obtaining results of tests on suspected infectious agents. The nation's laboratories are generally classified as Level A, B, C, or D. Level A laboratories are those typically found in community hospitals and are designated to perform initial testing on all clinical specimens. Public health laboratories are usually Level B; these laboratories can confirm or refute preliminary test results and can usually perform antimicrobial susceptibility tests. Level C laboratories, which are reference facilities and can be public health laboratories, perform more rapid identification tests. Level D laboratories are designed to perform the most sophisticated tests and are located in federal facilities such as CDC. CDC is currently working with public and private laboratory partners to develop a formal a National Laboratory System linking all four Levels.

Every state has a Laboratory Response Network (LRN) contact. The LRN links state and local public health laboratories with advanced-capacity laboratories, including clinical, military, veterinary, agricultural, water, and food-testing laboratories. Laboratorians should contact their state public health laboratory to identify their local LRN representative.

With all this talk about possible biochemical agents, just how safe is our water? Should I be disinfecting my water just in case?

The United States public water supply system is one of the safest in the world. The general public should continue to drink and use water just as they would under normal conditions. Your local water treatment supplier and local governments are on the alert for any unusual activity and will notify you immediately in the event of any public health threat. At this point, we have no reason to believe that additional measures need to be taken.

The U.S. Environmental Protection Agency (EPA) is the lead federal agency that makes recommendations about water utility issues. The EPA is working closely with the CDC and the U.S. Departments of Defense and Energy to help water agencies assess their systems, determine actions that need to be taken to guard against possible attack, and develop emergency response plans. For more information, visit http://www.epa.gov/safewater.

Biothreats—Are Claims To Treat Really Just A Trick?

In the aftermath of the anthrax scare last fall (2001), some marketers are trying to cash in on consumers' heightened fears and vulnerabilities, plying products that claim to detect, prevent, protect against, or treat biological and chemical agents.

The Federal Trade Commission (FTC) and other law enforcement authorities have examined hundreds of sites marketing gas masks, protective suits, biohazard test kits, colloidal silver, oregano oil, and similar products that claim to be safe and effective against biological or chemical contamination. But according to the FTC, consumers should greet these claims with a healthy dose of skepticism.

Officials at the nation's consumer protection agency say many of these products simply can't do what they claim. For example, kits marketed to detect the presence of anthrax in your surroundings have almost never been tested on actual anthrax spores. At best, says the agency, that would make them ineffective. But the products also can be inaccurate and unreliable. False positive results could create unnecessary anxiety for consumers, and even worse, a false negative result could delay medical treatment in the unlikely event a consumer was exposed to anthrax spores.

Fraudulent promoters also are offering dietary supplements, like colloidal silver, zinc mineral water, and oregano oil, as treatments for contamination from biological agents. The FTC is not aware of any scientific basis for these self-treatment alternatives. Indeed, the leading dietary supplement industry trade associations have urged dietary supplement sellers not to promote any dietary supplement for the prevention, cure, or treatment of anthrax.

For consumers who are worried about preventing, detecting, or treating biological or chemical threats, the FTC suggests that you:

- Consult your physician immediately if you believe you have been exposed to anthrax or any other biological or chemical agent.

- Cut claims down to size. When you see claims that a product can, say, "eliminate all pathogens in the human body in six minutes or less," it's time for a reality check. If any product really did that, wouldn't you have heard it first on the news—not in an ad?

- Check out your source. Appearances can be deceiving. Many fraudulent businesses either use names that sound like established legitimate organizations or sell products that imitate respected, well-known brands. How can you know if a business is legitimate? It can be tricky. Ask questions, do some research and check with local consumer protection agencies.

The FTC works for the consumer to prevent fraudulent, deceptive and unfair business practices in the marketplace and to provide information to help consumers spot, stop, and avoid them. To file a complaint or to get free information on consumer issues, visit http://www.ftc.gov or call toll-free, 1-877-FTC-HELP (1-877-382-4357); TTY:

1-866-653-4261. The FTC enters internet, telemarketing, identity theft, and other fraud-related complaints into Consumer Sentinel, a secure, online database available to hundreds of civil and criminal law enforcement agencies in the U.S. and abroad.

Chapter 62

Biological Weapons: Agents of Special Concern

Anthrax

The October 2001 anthrax attacks were conducted via five envelopes containing *B. anthracis* that were sent through the U.S. postal system. All were mailed from Trenton, New Jersey, and all letters contained spores identified as the Ames strain. Twenty-two cases of anthrax resulted—eleven inhalational, eleven cutaneous. In all, five people died from inhalational anthrax.

For those who developed inhalational anthrax following the October 2001 attacks, common symptoms included fever, shortness of

This chapter includes "Anthrax Fact Sheet, 2002," © 2002 Center for Biosecurity of the University of Pittsburgh Medical Center, "Botulinum Toxin Fact Sheet," © 2001 Center for Biosecurity of the University of Pittsburgh Medical Center, "Plague Fact Sheet," © 2000 Center for Biosecurity of the University of Pittsburgh Medical Center, "Smallpox Fact Sheet," © 1999 Center for Biosecurity of the University of Pittsburgh Medical Center, "Tularemia Fact Sheet," © 2001 Center for Biosecurity of the University of Pittsburgh Medical Center, and "Viral Hemorrhagic Fevers Fact Sheet" © 2002 Center for Biosecurity of the University of Pittsburgh Medical Center. These factsheets are reprinted with permission of the Center for Biosecurity of the University of Pittsburgh Medical Center, www.upmcbiosecurity.org. All rights reserved. This chapter also includes "Glanders," reviewed 2001; "Melioidosis (*Burkholderia pseudomallei*)," reviewed 2000; and "Q Fever," reviewed 2003 which are from the Division of Bacterial and Mycotic Diseases, National Center for Infectious Diseases, Centers for Disease Control and Prevention (CDC), www.cdc.gov/ncidod/dbmd/diseaseinfo. For comprehensive CDC information about bioterrorism and related issues, please visit http://www.bt.cdc.gov.

breath, cough, nausea, malaise, headache, sweats, chest pain. All of the first ten patients who presented with inhalational anthrax in October 2001 had abnormal chest x-ray film results, and CT scans were abnormal for the eight patients on whom scans were conducted. Blood cultures were positive in all those patients who had cultures obtained prior to the initiation of antibiotics.

The diagnosis of cutaneous anthrax proved difficult to make in a number of cases following the October 2001 attacks. One case has been reported in great detail and is particularly instructive. This was the case of a seven month old infant who presented with a depressed black eschar on the skin. The diagnosis was initially unclear, and the infection progressed rapidly into severe systemic illness. Following recognition of cutaneous anthrax and initiation of proper therapy, the child made a full clinical recovery. Although the mortality rate from cutaneous anthrax has been reported to be as high as 20% without antibiotics, death due to cutaneous anthrax following initiation of antibiotic treatment is reported to be rare. None of cutaneous anthrax cases that followed the October 2001 attacks were fatal. No gastrointestinal anthrax cases were reported in connection with the October 2001 attacks.

As of 2002, there is a limited supply of the licensed anthrax vaccine AVA currently available. However there is only one anthrax vaccine manufacturer in the U.S., and supplies remain too limited to consider widespread vaccination programs. The Institute of Medicine recently concluded that AVA is safe and efficacious against aerosol challenge of anthrax spores. There are a number of studies underway with AVA to determine if the vaccine can be administered with a lower side effect profile and whether protection can be achieved with less than the currently recommended 6 inoculations. Research is also underway to develop a recombinant anthrax vaccine.

The Working Group recommends that treatment for inhalational anthrax include either ciprofloxacin (or other fluoroquinolone antibiotics) or doxycycline in addition to a second antibiotic with efficacy against *B. anthracis*. For details regarding treatment and post-exposure prophylaxis recommendations of the Working Group, please see Inglesby TV, et al. 2002. Anthrax as a biological weapon 2002: Updated recommendations for management. *JAMA.* 287(17).

Note: "Anthrax Fact Sheet" http://www.upmcbiosecurity.org/pages/agents/anthrax_facts_2002.html Source: Inglesby TV, O'Toole T, Henderson, DA Bartlett JG, Ascher, MS, Eitzen E, Friedlander AM, Gerberding J, Hauer J, Hughes J, McDade J, Osterholm MT, Parker G, Perl TM, Russell PK, Tonat K, for the Working Group on Civilian

Biodefense 2002. Anthrax as a biological weapon, 2002: Updated recommendations for management. *JAMA*.287(17).

Botulinum Toxin

Botulinum toxin poses a major bioweapons threat because of its extreme potency and lethality; its ease of production, transport and misuse; and the potential need for prolonged intensive care in affected persons. Botulinum toxin is the single most poisonous substance known.

A number of states named by the U.S. State Department as "state sponsors of terrorism" have developed or are developing botulinum toxin as a biological weapon. Aum Shinrikyo tried but failed to use botulinum toxin as a biological weapon.

Botulinum toxin is derived from the genus of anaerobic bacteria named *Clostridia*. Seven antigenic types of botulinum toxin exist, designated from A through G. They can be identified based on antibody cross reactivity studies—i.e., anti-A toxin antibodies do not neutralize the B through G toxins.

Naturally occurring botulism is the disease that results from the absorption of botulinum toxin into the circulation from a mucosal surface (gut, lung) or a wound. It does not penetrate intact skin. The toxin irreversibly binds to peripheral cholinergic synapses, preventing the release of the neurotransmitter acetylcholine from the terminal end of motor neurons. This leads to muscle paralysis, and in severe cases, can lead to a need for mechanical respiration.

The incubation period for food-borne botulism can be from 2 hours to 8 days after ingestion, depending on the dose of the bacteria or the toxin. The average incubation period is 12–72 hours after ingestion. Patients with botulism typically present with difficulty speaking, seeing and/or swallowing. Prominent neurologic findings in all forms of botulism include ptosis, diplopia, blurred vision, dysarthria and dysphagia. Patients typically are afebrile and do not have an altered level of consciousness. Patients may initially present with gastrointestinal distress, nausea, and vomiting preceding neurological symptoms. Symptoms are similar for all toxin types, but the severity of illness can vary widely, in part depending on the amount of toxin absorbed. Recovery from paralysis can take from weeks to months and requires the growth of new motor nerve endings. **In the event botulism is suspected, the hospital epidemiologist and local and state health departments should be contacted immediately.**

Natural cases of botulism are rare and typically result from food contamination. Many types of food have been associated in outbreaks in the past, with the common factor being that implicated food items were not heated or were incompletely heated. Heat > 85°C inactivates the toxin. The largest botulism outbreak in the U.S. in the past century occurred in 1977, when 59 people became ill from poorly preserved jalapeño peppers.

No cases of waterborne botulism have ever been reported. This is likely due to the large amount of toxin needed, and the fact that the toxin is easily neutralized by common water treatment techniques.

A deliberate aerosol or food-borne release of botulinum toxin could be detected by several features including: a large number of acute cases presenting all at once; cases involving an uncommon toxin type (C, D, F, G, or non-aquatic food associated E); patients with a common geographic factor but without a common dietary exposure; and, multiple simultaneous outbreaks without a common source.

Diagnosis and testing are available at the CDC and some local and state laboratories. The standard test for the toxin is the mouse bioassay. Unfortunately, this assay is time consuming. Future development is focused on rapid diagnosis/detection. Polymerase Chain Reaction (PCR) assays that can detect the *Clostridia spp.* bacterial DNA toxin sequences are currently under development. Enzyme Linked Immuno-Sorbent Assays (ELISAs) are being developed to detect functionally active toxins.

In the event that there is a clinical suspicion of botulinum toxin, treatment with antitoxin should not be delayed for microbiological testing. In the U.S., licensed botulinum antitoxin is available from the CDC via state and local health departments. An investigational heptavalent antitoxin is held by the U.S. Army. Optimal therapy for botulism requires early suspicion of the disease and prompt administration of antitoxin in conjunction with supportive care. Supportive care for patients with botulism may include mechanical ventilators in the intensive care unit, parenteral nutrition, and treatment of secondary infections.

An investigational botulinum toxoid is used to provide immunity for laboratory workers. It has been used to provide immunity against botulinum toxin over the past 30 years. However, supply of the toxoid is limited, and use of it would eliminate possible beneficial uses of toxoid for medical purposes. The toxoid induces immunity over several months and so would not be effective for rapid, post-exposure prophylaxis.

Existing technologies could produce large reserves of human antibody against the botulinum toxin. Administration of such a therapy could provide immunity of up to a month or greater and obviate the need for rationing the equine antitoxin. The development of such a human antibody reserve would require sufficient resources be dedicated to this problem.

Note: "Botulinum Toxin" http://www.upmcbiosecurity.org/pages/ agents/botulism_facts.html Source: Amon SS, Scheehter R, Inglesby TV, Henderson DA, Bartlett JG, Ascher MS, Eitzen E, Fine AD, Hauer J, Layton M, Lillibridge S, Osterholm MT, O'Tolle T, Parker G, Perl TM, Russell PK, Swerdlow DL, Tonat K, for the Working Group on Civilian Biodefense. 2001. Botulinum toxin as a biological weapon: Medical and public health management. *JAMA*. 285(8). Reprinted with permission of the Center for Biosecurity of the University of Pittsburgh Medical Center, www.upmc-biosecurity.org © February 2001 Center for Biosecurity of the University of Pittsburgh Medical Center. All rights reserved.

*Glanders (*Burkholderia mallei*)*

What is glanders?

Glanders is an infectious disease that is caused by the bacterium *Burkholderia mallei*. Glanders is primarily a disease affecting horses, but it also affects donkeys and mules and can be naturally contracted by goats, dogs, and cats. Human infection, although not seen in the United States since 1945, has occurred rarely and sporadically among laboratory workers and those in direct and prolonged contact with infected, domestic animals.

Why has glanders become a current issue?

Burkholderia mallei is an organism that is associated with infections in laboratory workers because so very few organisms are required to cause disease. The organism has been considered as a potential agent for biological warfare and of biological terrorism.

How common is glanders?

The United States has not seen any naturally occurring cases since the 1940s. However, it is still commonly seen among domestic animals in Africa, Asia, the Middle East, and Central and South America.

How is glanders transmitted and who can get it?

Glanders is transmitted to humans by direct contact with infected animals. The bacteria enter the body through the skin and through mucosal surfaces of the eyes and nose. The sporadic cases have been documented in veterinarians, horse caretakers, and laboratorians.

What are the symptoms of glanders?

The symptoms of glanders depend upon the route of infection with the organism. The types of infection include localized, pus-forming cutaneous infections, pulmonary infections, bloodstream infections, and chronic suppurative infections of the skin. Generalized symptoms of glanders include fever, muscle aches, chest pain, muscle tightness, and headache. Additional symptoms have included excessive tearing of the eyes, light sensitivity, and diarrhea.

- Localized infections: If there is a cut or scratch in the skin, a localized infection with ulceration will develop within 1 to 5 days at the site where the bacteria entered the body. Swollen lymph nodes may also be apparent. Infections involving the mucous membranes in the eyes, nose, and respiratory tract will cause increased mucus production from the affected sites.

- Pulmonary infections: In pulmonary infections, pneumonia, pulmonary abscesses, and pleural effusion can occur. Chest x-rays will show localized infection in the lobes of the lungs.

- Bloodstream infections: Glanders bloodstream infections are usually fatal within 7 to 10 days.

- Chronic infections: The chronic form of glanders involves multiple abscesses within the muscles of the arms and legs or in the spleen or liver.

Where is glanders usually found?

Geographically, the disease is endemic in Africa, Asia, the Middle East, and Central and South America.

How is glanders diagnosed?

The disease is diagnosed in the laboratory by isolating *Burkholderia mallei* from blood, sputum, urine, or skin lesions. Serologic assays are not available.

Can glanders spread from person to person?

In addition to animal exposure, cases of human-to-human transmission have been reported. These cases included two suggested cases of sexual transmission and several cases in family members who cared for the patients.

Is there a way to prevent infection?

There is no vaccine available for glanders. In countries where glanders is endemic in animals, prevention of the disease in humans involves identification and elimination of the infection in the animal population. Within the health care setting, transmission can be prevented by using common blood and body fluid precautions.

Is there a treatment for glanders?

Because human cases of glanders are rare, there is limited information about antibiotic treatment of the organism in humans. Sulfadiazine has been found to be an effective in experimental animals and in humans. *Burkholderia mallei* is usually sensitive to tetracyclines, ciprofloxacin, streptomycin, novobiocin, gentamicin, imipenem, ceftazidime, and the sulfonamides. Resistance to chloramphenicol has been reported.

*Melioidosis (*Burkholderia pseudomallei*)*

What is melioidosis?

Melioidosis, also called Whitmore's disease, is an infectious disease caused by the bacterium *Burkholderia pseudomallei*. Melioidosis is clinically and pathologically similar to glanders disease, but the ecology and epidemiology of melioidosis are different from glanders. Melioidosis is predominately a disease of tropical climates, especially in Southeast Asia where it is endemic. The bacteria causing melioidosis are found in contaminated water and soil and are spread to humans and animals through direct contact with the contaminated source. Glanders is contracted by humans from infected domestic animals.

Why has melioidosis become a current issue?

Burkholderia pseudomallei is an organism that has been considered as a potential agent for biological warfare and biological terrorism.

How common is melioidosis and where is it found?

Melioidosis is endemic in Southeast Asia, with the greatest concentration of cases reported in Vietnam, Cambodia, Laos, Thailand,

Malaysia, Myanmar (Burma), and northern Australia. Additionally, it is seen in the South Pacific, Africa, India, and the Middle East. In many of these countries, *Burkholderia pseudomallei* is so prevalent that it is a common contaminate found on laboratory cultures. Moreover, it has been a common pathogen isolated from troops of all nationalities that have served in areas with endemic disease. A few isolated cases of melioidosis have occurred in the Western Hemisphere in Mexico, Panama, Ecuador, Haiti, Brazil, Peru, Guyana, and in the states of Hawaii and Georgia. In the United States, confirmed cases range from none to five each year and occur among travelers and immigrants.

How is melioidosis transmitted and who can get it?

Besides humans, many animal species are susceptible to melioidosis. These include sheep, goats, horses, swine, cattle, dogs, and cats. Transmission occurs by direct contact with contaminated soil and surface waters. In Southeast Asia, the organism has been repeatedly isolated from agriculture fields, with infection occurring primarily during the rainy season. Humans and animals are believed to acquire the infection by inhalation of dust, ingestion of contaminated water, and contact with contaminated soil especially through skin abrasions, and for military troops, by contamination of war wounds. Person-to-person transmission can occur. There is one report of transmission to a sister with diabetes who was the caretaker for her brother who had chronic melioidosis. Two cases of sexual transmission have been reported. Transmission in both cases was preceded by a clinical history of chronic prostatitis in the source patient.

What are the symptoms of melioidosis?

Illness from melioidosis can be categorized as acute or localized infection, acute pulmonary infection, acute bloodstream infection, and chronic suppurative infection. Inapparent infections are also possible. The incubation period (time between exposure and appearance of clinical symptoms) is not clearly defined, but may range from 2 days to many years.

- Acute, localized infection: This form of infection is generally localized as a nodule and results from inoculation through a break in the skin. The acute form of melioidosis can produce fever and general muscle aches, and may progress rapidly to infect the bloodstream.

- Pulmonary infection: This form of the disease can produce a clinical picture of mild bronchitis to severe pneumonia. The onset of pulmonary melioidosis is typically accompanied by a high fever, headache, anorexia, and general muscle soreness. Chest pain is common, but a nonproductive or productive cough with normal sputum is the hallmark of this form of melioidosis.

- Acute bloodstream infection: Patients with underlying illness such as HIV, renal failure, and diabetes are affected by this type of the disease, which usually results in septic shock. The symptoms of the bloodstream infection vary depending on the site of original infection, but they generally include respiratory distress, severe headache, fever, diarrhea, development of pus-filled lesions on the skin, muscle tenderness, and disorientation. This is typically an infection of short duration, and abscesses will be found throughout the body.

- Chronic suppurative infection: Chronic melioidosis is an infection that involves the organs of the body. These typically include the joints, viscera, lymph nodes, skin, brain, liver, lung, bones, and spleen.

How is melioidosis diagnosed?

Melioidosis is diagnosed by isolating *Burkholderia pseudomallei* from the blood, urine, sputum, or skin lesions. Detecting and measuring antibodies to the bacteria in the blood is another means of diagnosis.

Can melioidosis be spread from person to person?

Melioidosis can spread from person to person by contact with the blood and body fluids of an infected person. Two documented cases of male-to-female sexual transmission involved males with chronic prostatic infection due to melioidosis.

Is there a way to prevent infection?

There is no vaccine for melioidosis. Prevention of the infection in endemic-disease areas can be difficult since contact with contaminated soil is so common. Persons with diabetes and skin lesions should avoid contact with soil and standing water in these areas. Wearing boots during agricultural work can prevent infection through the feet and lower legs. In health care settings, using common blood and body fluid precautions can prevent transmission.

Is there a treatment for melioidosis?

Most cases of melioidosis can be treated with appropriate antibiotics. *Burkholderia pseudomallei,* the organism that causes melioidosis, is usually sensitive to imipenem, penicillin, doxycycline, amoxicillin-clavulanic acid, azlocillin, ceftazidime, ticarcillin-vulanic acid, ceftriaxone, and aztreonam. Treatment should be initiated early in the course of the disease. Although bloodstream infection with melioidosis can be fatal, the other types of the disease are nonfatal. The type of infection and the course of treatment can predict any long-term sequelae.

Plague

Plague, the disease caused by the bacteria *Yersinia pestis* (*Y. pestis*), has had a profound impact on human history. In AD 541, the first great plague pandemic began in Egypt and swept over the world in the next four years.

Population losses attributable to plague during those years were between 50 and 60 percent. In 1346, the second plague pandemic, also known as the Black Death or the Great Pestilence, erupted and within 5 years had ravaged the Middle East and killed more than 13 million in China and 20–30 million in Europe, one third of the European population.

Advances in living conditions, public health and antibiotic therapy make such natural pandemics improbable, but plague outbreaks following an attack with a biological weapon do pose a serious threat.

Plague is one of very few diseases that can create widespread panic following the discovery of even a small number of cases. This was apparent in Surat, India, in 1994, when an estimated 500,000 persons fled the city in fear of a plague epidemic.

In the 1950s and 1960s, the U.S. and Soviet biological weapons programs developed techniques to directly aerosolize plague particles, a technique that leads to pneumonic plague, an otherwise uncommon, highly lethal and potentially contagious form of plague. A modern attack would most probably occur via aerosol dissemination of *Y. pestis,* and the ensuing outbreak would be almost entirely pneumonic plague.

More than 10 institutes and thousands of scientists were reported to have worked with plague in the former Soviet Union.

Given the availability of *Y. pestis* in microbe banks around the world, reports that techniques for mass production and aerosol dissemination of plague have been developed, the high fatality rate in untreated cases and the potential for secondary spread, a biological attack with plague is a serious concern.

An understanding of the epidemiology, clinical presentation and the recommended medical and public health response following a biological attack with plague could substantially decrease the morbidity and mortality of such an event.

A plague outbreak developing after the use of a biological weapon would follow a very different epidemiologic pattern than a naturally occurring plague epidemic.

The size of a pneumonic plague epidemic following an aerosol attack would depend on a number of factors, including the amount of agent used, the meteorological conditions and methods of aerosolization and dissemination.

A group of initial pneumonic cases would appear in about 1–2 days following the aerosol cloud exposure, with many people dying quickly after symptom onset. Human experience and animal studies suggest that the incubation period in this setting is 1 to 6 days.

A 1970 World Health Organization assessment asserted that, in a worst case scenario, a dissemination of 50 kg of *Y. pestis* in an aerosol cloud over a city of 5 million might result in 150,000 cases of pneumonic plague, 80,000–100,000 of which would require hospitalization, and 36,000 of which would be expected to die.

There are no effective environmental warning systems to detect an aerosol cloud of plague bacilli, and there are no widely available rapid, diagnostic tests of utility. The first sign of a bioterrorist attack with plague would most likely be a sudden outbreak of patients presenting with severe symptoms.

A U.S. licensed vaccine exists and in a pre-exposure setting appears to have some efficacy in preventing or ameliorating bubonic disease. The mortality of untreated pneumonic plague approaches 100%.

Research and development efforts for a vaccine that protects against inhalationally acquired pneumonic plague are ongoing. A number of promising antibiotics and intervention strategies in the treatment and prevention of plague infection have yet to be fully explored experimentally.

Given that naturally occurring antibiotic resistance is rare and the lack of confirmation of engineered antibiotic resistance, the Working Group believes initial treatment recommendations should be based on known drug efficacy, drug availability and ease of administration.

People with household or face-to-face contacts with known pneumonic cases should immediately initiate antibiotic prophylaxis and, if exposure is ongoing, should continue it for 7 days following the last exposure.

In addition to antibiotic prophylaxis, people with established ongoing exposure to a patient with pneumonic plague should wear simple masks and should have patients do the same.

Note: "Plague" http://www.upmcbiosecurity.org/pages/agents/plague_facts.html. Source: Inglesby TV, Dennis DT, Henderson DA, Bartlett JG, Ascher MS, Fitzen E, Fine AD, Friedlander AM, Hauer J, Koerner JF, Layton M, McDade J, Osterholm MT, O'Toole T, Parker G, Perl TM, Russell PK, Schoch-Spana M, Tonat K, for the Working Group of Civilian Biodefense, 2000. Plague as a biological weapon: Medical and public health management. *JAMA*. 283(17).

Q Fever

Overview

Q fever is a zoonotic disease caused by *Coxiella burnetii*, a species of bacteria that is distributed globally. In 1999, Q fever became a notifiable disease in the United States but reporting is not required in many other countries. Because the disease is underreported, scientists cannot reliably assess how many cases of Q fever have actually occurred worldwide. Many human infections are inapparent.

Cattle, sheep, and goats are the primary reservoirs of *C. burnetii*. Infection has been noted in a wide variety of other animals, including other breeds of livestock and in domesticated pets. *Coxiella burnetii* does not usually cause clinical disease in these animals, although abortion in goats and sheep has been linked to *C. burnetii* infection. Organisms are excreted in milk, urine, and feces of infected animals. Most importantly, during birthing the organisms are shed in high numbers within the amniotic fluids and the placenta. The organisms are resistant to heat, drying, and many common disinfectants. These features enable the bacteria to survive for long periods in the environment. Infection of humans usually occurs by inhalation of these organisms from air that contains airborne barnyard dust contaminated by dried placental material, birth fluids, and excreta of infected herd animals. Humans are often very susceptible to the disease, and very few organisms may be required to cause infection.

Ingestion of contaminated milk, followed by regurgitation and inspiration of the contaminated food, is a less common mode of transmission. Other modes of transmission to humans, including tick bites and human to human transmission, are rare.

Signs and Symptoms in Humans

Only about one-half of all people infected with *C. burnetii* show signs of clinical illness. Most acute cases of Q fever begin with sudden onset of one or more of the following: high fevers (up to 104–105° F), severe headache, general malaise, myalgia, confusion, sore throat, chills, sweats, non-productive cough, nausea, vomiting, diarrhea, abdominal pain, and chest pain. Fever usually lasts for 1 to 2 weeks. Weight loss can occur and persist for some time. Thirty to fifty percent of patients with a symptomatic infection will develop pneumonia. Additionally, a majority of patients have abnormal results on liver function tests and some will develop hepatitis. In general, most patients will recover to good health within several months without any treatment. Only 1%–2% of people with acute Q fever die of the disease.

Chronic Q fever, characterized by infection that persists for more than 6 months is uncommon but is a much more serious disease. Patients who have had acute Q fever may develop the chronic form as soon as 1 year or as long as 20 years after initial infection. A serious complication of chronic Q fever is endocarditis, generally involving the aortic heart valves, less commonly the mitral valve. Most patients who develop chronic Q fever have pre-existing valvular heart disease or have a history of vascular graft. Transplant recipients, patients with cancer, and those with chronic kidney disease are also at risk of developing chronic Q fever. As many as 65% of persons with chronic Q fever may die of the disease.

The incubation period for Q fever varies depending on the number of organisms that initially infect the patient. Infection with greater numbers of organisms will result in shorter incubation periods. Most patients become ill within 2–3 weeks after exposure. Those who recover fully from infection may possess lifelong immunity against re-infection.

Diagnosis

Because the signs and symptoms of Q fever are not specific to this disease, it is difficult to make an accurate diagnosis without appropriate laboratory testing. Results from some types of routine laboratory tests in the appropriate clinical and epidemiologic settings may suggest a diagnosis of Q fever. For example, a platelet count may be suggestive because persons with Q fever may show a transient thrombocytopenia. Confirming a diagnosis of Q fever requires serologic testing to detect the presence of antibodies to *Coxiella burnetii* antigens. In most laboratories, the indirect immunofluorescence assay (IFA) is the most dependable and widely used method. *Coxiella burnetii* may also be identified in infected tissues by using immunohistochemical staining and DNA detection methods.

Coxiella burnetii exists in two antigenic phases called phase I and phase II. This antigenic difference is important in diagnosis. In acute cases of Q fever, the antibody level to phase II is usually higher than that to phase I, often by several orders of magnitude, and generally is first detected during the second week of illness. In chronic Q fever, the reverse situation is true. Antibodies to phase I antigens of *C. burnetii* generally require longer to appear and indicate continued exposure to the bacteria. Thus, high levels of antibody to phase I in later specimens in combination with constant or falling levels of phase II antibodies and other signs of inflammatory disease suggest chronic Q fever. Antibodies to phase I and II antigens have been known to persist for months or years after initial infection.

Recent studies have shown that greater accuracy in the diagnosis of Q fever can be achieved by looking at specific levels of classes of antibodies other than IgG, namely IgA and IgM. Combined detection of IgM and IgA in addition to IgG improves the specificity of the assays and provides better accuracy in diagnosis. IgM levels are helpful in the determination of a recent infection. In acute Q fever, patients will have IgG antibodies to phase II and IgM antibodies to phases I and II. Increased IgG and IgA antibodies to phase I are often indicative of Q fever endocarditis.

Treatment

Doxycycline is the treatment of choice for acute Q fever. Antibiotic treatment is most effective when initiated within the first 3 days of illness. A dose of 100 mg of doxycycline taken orally twice daily for 15–21 days is a frequently prescribed therapy. Quinolone antibiotics have demonstrated good in vitro activity against *C. burnetii* and may be considered by the physician. Therapy should be started again if the disease relapses.

Chronic Q fever endocarditis is much more difficult to treat effectively and often requires the use of multiple drugs. Two different treatment protocols have been evaluated: 1) doxycycline in combination with quinolones for at least 4 years and 2) doxycycline in combination with hydroxychloroquine for 1.5 to 3 years. The second therapy leads to fewer relapses, but requires routine eye exams to detect accumulation of chloroquine. Surgery to remove damaged valves may be required for some cases of *C. burnetii* endocarditis.

Prevention

In the United States, Q fever outbreaks have resulted mainly from occupational exposure involving veterinarians, meat processing plant workers, sheep and dairy workers, livestock farmers, and researchers at facilities housing sheep. Prevention and control efforts should be directed primarily toward these groups and environments.

The following measures should be used in the prevention and control of Q fever:

- Educate the public on sources of infection.

- Appropriately dispose of placenta, birth products, fetal membranes, and aborted fetuses at facilities housing sheep and goats.

- Restrict access to barns and laboratories used in housing potentially infected animals.

- Use only pasteurized milk and milk products.

- Use appropriate procedures for bagging, autoclaving, and washing of laboratory clothing.

- Vaccinate (where possible) individuals engaged in research with pregnant sheep or live *C. burnetii*.

- Quarantine imported animals.

- Ensure that holding facilities for sheep should be located away from populated areas. Animals should be routinely tested for antibodies to *C. burnetii*, and measures should be implemented to prevent airflow to other occupied areas.

- Counsel persons at highest risk for developing chronic Q fever, especially persons with pre-existing cardiac valvular disease or individuals with vascular grafts.

A vaccine for Q fever has been developed and has successfully protected humans in occupational settings in Australia. However, this vaccine is not commercially available in the United States. Persons wishing to be vaccinated should first have a skin test to determine a history of previous exposure. Individuals who have previously been exposed to *C. burnetii* should not receive the vaccine because severe reactions, localized to the area of the injected vaccine, may occur. A vaccine for use in animals has also been developed, but it is not available in the United States.

461

Significance for Bioterrorism

Coxiella burnetii is a highly infectious agent that is rather resistant to heat and drying. It can become airborne and inhaled by humans. A single *C. burnetii* organism may cause disease in a susceptible person. This agent could be developed for use in biological warfare and is considered a potential terrorist threat.

Smallpox

Smallpox, because of its high case-fatality rates and transmissibility, now represents one of the most serious bioterrorist threats to the civilian population. Over the centuries, naturally occurring smallpox, with its case-fatality rate of 30 percent or more and its ability to spread in any climate and season, has been universally feared as the most devastating of all the infectious diseases.

Smallpox was once worldwide in scope; before vaccination was practiced almost everyone eventually contracted the disease. In 1980, the World Health Assembly announced that smallpox had been eradicated and recommended that all countries cease vaccination. That same year, the Soviet government embarked on an ambitious program to grow smallpox in large quantities and adapt it for use in bombs and intercontinental ballistic missiles. That initiative succeeded.

Russia still possesses an industrial facility that is capable of producing tons of smallpox virus annually and also maintains a research program that is thought to be seeking to produce more virulent and contagious strains.

An aerosol release of smallpox virus would disseminate readily given its considerable stability in aerosol form and epidemiological evidence suggesting the infectious dose is very small. Even as few as 50–100 cases would likely generate widespread concern or panic and a need to invoke large-scale, perhaps national emergency control measures.

Several factors fuel the concern: the disease has historically been feared as one of the most serious of all pestilential diseases; it is physically disfiguring; it bears a 30 percent case-fatality rate; there is no treatment; it is communicable from person to person; and no one in the U.S. has been vaccinated during the past 25 years. Vaccination ceased in this country in 1972, and vaccination immunity acquired before that time has undoubtedly waned.

Smallpox spreads directly from person to person, primarily by droplet nuclei expelled from the oropharynx of the infected person or by aerosol. Natural infection occurs following implantation of the virus on the oropharyngeal or respiratory mucosa.

Contaminated clothing or bed linen could also spread the virus. Special precautions need to be taken to insure that all bedding and clothing of patients are autoclaved. Disinfectants such as hypochlorite and quaternary ammonia should be used for washing contaminated surfaces.

A smallpox outbreak poses difficult problems because of the ability of the virus to continue to spread throughout the population unless checked by vaccination and/or isolation of patients and their close contacts.

Between the time of an aerosol release of smallpox and diagnosis of the first cases, an interval of as much as two weeks is apt to occur. This is because there is an average incubation period of 12 to 14 days.

After the incubation period, the patient experiences high fever, malaise, and prostration with headache and backache. Severe abdominal pain and delirium are sometimes present. A mascopapular rash then appears, first on the mucosa of the mouth and pharynx, face and forearms, spreading to the trunk and legs. Within one or two days, the rash becomes vesicular and later pustular. The pustules are characteristically round, tense and deeply embedded in the dermis; crusts begin to form about the eighth or ninth day. When the scabs separate, pigment-free skin remains, and eventually pitted scars form.

Approximately 140,000 vials of vaccine are in storage at the Centers for Disease Control and Prevention, each with doses for 50–60 people, and an additional 50–100 million doses are estimated to exist worldwide. This stock cannot be immediately replenished, since all vaccine production facilities were dismantled after 1980, and renewed vaccine production is estimated to require at least 24–36 months.

In 2000, CDC awarded a contract to Oravax of Cambridge, Massachusetts to produce smallpox vaccine. Initially producing 40 million doses, Oravax anticipates delivery of the first full scale production lots in 2004.

Treatment of smallpox is limited to supportive therapy and antibiotics as required for treating secondary bacterial infections. There are no proven antiviral agents effective in treating smallpox.

Recommendations of the Working Group include testing and ultimate consideration for FDA approval of a vaccinia strain grown in tissue culture rather than on calves, finding a rapid diagnostic test for smallpox virus in the asymptomatic early stages, and developing a more attenuated strain of vaccine.

Note: "Smallpox" http://www.upmc_biosecurity.org/pages/agents/smallpox_facts.html. Source: Henderson DA, Inglesby TV, Bartlett JG,

Ascher MS, Eitzen E, Jahrling PB, Hauer J, Layton M, McDage J, Osterholm MT, O'Tolle T, Parker G, Perl T, Russell PK, Tonat K, for the Working Group on Civilian Biodefense. 1999. Smallpox as a biological weapon: Medical and public health management. *JAMA*. 281(22).

Tularemia

Francisella tularensis, the organism that causes tularemia, is one of the most infectious pathogenic bacteria known, requiring inoculation or inhalation of as few as 10 organisms to cause disease. It is considered to be a dangerous potential biological weapon because of its extreme infectivity, ease of dissemination, and substantial capacity to cause illness and death.

During World War II, the potential of *F. tularensis* as a biological weapon, was studied by the Japanese as well as by the U.S. and its allies.

Tularemia was one of several biological weapons that were stockpiled by the U.S. military in the late 1960s, all of which were destroyed by 1973. The Soviet Union continued weapons production of antibiotic and vaccine resistant strains into the early 1990s.

Francisella tularensis is a hardy non-spore forming organism that is capable of surviving for weeks at low temperatures in water, moist soil, hay, straw or decaying animal carcasses.

F. tularensis has been divided into two subspecies: *F. tularensis* biovar tularensis (type A), which is the most common biovar isolated in North America and may be highly virulent in humans and animals; *F. tularensis* biovar palaearctica (type B) which is relatively avirulent and thought to the cause of all human tularemia in Europe and Asia.

Tularemia is a zoonosis. Natural reservoirs include small mammals such as voles, mice, water rats, squirrels, rabbits and hares. Naturally acquired human infection occurs through a variety of mechanisms such as: bites of infected arthropods; handling infectious animal tissues or fluids; direct contact or ingestion of contaminated water, food, or soil; and inhalation of infective aerosols. *F. tularensis* is so infective that examining an open culture plate can cause infection.

Human to human transmission has not been documented.

In the natural setting, tularemia is noted to be a predominately rural disease with clinical presentations including ulceroglandular, glandular, oculoglandular, oropharyngeal, pneumonic, typhoidal and septic forms.

The Working Group on Civilian Biodefense believes that of the various possible ways that *F. tularensis* could be used as a weapon, an aerosol release would cause the greatest adverse medical and public health consequences.

A World Health Organization (WHO) expert committee reported in 1970 that if 50 kg of virulent *F. tularensis* was dispersed as an aerosol over a metropolitan area with a population of 5 million there would an estimated 250,000 incapacitating casualties, including 19,000 deaths.

Aerosol dissemination of *F. tularensis* in a populated area would be expected to result in the abrupt onset of large numbers of cases of acute, non-specific febrile illness beginning 3 to 5 days later (incubation range, 1–14 days), with pleuropneumonitis developing in a significant proportion of cases over the ensuing days and weeks. Without antibiotic treatment, the clinical course could progress to respiratory failure, shock and death.

The overall mortality rate for severe Type A strains has been 5–15%, but in pulmonic or septicemic cases of tularemia without antibiotics treatment the mortality rate has been as high as 30–60%. With treatment, the most recent mortality rates in the U.S. have been 2%. Aminoglycosides, macrolides, chloramphenicol and fluoroquinolones have each been with used with success in the treatment of tularemia.

In the United States, a live-attenuated vaccine derived from the avirulent Live Vaccine Strain (LVS) has been used to protect laboratory personnel routinely working with *F. tularensis*. Given the short incubation period of tularemia and incomplete protection of current vaccines against inhalational tularemia, vaccination is not recommended for post-exposure prophylaxis.

Given the lack of human-to-human transmission, isolation is not recommended for tularemia patients.

The Working Group lacks information on survival of intentionally-dispersed particles, but would expect a short half-life due to desiccation, solar radiation, oxidation and other environmental factors, and a very limited risk from secondary dispersal.

Simple, rapid and reliable diagnostic tests that could be used to identify persons infected with *F. tularensis* in the mass exposure setting need to be developed. Research is also needed to develop accurate and reliable procedures to rapidly detect *F. tularensis* in environmental samples.

Note: "Tularemia" http://www.upmcbiosecurity.org/pages/agents/tularemia_facts.html Source: Dennis DT, Inglesby TV, Henderson DA, Bartlett JG, Ascher MS, Eitzen E, Fine AD, Friedlander AM, Hauer J, Layton M, Lillibridge SR, McDade J, Osterholm MT, O'Tolle T, Parker G, Perl T, Russell PK, Tonat K, for the Working Group on Civilian Biodefense. 2001. *JAMA*. 285(21).

Viral Hemorrhagic Fevers

Background

Hemorrhagic fever viruses (HFVs) are a diverse group of organisms, each of which belong to one of four distinct families:

1. **Filoviridae:** Ebola and Marburg viruses

2. **Arenaviridae:** Lassa fever virus and a group of viruses referred to as the New World arenaviruses

3. **Bunyaviridae:** Crimean Congo hemorrhagic fever virus, Rift Valley fever virus, and a group of viruses known as the 'agents of hemorrhagic fever with renal syndrome'

4. **Flaviviridae:** dengue, yellow fever, Omsk hemorrhagic fever, and Kyasanur Forest disease virus

Hemorrhagic fever viruses are all capable of causing clinical diseases associated with fever and bleeding disorder, classically referred to as viral hemorrhagic fever (VHF). None of these viruses occurs naturally in the United States. Risk factors for these diseases include travel to certain geographic areas where these diseases may naturally occur (such as certain areas of Africa, Asia, the Middle East, and South America), handling of animal carcasses, contact with sick animals or people with the disease, and arthropod bites. The Working Group for Civilian Biodefense identified a subset of these viruses that pose particularly serious threats as biological weapons, based on, among other characteristics, their infectious properties, morbidity and mortality, transmissibility by way of aerosol dissemination, and prior research and development as biological weapons. Specifically, these viruses are: Ebola, Marburg, Lassa fever, New World arenaviruses, Rift Valley fever, yellow fever, Omsk hemorrhagic fever, and Kyasanur Forest disease. The history and characteristics of these viruses are described in detail in the full consensus statement.

Epidemiology

An understanding of the epidemiology, clinical presentation, and the recommended medical and public health response following a biological attack with any of the HFVs of greatest concern could substantially decrease the morbidity and mortality of such an event.

There is the potential for significant morbidity and mortality if hemorrhagic fever viruses were disseminated by aerosol dispersal, given the lack of readily available therapy and vaccines. Some of these viruses (namely, Ebola, Marburg, Lassa fever, New World arenaviruses, and Crimean-Congo hemorrhagic fever viruses) are also transmissible from person-to-person; this characteristic has the potential to amplify disease outbreaks.

Most of what is known regarding the epidemiology of these diseases is derived from naturally occurring outbreaks. Rift Valley fever and the Flaviviridae are not transmissible from person-to-person. For the remaining HFVs of concern, the major mode of transmission appears to be from direct contact with a sick person or contaminated items, such as syringes. Transmission via the airborne route appears to be rare but cannot be conclusively ruled out. All of these viruses, including Rift Valley fever and the Flaviviridae, may be transmitted to laboratory personnel by way of aerosol generated during specimen processing. For that reason, attempts to culture these viruses must be conducted in high containment (BSL-4) laboratories. There are two such labs in the U.S.; one is located at the Centers for Disease Control and Prevention, and the other at the United States Army Medical Research Institute of Infectious Diseases.

Clinical Manifestations

Following an aerosol dissemination of any of these HFVs of concern, cases would likely appear 2–21 days following exposure. Patients would present with fever, rashes, body aches, headaches, and fatigue, and bleeding manifestations could occur later in the disease course. Suspected cases of viral hemorrhagic fevers should be immediately reported to local or state health department. These illnesses are not endemic in the U.S.; thus, were a case of VHF to be detected domestically in a person who does not have any of the risk factors for the disease, bioterrorism should be considered as a potential cause.

Health-care workers caring for patients with suspected or confirmed VHF should take special protective measures. The Working Group recommends adherence to strict hand hygiene and the donning of double-gloves, impermeable gowns, leg and shoe coverings, face shields or goggles for eye protection, and either N-95 masks or powered air-purifying respirators (for airborne precautions). In addition, if resources are available, patients should be cared for in a negative pressure isolation room (used for the care of patients with tuberculosis).

Prophylaxis and Treatment

Currently, there is no approved antiviral medication for the treatment of any of these diseases. Ribavirin, an antiviral medication which, when used in combination with interferon, is approved for the treatment of chronic hepatitis C, is active against some of these viruses (the Arenaviridae and Bunyaviridae). Unfortunately, no antiviral medications have been shown to be useful in the treatment of the other families of viruses (the Filoviridae and Flaviviridae).

A vaccine exists for only one of these viruses: yellow fever. The vaccine is very effective in protecting travelers to areas where the disease is endemic from acquiring yellow fever. This vaccine would not be useful following a bioterrorist attack because yellow fever has a very short incubation period, so that even if victims were vaccinated subsequent to a known exposure, they would likely develop the disease before they develop protective antibodies.

The Working Group recommends that ribavirin be administered to individuals believed to have VHF after a bioterrorist attack, and to those who develop symptoms after a VHF contact with other sick persons. However, if the causative virus is ultimately identified as a Filoviridae or a Flaviviridae, ribavirin will not be useful and should not be continued. Persons who may have been infected by a bioweapon disseminating HFVs should be followed closely by a designated medical expert or public health official so they may be immediately treated if they develop symptoms. There is an urgent need for the development of rapid diagnostic tests, effective vaccines and drug therapy for the HFVs of greatest concern.

Note: "Viral Hemorrhagic Fevers" http://www.upmcbiosecurity.org/pages/agents/vhf_facts.html. Source: Borio L, Inglesby TV, Peters CJ, Schmaljohn AL, Hughes JM, Jahrling PB, Ksiazek T, Johnson KM, Meyerhoff A, O'Toole T, Ascher MS, Bartlett J, Breman JG, Fitzen EM, Hamburg M, Hauer J, Henderson DA, Johnson RT, Kwik G, Layton M, Lillibridge s, Nabel GJ, Osterholm MT, Perl TM, Russell P, Tonat K for the Working Group on Civilian Biodefense. 2002. Hemorrhagic fever viruses as biological weapons: Medical and public health management *JAMA*. 287(18).

Chapter 63

Food Safety and Terrorism

***What is the Food and Drug Administration (FDA) doing to
protect the food supply against terrorism?***

Over the last few years, FDA has worked with food safety agencies at federal, state and local levels to significantly strengthen the Nation's food safety system across the entire distribution chain—from the farm to the table. The main results of this cooperation—more effective prevention programs, new surveillance systems, and faster foodborne illness outbreak response capabilities—have already enabled the agency to protect the safety of our food supply against natural and accidental threats.

In addition, since the September 11 attack, FDA has increased its emergency response capability by realigning resources for possible use to counter terrorism, and by reassessing and strengthening its emergency response plans. The agency also continues to work closely with other federal, state, and local food safety authorities and with regulatory agencies abroad to maximize coordination of efforts to protect food and to respond rapidly to evidence of threats to the food supply.

All of these provisions and systems can be employed to prevent or respond to a terrorist assault on our food supply.

"Frequently Asked Consumer Questions about Food Safety and Terrorism," Center for Food Safety and Applied Nutrition, U.S. Food and Drug Administration (FDA), November 15, 2001.

Does FDA cooperate with industry in the defense against food terrorism?

FDA is working with a broad spectrum of industries that has formed the Food Security Alliance, a group dedicated to strengthening the physical security of industrial food production. With help from the industry, FDA is developing a Food Security Guidance that food producers can use to improve the protection of their products against tampering or terrorist actions. The guide will be primarily focused on the management of food security as it applies to the plant, employees, raw materials, packaging, and finished products.

Is anything being done to intensify the FDA surveillance of food imports and food production?

The Administration has asked Congress for increased FDA resources to build up its food surveillance of both domestic and imported foods through these major actions:

- it will hire 210 additional import inspectors to monitor food as it enters the United States;

- add 100 inspectors to survey points that are critical for product safety in the domestic food production and distribution system;

- add 100 technical analysts to multiply the number of food samples tested for possible contamination.

In addition to a request for increased resources for surveillance, the Administration is seeking further authority to strengthen FDA's oversight of food in the case of an emergency. The increased authority will allow FDA to require information from food producers that will enable the agency to rapidly address possible health hazards by quickly tracing the source and distribution of both domestic and imported food.

What can consumers do to protect themselves and their families from food tampering or other kinds of food contamination?

Consumers are the final judges of the safety of the food they buy. The essential step for their protection is to check whether the food package or can is intact before opening it. If it has been damaged, dented or opened prior to purchase, the contents should not be used.

Consumers need to be alert also to abnormal odor, taste, and appearance of a food item. If there is any doubt about its safety, don't eat it. If the food appears to have been tampered with, report it to one of the authorities listed below.

What should consumers do if they suspect a food product has been contaminated or tampered with?

If the suspected food product does NOT contain meat or poultry—such as seafood, produce, or eggs—consumers should notify the FDA 24-hour emergency number at 301-443-1240 or call the consumer complaint coordinator at their nearest FDA District Office.

If the food product DOES contain meat or poultry, call the U.S. Department of Agriculture's Meat and Poultry Hotline at 1-800-535-4555.

Should consumers take antibiotics for protection against contaminated food?

Antibiotics should not be taken preventively unless prescribed by a physician. Although antibiotics can be effective against some bacterial contaminants, they are not effective against viruses, chemicals, or radiological substances.

What food handling practices should consumers follow on a day-to-day basis to help prevent foodborne illness?

Consumers can protect themselves by following basic safe food handling practices:

- Wash all raw food products such as fruits and vegetables before eating them to help eliminate bacteria that may be on the food.

- Wash hands, cutting boards, knives, and utensils in hot, soapy water before and after handling each raw food item and before touching another food or a surface that will come into contact with food. This will prevent bacteria from spreading and contaminating other food.

- Separate raw foods such as meat, poultry, and seafood from foods that are ready-to-eat.

- Cook foods thoroughly to kill harmful bacteria that may be present.

- Refrigerate foods promptly. Cold temperatures keep most harmful bacteria from growing and multiplying.

Where can I get more information about food safety?

For more information about food safety, call FDA's toll free consumer information line at 1-888-SAFEFOOD, or visit the World Wide Web at http://www.foodsafety.gov.

Chapter 64

National Pharmaceutical Stockpile

The mission of CDC's (Centers for Disease Control and Prevention) National Pharmaceutical Stockpile (NPS) Program is to ensure the availability and rapid deployment of life-saving pharmaceuticals, antidotes, other medical supplies, and equipment necessary to counter the effects of nerve agents, biological pathogens, and chemical agents. The NPS Program stands ready for immediate deployment to any U.S. location in the event of a terrorist attack using a biological toxin or chemical agent directed against a civilian population.

Synopsis

CDC's Bioterrorism Preparedness and Response Program

A release of selected biological or chemical agents targeting the U.S. civilian population will require rapid access to large quantities of pharmaceuticals and medical supplies. Such quantities may not be readily available unless special stockpiles are created. No one can anticipate exactly where a terrorist will strike and few state or local governments have the resources to create sufficient stockpiles on their own. Therefore, a national stockpile has been created as a resource for all. As part of the Department of Health and Human Services (HHS) 1999 Bioterrorism Initiative, CDC was designated to lead an effort working with governmental and non-governmental partners to upgrade the nations'

"National Pharmaceutical Stockpile," Centers for Disease Control and Prevention (CDC), December 18, 2002.

public health capacity to respond to biological and chemical terrorism and establish a Bioterrorism Preparedness and Response Program. Critical to success of this initiative is to ensure capacity is developed at federal, state, and local levels. The National Pharmaceutical Stockpile (NPS) Program is an essential response component of CDC's larger Bioterrorism Preparedness and Response Initiative.

A National Repository of Life-Saving Pharmaceuticals and Medical Supplies

The mission of CDC's National Pharmaceutical Stockpile (NPS) Program is to ensure the availability of life-saving pharmaceuticals, antidotes, and other medical supplies and equipment necessary to counter the effects of nerve agents, biological pathogens, and chemical agents. The NPS Program stands ready for immediate deployment to any U.S. location in the event of a terrorist attack using a biological, toxin, or chemical agent directed against a civilian population. The NPS is comprised of pharmaceuticals, vaccines, medical supplies, and medical equipment that exist to augment depleted state and local resources for responding to terrorist attacks and other emergencies. These packages are stored in strategic locations around the U.S. to ensure rapid delivery anywhere in the country.

Following the federal decision to deploy, the NPS will typically arrive by air or ground in two phases. The first phase shipment is called a 12-hour Push Package. "12" because it will arrive in 12-hours or less, "push" because a state need only ask for help—not for specific items, and "package" because the Program will ship a complete package of medical materiel—to include nearly everything a state will need to respond to a broad range of threats. Also available are inventory supplies known as Vendor Managed Inventory, or VMI packages. VMI packages can be tailored to provide pharmaceuticals, vaccines, medical supplies, and/or medical products specific to the suspected or confirmed agent or combination of agents.

A CDC team of five or six technical advisors will also deploy at the same time as the first shipment. Known as a Technical Advisory Response Unit (TARU), this team is comprised of pharmacists, emergency responders, and logistics experts that will advise local authorities on receiving, distributing, dispensing, replenishing, and recovering NPS materiel.

The NPS Program was tested in a real-life terrorist attack in response to the tragic events of September 11th when New York State and local officials requested large quantities of medical materiel and logistical assistance. With the support of local and state public health and emergency response officials, all facets of the New York operation performed exactly as intended. The NPS Program has also assisted many states and cities by providing pharmaceutical and logistical support to areas affected by the anthrax attacks in October and November 2001.

Determining and Maintaining NPS Assets

The CDC, in consultation with other partners in chemical/biological preparedness, have developed a stockpile to respond to biological or chemical terrorism emergencies. To determine and review the composition of the NPS, CDC considers many factors, such as current biological and/or chemical threats, the availability of medical materiel, and the ease of dissemination of pharmaceuticals. One of the most significant factors in determining NPS composition, however, is the medical vulnerability of the U.S. civilian population.

NPS assets are stored at strategic locations throughout the U.S. to assure the most rapid response possible. CDC ensures that the medical materiel in these NPS storage facilities is rotated and kept within potency shelf life limits.

Supplementing State and Local Resources

In a biological or chemical terrorism event, state, local, and private stocks of medical materiel will deplete quickly. The NPS can support local first response efforts with a Push Package followed by quantities of materiel specific to the terrorist agent used (utilizing VMI). The NPS is not a first response tool. State and local first responders and health officials can use the NPS to bolster their response to a biological or chemical terrorism attack—thereby increasing their capacity to more rapidly mitigate the results of this type of terrorism.

Transfer of NPS Assets to State and/or Local Authorities

As part of CDC's Bioterrorism Response, CDC will transfer authority for the NPS materiel to the state and/or local authorities once it arrives at the airfield. State and/or local authorities will then repackage and label bulk medicines and other NPS materiel according to their state terrorism contingency plan. CDC's technical advisors will accompany the NPS in order to assist and advise state/local officials in putting the NPS assets to prompt, effective use.

When and How is the NPS Deployed?

The decision to deploy NPS assets may be based on evidence showing the overt release of an agent that might adversely affect public health. It is more likely, however, that subtle indicators, such as unusual morbidity and/or mortality identified through the Nation's disease outbreak surveillance and epidemiology network, will alert health officials to the possibility (and confirmation) of a biological or chemical terrorism incident. To receive NPS assets, the affected state can directly request the deployment of the NPS from the Director of CDC. Once requested, the Director of CDC has the authority, in consultation with the Surgeon General, and the Secretary of Health and Human Services, to order the deployment of the NPS.

Training and Education

CDC is charged with leading a nationwide preparedness training and education program for state and local health care providers, first responders, and governments (to include Federal officials, Governors' offices, state/local health departments, and emergency management agencies). This training not only explains CDC's mission and operations, it alerts state and local emergency response officials to the important issues they must plan for in order to receive, secure, and distribute NPS assets. To conduct this outreach and training, CDC Program staff are currently working with HHS agencies, Regional Emergency Response Coordinators at all ten U.S. Public Health Service regional offices as well as state and local departments of health, state emergency management offices, and the Metro Medical Response System, the Federal Emergency Management Agency, the Department of Veterans' Affairs, and the Department of Defense.

Key Activities of the NPS Program

- Procurement and management of NPS Inventory;
- Ensuring rapid transport of NPS assets in response to a terrorism incident;
- Coordination with state, local, and Federal emergency responders;
- Provision of CDC technical consultants to accompany pharmaceuticals, vaccines, or other medical materiel to the area of need;
- Operational research and program evaluation; and
- Education and training for state, local, and Federal partners.

Contact Information

For further information about the National Pharmaceutical Stockpile, contact the NPS Program at 404-639-0459.

Chapter 65

Sheltering in Place

Chemical Agents: Facts about Sheltering in Place

What "Sheltering in Place" Means

Some kinds of chemical accidents or attacks may make going outdoors dangerous. Leaving the area might take too long or put you in harm's way. In such a case it may be safer for you to stay indoors than to go outside.

"Shelter in place" means to make a shelter out of the place you are in. It is a way for you to make the building as safe as possible to protect yourself until help arrives. You should not try to shelter in a vehicle unless you have no other choice. Vehicles are not airtight enough to give you adequate protection from chemicals.

How to Prepare to Shelter in Place

Choose a room in your house or apartment for your shelter. The best room to use for the shelter is a room with as few windows and doors as possible. A large room, preferably with a water supply, is desirable—something like a master bedroom that is connected to a bathroom. For chemical events, this room should be as high in the

---

"Chemical Agents: Facts about Sheltering in Place," reviewed on May 21, 2003, and "Sheltering in Place During a Radiation Emergency," modified April 30, 2003, Public Health Emergency Preparedness and Response, Centers for Disease Control and Prevention (CDC).

structure as possible to avoid vapors (gases) that sink. This guideline is different from the sheltering-in-place technique used in tornadoes and other severe weather, when the shelter should be low in the home.

You might not be at home if the need to shelter in place ever arises, but if you are at home, the following items would be good to have on hand. (Ideally, all of these items would be stored in the shelter room to save time.)

- First aid kit
- Food and bottled water. Store 1 gallon of water per person in plastic bottles as well as ready-to-eat foods that will keep without refrigeration at the shelter-in-place location. If you do not have bottled water, or if you run out, you can drink water from a toilet tank (not from a toilet bowl).
- Flashlight, battery-powered radio, and extra batteries for both.
- Duct tape and scissors.
- Towels and plastic sheeting.
- A working telephone.

How to Know if You Need to Shelter in Place

- You will hear from the local police, emergency coordinators, or government on the radio and on television if you need to shelter in place.
- If there is a "code red" or "severe" terror alert, you should pay attention to radio and television broadcasts to know right away whether a shelter-in-place alert is announced for your area.
- If you are away from your shelter-in-place location when a chemical event occurs, follow the instructions of emergency coordinators to find the nearest shelter. If your children are at school, they will be sheltered there. Unless you are instructed to do so, do not try to get to the school to bring your children home.

What to Do

Act quickly and follow the instructions of your local emergency coordinators. Every situation can be different, so local emergency coordinators might have special instructions for you to follow. In general, do the following:

478

- Go inside as quickly as possible.

- If there is time, shut and lock all outside doors and windows. Locking them may provide a tighter seal against the chemical. Turn off the air conditioner or heater. Turn off all fans, too. Close the fireplace damper and any other place that air can come in from the outside.

- Go in the shelter-in-place room and shut the door.

- Tape plastic over any windows in the room. Use duct tape around the windows and doors and make an unbroken seal. Use the tape over any vents into the room and seal any electrical outlets or other openings. Sink and toilet drain traps should have water in them (you can use the sink and toilet as you normally would). If it is necessary to drink water, drink the stored water, not water from the tap.

- Turn on the radio. Keep a telephone close at hand, but don't use it unless there is a serious emergency.

Sheltering in this way should keep you safer than if you are outdoors. Most likely, you will be in the shelter for no more than a few hours. Listen to the radio for an announcement indicating that it is safe to leave the shelter. After you come out of the shelter, emergency coordinators may have additional instructions on how to make the rest of the building safe again.

How You Can Get More Information about Sheltering in Place

You can contact one of the following:

- State and local health departments
- Centers for Disease Control and Prevention Public Response Hotline (CDC)
  - Public Response Hotline (CDC)
    - English (888) 246-2675
    - Español (888) 246-2857
    - TTY (866) 874-2646
  - Emergency Preparedness and Response Web site
  - E-mail inquiries: cdcresponse@ashastd.org

479

- Mail inquiries:

  Public Inquiry c/o BPRP
  Bioterrorism Preparedness and Response Planning
  Centers for Disease Control and Prevention
  Mailstop C-18
  1600 Clifton Road
  Atlanta, GA 30333

Sheltering in Place During a Radiation Emergency

With recent terrorist events, many people have wondered about the possibility of a terrorist attack involving radioactive materials. People who live near but not in the immediate area of the attack may be asked to stay home and take shelter rather than try to evacuate. This action is called "sheltering in place." Because many radioactive materials rapidly decay and dissipate, staying in your home may protect your from exposure to radiation. The thick walls of your home may block much of the harmful radiation. Taking a few simple precautions can help you reduce your exposure to radiation. The Centers for Disease Control and Prevention (CDC) has prepared the information to help you protect yourself and your family and to help you prepare a safe and well-stocked shelter.

Preparing a Shelter in Your Home

The safest place in your home during an emergency involving radioactive materials is a centrally located room or basement. This area should have as few windows as possible. The further your shelter is from windows, the safer you will be.

Preparation is the key. Store emergency supplies in this area. An emergency could happen at any time, so it is best to stock supplies in advance and have everything that you need stored in the shelter.

Every 6 months, check the supplies in your shelter. Replace any expired medications, food, or batteries. Also, replace the water in your shelter every 6 months to keep it fresh.

Make sure that all family members know where the shelter is and what it is for. Caution them not to take any items from that area. If someone "borrows" items from your shelter, you may find that important items are missing when they are most needed.

If you have pets, prepare a place for them to relieve themselves in the shelter. Pets should not go outside during a radiation emergency because they may track radioactive materials from fallout into the shelter. Preparing a place for pets will keep the radioactive materials from getting inside the shelter.

Preparing Emergency Supplies

Stock up on supplies, just as you would in case of severe weather conditions or other emergencies. Following is a list of things to consider when preparing your emergency kit.

- Food with a long shelf life. Examples of this include canned, dried, and packaged food products. Store enough food for each member of the household for at least 3 days.

- Water. In preparation for an emergency, purchase and store bottled water or simply store water from the tap. Each person in the household will need about 1 gallon per day; plan on storing enough water for at least 3 days.

- A change of clothes and shoes. Check clothing every 6 months and remove clothes that no longer fit or are unsuitable for seasonal weather. Remember to include underwear, socks, sturdy shoes or work boots, and winter or summer clothes as needed.

- Paper plates, paper towels, and plastic utensils. Store disposable dishware and utensils because you will not have enough water to wash dishes and because community water sources may be contaminated.

- Plastic bags. Because you may not be able to leave your shelter for several days, you will need to collect your waste in plastic bags until it can be removed.

- Bedding. Store sheets, blankets, towels, and cots for use during the time that you cannot leave your shelter.

- Battery-operated radio and batteries. Electrical power may not be on for several days. A battery-operated radio will allow you to listen to emergency messages.

- Medicines. Have 2-3 days' dose of your current prescription medicines in a childproof bottle for your shelter medical kit; label with the name and expiration date of the medicine. (Discuss with your doctor the best way to obtain this small amount of extra medicine.) Be sure to check medicines in your kit every 6 months to make sure they are not past the expiration date.

- Toiletries. Keep a supply of soap, hand sanitizer, toilet paper, deodorant, disinfectants, etc.

- Flashlight and batteries. Electrical power may be out for several days. A flashlight will help you see in your shelter.

- A telephone or cell phone. Although cell phone or ground phone service may be interrupted, there is still a chance that you will be able to use a phone to call outside for information and advice from emergency services.

- Extra eyeglasses or contact lenses and cleaning supplies.

- Duct tape and heavy plastic sheeting. You can use these items to seal the door to your shelter and to seal any vents that open into your shelter for a short period of time if a radiation plume is passing over.

- Pet food, baby formula, diapers, etc. Don't forget the other members of your family. If you have an infant, store extra formula and diapers. If you have pets keep a 3-day supply of pet food.

- First aid kit. You can purchase a first-aid kit or prepare one yourself. Be sure to include the following items:
  - Sterile adhesive bandages
  - Sterile gauze pads in 2 inch and 4 inch sizes
  - Adhesive tape
  - Sterile rolled bandages
  - Scissors
  - Tweezers
  - Needle
  - Thermometer
  - Moistened towelettes
  - Antiseptic ointment
  - Tube of petroleum jelly or other lubricant
  - Soap or hand sanitizer
  - Latex or vinyl gloves
  - Safety pins
  - Aspirin or aspirin free pain reliever
  - Antidiarrhea medication

- Laxatives

- Antacids for stomach upset

- Syrup of ipecac to cause vomiting if advised by the Poison Control Center

- Activated charcoal to stop vomiting if advised by the Poison Control Center

- Games, books and other entertainment. Because you may be in your shelter for several days, keep items on hand to occupy your family during that time. Children are likely to get bored if they have to stay in one place for long periods. Think of activities that they will enjoy doing while in the shelter—finger painting, coloring, playing games, etc.

Tips Before Entering a Shelter

If you are outside when the alert is given, try to remove clothing and shoes and place them in a plastic bag before entering the house. During sever weather, such as extreme cold, remove at least the outer layer of clothes before entering the home to avoid bringing radioactive material into your shelter. Leave clothing and shoes outside. Shower and wash your body with soap and water. Removing clothing will eliminate 90% of radioactive contamination. By taking this simple step, you will reduce the time that you are exposed and also your risk of injury from the radiation.

Before entering the shelter, turn off fans, air conditioners, and forced-air heating units that bring air in from the outside. Close and lock all windows and doors, and close fireplace dampers.

When you move to your shelter, use duct tape and plastic sheeting to seal any doors, windows, or vents for a short period of time in case a radiation plume is passing over (listen to your radio for instructions). Within a few hours, you should remove the plastic and duct tape and ventilate the room. Suffocation could occur if you keep the shelter tightly sealed for more than a few hours.

Keep your radio tuned to an emergency response network at all times for updates on the situation. The announcers will provide information about when you may leave your shelter and whether you need to take other emergency measures.

Chapter 66

Radiation Emergencies

Radiation Facts

What is radiation and how can I be exposed?

Radiation is a form of energy. It comes from man-made sources such as x-ray machines, from the sun and outer space, and from some radioactive materials such as uranium in soil.

Small quantities of radioactive materials occur naturally in the air we breathe, the water we drink, the food we eat, and in our own bodies. Radiation that goes inside our bodies causes what we refer to as internal exposure. The exposure that is referred to as external comes from sources outside the body, such as radiation from sunlight and man-made and naturally occurring radioactive materials.

Radiation doses that people receive are measured in units called "rem" or "sievert." (One sievert is equal to 100 rem.) Scientists estimate that the average person in the United States receives a dose of about one-third of a rem per year. Eighty percent of typical human exposure comes from natural sources and the remaining 20 percent comes from artificial radiation sources, primarily medical x-rays.

This chapter includes text excerpted from the following fact sheets developed by Public Health Emergency Preparedness and Response, Centers for Disease Control and Prevention (CDC): "Radiation Facts," modified April 2003; "Frequently Asked Questions (FAQs) About a Radiation Emergency," modified March 2003; "Dirty Bombs," modified April 2003; "Acute Radiation Syndrome," modified April 2003, "Potassium Iodide (KI)," modified June 2003, and "Prussian Blue," modified May 2003.

How can I protect myself from radiation?

The three basic ways to reduce your exposure are through:

- **Time:** Decrease the amount of time you spend near the source of radiation.

- **Distance:** Increase your distance from a radiation source.

- **Shielding:** Increase the shielding between you and the radiation source. Shielding is anything that creates a barrier between people and the radiation source. Depending on the type of radiation, the shielding can range from something as thin as a plate of window glass or as thick as several feet of concrete. Being inside a building or a vehicle can provide shielding from some kinds of radiation.

Frequently Asked Questions (FAQs) About a Radiation Emergency

What happens when people are exposed to radiation?

Radiation can affect the body in a number of ways, and the adverse health effects of exposure may not be apparent for many years. These adverse health effects can range from mild effects, such as skin reddening, to serious effects such as cancer and death, depending on the amount of radiation absorbed by the body (the dose), the type of radiation, the route of exposure, and the length of time a person was exposed. Exposure to very large doses of radiation may cause death within a few days or months. Exposure to lower doses of radiation may lead to an increased risk of developing cancer or other adverse health effects later in life.

What types of terrorist events might involve radiation?

Possible terrorist events could involve introducing radioactive material into the food or water supply, using explosives (like dynamite) to scatter radioactive materials (called a "dirty bomb"), bombing or destroying a nuclear facility, or exploding a small nuclear device.

Although introducing radioactive material into the food or water supply most likely would cause great concern or fear, it probably would not cause much contamination or increase the danger of adverse health effects.

Although a dirty bomb could cause serious injuries from the explosion, it most likely would not have enough radioactive material in a form that would cause serious radiation sickness among large numbers of people. However, people who were exposed to radiation scattered by the bomb could have a greater risk of developing cancer later in life, depending on their dose.

A meltdown or explosion at a nuclear facility could cause a large amount of radioactive material to be released. People at the facility would probably be contaminated with radioactive material and possibly be injured if there was an explosion. Those people who received a large dose might develop acute radiation syndrome. People in the surrounding area could be exposed or contaminated.

Clearly, an exploded nuclear device could result in a lot of property damage. People would be killed or injured from the blast and might be contaminated by radioactive material. Many people could have symptoms of acute radiation syndrome. After a nuclear explosion, radioactive fallout would extend over a large region far from the point of impact, potentially increasing people's risk of developing cancer over time.

What preparations can I make for a radiation emergency?

Your community should have a plan in place in case of a radiation emergency. Check with community leaders to learn more about the plan and possible evacuation routes. Check with your child's school, the nursing home of a family member, and your employer to see what their plans are for dealing with a radiation emergency. Develop your own family emergency plan so that every family member knows what to do. At home, put together an emergency kit that would be appropriate for any emergency. The kit should include the following items:

- A flashlight with extra batteries
- A portable radio with extra batteries
- Bottled water
- Canned and packaged food
- A hand-operated can opener
- A first-aid kit and essential prescription medications
- Personal items such as paper towels, garbage bags, and toilet paper

How can I protect myself during a radiation emergency?

After a release of radioactive materials, local authorities will monitor the levels of radiation and determine what protective actions to take. The most appropriate action will depend on the situation. Tune to the local emergency response network or news station for information and instructions during any emergency.

If a radiation emergency involves the release of large amounts of radioactive materials, you may be advised to "shelter in place," which means to stay in your home or office; or you may be advised to move to another location. If you are advised to shelter in place, you should do the following:

- Close and lock all doors and windows.

- Turn off fans, air conditioners, and forced-air heating units that bring in fresh air from the outside. Only use units to recirculate air that is already in the building.

- Close fireplace dampers.

- If possible, bring pets inside.

- Move to an inner room or basement.

- Keep your radio tuned to the emergency response network or local news to find out what else you need to do.

If you are advised to evacuate, follow the directions that your local officials provide. Leave the area as quickly and orderly as possible. In addition:

- Take a flashlight, portable radio, batteries, first-aid kit, supply of sealed food and water, hand-operated can opener, essential medicines, and cash and credit cards.

- Take pets only if you are using your own vehicle and going to a place you know will accept animals. Emergency vehicles and shelters usually will not accept animals.

Dirty Bombs

What Is a "dirty bomb"?

A dirty bomb, or radiological dispersion device, is a bomb that combines conventional explosives, such as dynamite, with radioactive materials in the form of powder or pellets. The idea behind a dirty bomb is to blast radioactive material into the area around the explosion. This could possibly cause buildings and people to be exposed to radioactive material. The main purpose of a dirty bomb is to frighten people and make buildings or land unusable for a long period of time.

The atomic explosions that occurred in Hiroshima and Nagasaki were conventional nuclear weapons involving a fission reaction. A dirty bomb is designed to spread radioactive material and contaminate a small area. It does not include the fission products necessary to create a large blast like those seen in Hiroshima and Nagasaki.

There has been a lot of speculation about where terrorists could get radioactive material to place in a dirty bomb. The most harmful radioactive materials are found in nuclear power plants and nuclear weapons sites. However, increased security at these facilities makes obtaining materials from them more difficult.

Because of the dangerous and difficult aspects of obtaining high-level radioactive materials from a nuclear facility, there is a greater chance that the radioactive materials used in a dirty bomb would come from low-level radioactive sources. Low-level radioactive sources are found in hospitals, on construction sites, and at food irradiation plants. The sources in these areas are used to diagnose and treat illnesses, sterilize equipment, inspect welding seams, and irradiate food to kill harmful microbes.

What are the dangers of a dirty bomb?

If low-level radioactive sources were to be used, the primary danger from a dirty bomb would be the blast itself. Gauging how much radiation might be present is difficult when the source of the radiation is unknown. However, at the levels created by most probable sources, not enough radiation would be present in a dirty bomb to cause severe illness from exposure to radiation.

Radiation cannot be seen, smelled, felt, or tasted by humans. Therefore, if people are present at the scene of an explosion, they will not know whether radioactive materials were involved at the time of the explosion. If people are not too severely injured by the initial blast, they should:

- Leave the immediate area on foot. Do not panic. Do not take public or private transportation such as buses, subways, or cars because if radioactive materials were involved, they may contaminate cars or the public transportation system.

- Go inside the nearest building. Staying inside will reduce people's exposure to any radioactive material that may be on dust at the scene.

- Remove their clothes as soon as possible, place them in a plastic bag, and seal it. Removing clothing will remove most of the contamination caused by external exposure to radioactive materials. Saving the contaminated clothing would allow testing for exposure without invasive sampling.

- Take a shower or wash themselves as best they can. Washing will reduce the amount of radioactive contamination on the body and will effectively reduce total exposure.

- Be on the lookout for information. Once emergency personnel can assess the scene and the damage, they will be able to tell people whether radiation was involved.

Even if people do not know whether radioactive materials were present, following these simple steps can help reduce their injury from other chemicals that might have been present in the blast.

Keep televisions or radios tuned to local news networks. If a radioactive material was released, people will be told where to report for radiation monitoring and blood tests to determine whether they were exposed to the radiation as well as what steps to take to protect their health.

Acute Radiation Syndrome

Radiation sickness, known as acute radiation sickness (ARS), is a serious illness that occurs when the entire body (or most of it) receives a high dose of radiation, usually over a short period of time. Many survivors of the Hiroshima and Nagasaki atomic bombs in the 1940s and many of the firefighters who first responded after the Chernobyl Nuclear Power Plant accident in 1986 became ill with ARS. People exposed to radiation will get ARS only if:

- The radiation dose was high (doses from medical procedures such as chest x-rays are too low to cause ARS; however, doses from radiation therapy to treat cancer may be high enough to cause some ARS symptoms),

- The radiation was penetrating (that is, able to reach internal organs),

- The person's entire body, or most of it, received the dose, and

- The radiation was received in a short time, usually within minutes.

The first symptoms of ARS typically are nausea, vomiting, and diarrhea. These symptoms will start within minutes to days after the exposure, will last for minutes up to several days, and may come and go. Then the person usually looks and feels healthy for a short time, after which he or she will become sick again with loss of appetite, fatigue, fever, nausea, vomiting, diarrhea, and possibly even seizures and coma. This seriously ill stage may last from a few hours up to several months.

People with ARS typically also have some skin damage. This damage can start to show within a few hours after exposure and can include swelling, itching, and redness of the skin (like a bad sunburn). There also can be hair loss. As with the other symptoms, the skin may heal for a short time, followed by the return of swelling, itching, and redness days or weeks later. Complete healing of the skin may take from several weeks up to a few years depending on the radiation dose the person's skin received.

The chance of survival for people with ARS decreases with increasing radiation dose. Most people who do not recover from ARS will die within several months of exposure. The cause of death in most cases is the destruction of the person's bone marrow, which results in infections and internal bleeding. For the survivors, the recovery process may last from several weeks up to 2 years.

If a radiation emergency occurs that exposes people to high doses of radiation in a short period of time, they should immediately seek medical care from their doctor or local hospital.

Potassium Iodide (KI)

How might a nuclear incident cause thyroid damage?

Some types of radioactive incidents release radioactive iodine. The thyroid gland, which will use any iodine that is in a person's bloodstream, cannot tell the difference between radioactive and nonradioactive forms of iodine. Because of this, the thyroid would rapidly absorb radioactive iodine just as it does iodine from a person's diet. The radioactive iodine releases energy (radiation) that, in high concentrations, can damage the cells of the thyroid gland. In some people, especially young children, this damage can cause thyroid cancer or other diseases of the thyroid within a few years of the exposure.

What is KI?

KI is a salt of iodine. It is one of several ingredients that can be added to table salt to make it iodized. KI has also been approved by the FDA as a nonprescription drug for use as a "blocking agent" to prevent the human thyroid gland from absorbing radioactive iodine. However, KI may not provide people with 100% protection against all radioactive iodine. Its effectiveness will depend on a variety of factors, including when a person takes it, how much iodine is already in the person's thyroid, how fast the person's body processes it, and the amount of radioactive iodine the person is exposed to. Iodized table salt will not provide enough iodine to protect the thyroid and should not be used as a substitute.

Why would KI be important in the event of a nuclear incident?

Because the thyroid will rapidly absorb any iodine that is in the body, people may need to take KI tablets soon after an incident that involves radioactive iodine. The KI will saturate the thyroid gland with iodine and help prevent it from absorbing radioactive iodine. However, KI does not prevent the effects of other radioactive elements. Using KI will only protect the thyroid gland from radioactive iodine. It will not protect other parts of the body from radioactive iodine, and it will not protect a person from other radioactive materials that may be released.

Who should or should not take KI if the public is told to do so?

If a nuclear incident occurs, officials will have to find out which radioactive substances are present before recommending that people take KI. If radioactive iodine is not present, then taking KI will not protect people.

Children are the most susceptible to the dangerous effects of radioactive iodine. The FDA and the World Health Organization (WHO) recommend that children from newborn to 18 years of age all take KI unless they have a known allergy to iodine.

Women who are breastfeeding should also take KI, according to the FDA and WHO, to protect both themselves and their breast milk. However, breastfeeding infants should still be given the recommended dosage of KI to protect them from any radioactive iodine that they may breathe in or drink in breast milk.

Young adults between the ages of 18 and 40 have a smaller chance of developing thyroid cancer or thyroid disease from exposure to radioactive iodine than do children. However, the FDA and WHO still recommend that people ages 18 to 40 take the recommended dose of KI. This includes pregnant and breast-feeding women, who should take the same dose as other young adults.

Adults over the age of 40 have the smallest chance of developing thyroid cancer or thyroid disease after an exposure to radioactive iodine, but they have a greater chance of having an allergic reaction to the high dose of iodine in KI. Because of this, they are not recommended to take KI unless a very large dose of radioactive iodine is expected. People should listen to emergency management officials for recommendations after an incident.

What medical conditions make it dangerous to take KI?

The high concentration of iodine in KI can be harmful to some people. People should not take KI if they:

- have ever had thyroid disease (such as hyperthyroidism, thyroid nodules, or goiter).

- know they are allergic to iodine (if you are allergic to shellfish, ask your doctor or pharmacist about taking KI).

- have certain skin disorders (such as dermatitis herpetiformis or urticaria vasculitis).

People should consult their doctor if they are unsure whether or not to take KI.

Prussian Blue

Prussian blue can remove select radioactive materials from people's bodies, but must be taken under the guidance of the Radiation Emergency Assistance Center/Training Site (REAC/TS) of the Oak Ridge Institute.

People may become internally contaminated (inside their bodies) with radioactive materials by accidentally ingesting (eating or drinking) or inhaling (breathing) them. The sooner that these materials are removed from the body, the fewer and less severe the health effects of the contamination will be. Prussian blue is a substance that can help remove certain radioactive materials from people's bodies. However, Prussian blue currently is available only when doctors have determined that a person is internally contaminated.

What is Prussian blue?

Prussian blue was first produced as a blue dye in 1704 and has been used by artists and manufacturers ever since. It got its name from its use as a dye for Prussian military uniforms. Prussian blue dye and paint are still available today from art supply stores.

How is Prussian blue used to treat radioactive contamination?

Since the 1960s, Prussian blue has been used to treat people who have been internally contaminated with radioactive cesium or thallium. Prussian blue can be given at any point after doctors have determined that a person is internally contaminated. Prussian blue will help speed up the removal of cesium and thallium from the body.

Radioactive cesium and thallium, whether ingested or inhaled, will end up in the intestines. Prussian blue traps these materials in the intestines and keeps them from being absorbed by the body. The radioactive materials then move through the intestines and are excreted in bowel movements. Prussian blue reduces the biological half-life of cesium in the body from about 115 days to about 40 days. Prussian blue reduces the biological half-life of thallium from about 8 days to about 3 days. Because Prussian blue reduces the time that radioactive cesium and thallium stay in the body, it helps limit the amount of time the body is exposed to radiation.

Who can take Prussian blue?

People may be prescribed Prussian blue during an emergency when cesium or thallium has entered their bodies. Because Prussian blue is only approved for limited use it must be taken under the guidance of REAC/TS. The drug is safe for all adults, children, and infants, including pregnant women and women who are breast-feeding their babies. Prussian blue may not be recommended for people who have had constipation or blockages in the intestines.

The most common side effects of Prussian blue are upset stomach and constipation. These side effects can easily be treated with other medications. People will have blue feces during the time that they are taking Prussian blue.

Prussian blue is not routinely available. When approved for use by REAC/TS it is supplied in 500-milligram capsules that can be swallowed whole or mixed in liquid for children to drink. The amount to be taken depends on how badly a person is contaminated. Prussian blue must be taken 3–4 times a day for up to 150 days, depending on the extent of the contamination, under the supervision of a doctor.

People **should not** take Prussian blue artist's dye in an attempt to treat themselves. This type of Prussian blue is not designed to treat radioactive contamination and is not manufactured in a germ-free arca. People who are concerned about the possibility of being contaminated with radioactive cesium or thallium should go to their doctors for advice and treatment.

Additional Information

For more information about health effects from radiation exposure, chcck the following websites:

- www.epa.gov/radiation
- www.orau.gov/reacts/injury.htm
- www.bt.cdc.gov/radiation/healthfacts.asp

For more information about radiation terrorist events, check the following websites:

- www.bt.cdc.gov/radiation/terrorismqa.asp
- www.orau.gov/reacts
- www.nrt.org
- www.energy.gov
- www.nrc.gov
- www.epa.gov

For more information about preparing for a radiation emergency event, check the following websites:

- ww.fema.gov
- www.redcross.org/services/disaster
- www.epa.gov/swercepp
- www.ojp.usdoj.gov/bja

Chapter 67

Other Toxic Agents

Sarin

Sarin is a human-made chemical warfare agent classified as a nerve agent. Nerve agents are the most toxic and rapidly acting of the known chemical warfare agents. They are similar to certain kinds of pesticides (insect killers) called organophosphates in terms of how they work and what kind of harmful effects they cause. However, nerve agents are much more potent than organophosphate pesticides.

Sarin is a clear, colorless, and tasteless liquid that has no odor in its pure form. However, sarin can evaporate into a vapor (gas) and spread into the environment. Sarin is also known as GB.

How does sarin work?

The extent of poisoning caused by sarin depends on the amount of sarin to which a person was exposed, how the person was exposed, and the length of time of the exposure. Symptoms will appear within a few seconds after exposure to the vapor form of sarin and within a few minutes up to 18 hours after exposure to the liquid form.

All the nerve agents cause their toxic effects by preventing the proper operation of the chemical that acts as the body's "off switch"

This chapter includes text excerpted from "Facts about Sarin," "Facts about Sulfur Mustard," "Frequently Asked Questions about Ricin," and "Facts about VX," Public Health Emergency Preparedness and Response, Centers for Disease control and Prevention (CDC), March 2003. The full text and additional information about bioterrorism is available online at www.bt.cdc.gov.

for glands and muscles. Without an "off switch," the glands and muscles are constantly being stimulated. They may tire and no longer be able to sustain breathing function.

Because it evaporates so quickly, sarin presents an immediate but short-lived threat. People may not know that they were exposed because sarin has no odor. People exposed to a low or moderate dose of sarin by breathing contaminated air, eating contaminated food, drinking contaminated water, or touching contaminated surfaces may experience some or all of the following symptoms within seconds to hours of exposure: runny nose; watery eyes; small, pinpoint pupils; eye pain; blurred vision; drooling and excessive sweating; cough; chest tightness; rapid breathing; diarrhea; increased urination; confusion; drowsiness; weakness; headache; nausea, vomiting, and/or abdominal pain; slow or fast heart rate; low or high blood pressure. Even a small drop of sarin on the skin can cause sweating and muscle twitching where sarin touched the skin.

Exposure to large doses of sarin by any route may result in the following harmful health effects: loss of consciousness; convulsions; paralysis; respiratory failure possibly leading to death. Showing these signs and symptoms does not necessarily mean that a person has been exposed to sarin.

Mild or moderately exposed people usually recover completely. Severely exposed people are not likely to survive. Unlike some organophosphate pesticides, nerve agents have not been associated with neurological problems lasting more than 1 to 2 weeks after the exposure.

Recovery from sarin exposure is possible with treatment, but the antidotes available must be used quickly to be effective. Therefore, the best thing to do is avoid exposure:

- Leave the area where the sarin was released and get to fresh air. Quickly moving to an area where fresh air is available is highly effective in reducing the possibility of death from exposure to sarin vapor.

- If the sarin release was outdoors, move away from the area where the sarin was released. Go to the highest ground possible, because sarin is heavier than air and will sink to low-lying areas.

- If the sarin release was indoors, get out of the building.

- If people think they may have been exposed, they should remove their clothing, rapidly wash their entire body with soap and water, and get medical care as quickly as possible.

- If sarin has been swallowed, do not induce vomiting or give fluids to drink.

- Seek medical attention immediately. Dial 911 and explain what has happened.

Treatment consists of removing sarin from the body as soon as possible and providing supportive medical care in a hospital setting. Antidotes are available for sarin. They are most useful if given as soon as possible after exposure.

Sulfur Mustard

Sulfur mustard is a type of chemical warfare agent. These kinds of agents are called vesicants or blistering agents, because they cause blistering of the skin and mucous membranes on contact. Sulfur mustard is also known as "mustard gas" or "mustard agent" or by the military designations H, HD, and HT. Sulfur mustard sometimes smells like garlic, onions, or mustard and sometimes has no odor. It can be a vapor (the gaseous form of a liquid), an oily-textured liquid, or a solid. Sulfur mustard can be clear to yellow or brown when it is in liquid or solid form.

How does sulfur mustard work?

Adverse health effects caused by sulfur mustard depend on the amount people are exposed to, the route of exposure, and the length of time that people are exposed. Sulfur mustard is a powerful irritant and blistering agent that damages the skin, eyes, and respiratory (breathing) tract. It damages DNA, a vital component of cells in the body. Sulfur mustard vapor is heavier than air, so it will settle in low-lying areas.

Exposure to sulfur mustard is usually not fatal. Depending on the severity of the exposure, symptoms may not occur for 2 to 24 hours. Some people are more sensitive to sulfur mustard than are other people, and may have symptoms sooner.

Sulfur mustard can have the following effects on specific parts of the body:

- **Skin:** redness and itching of the skin may occur 2 to 48 hours after exposure and change eventually to yellow blistering of the skin.

- **Eyes:** irritation, pain, swelling, and tearing may occur within 3 to 12 hours of a mild to moderate exposure. A severe exposure may cause symptoms within 1 to 2 hours and may include the symptoms of a mild or moderate exposure plus light sensitivity, severe pain, or blindness (lasting up to 10 days).

- **Respiratory tract:** runny nose, sneezing, hoarseness, bloody nose, sinus pain, shortness of breath, and cough within 12 to 24 hours of a mild exposure and within 2 to 4 hours of a severe exposure.

- **Digestive tract:** abdominal pain, diarrhea, fever, nausea, and vomiting.

The long-term health effects may be:

- Exposure to sulfur mustard liquid is more likely to produce second- and third- degree burns and later scarring than is exposure to sulfur mustard vapor. Extensive skin burning can be fatal.

- Extensive breathing in of the vapors can cause chronic respiratory disease, repeated respiratory infections, or death.

- Extensive eye exposure can cause permanent blindness.

- Exposure to sulfur mustard may increase a person's risk for lung and respiratory cancer.

What should people should do if they are exposed to sulfur mustard?

Because no antidote exists for sulfur mustard exposure, the best thing to do is avoid it. Immediately leave the area where the sulfur mustard was released. Try to find higher ground, because sulfur mustard is heavier than air and will settle in low-lying areas. If avoiding sulfur mustard exposure is not possible, rapidly remove the sulfur mustard from the body. Getting the sulfur mustard off as soon as possible after exposure is the only effective way to prevent or decrease tissue damage to the body.

Quickly remove any clothing that has liquid sulfur mustard on it. If possible, seal the clothing in a plastic bag, and then seal that bag inside a second plastic bag. Immediately wash any exposed part of the body (eyes, skin, etc.) thoroughly with plain, clean water. Eyes need to be flushed with water for 5 to 10 minutes. Do NOT cover eyes with bandages, but do protect them with dark glasses or goggles.

If someone has ingested sulfur mustard, do NOT induce vomiting. Give the person milk to drink. Seek medical attention right away. Dial 911 and explain what has happened.

The most important factor is removing sulfur mustard from the body. Exposure to sulfur mustard is treated by giving the victim supportive medical care to minimize the effects of the exposure. Though no antidote exists for sulfur mustard, exposure is usually not fatal.

Ricin

Ricin is a poison that can be made from the waste left over from processing castor beans. It can be in the form of a powder, a mist, or a pellet, or it can be dissolved in water or weak acid. It is a stable substance. For example, it is not affected much by extreme conditions such as very hot or very cold temperatures.

It takes a deliberate act to make ricin and use it to poison people. Accidental exposure to ricin is highly unlikely. People can breathe in ricin mist or powder and be poisoned. Ricin can also get into water or food and then be swallowed. Pellets of ricin, or ricin dissolved in a liquid, can be injected into people's bodies. Depending on the route of exposure (such as injection), as little as 500 micrograms of ricin could be enough to kill an adult. A 500-microgram dose of ricin would be about the size of the head of a pin. A much greater amount would be needed to kill people if the ricin were inhaled (breathed in) or swallowed. Ricin poisoning is not contagious. It cannot be spread from person to person through casual contact.

How does ricin work?

Ricin works by getting inside the cells of a person's body and preventing the cells from making the proteins they need. Without the proteins, cells die, and eventually the whole body can shut down and die. Specific effects of ricin poisoning depend on whether ricin was inhaled, swallowed, or injected. The signs and symptoms of ricin exposure are:

- **Inhalation:** Within a few hours of inhaling significant amounts of ricin, the likely symptoms would be coughing, tightness in the chest, difficulty breathing, nausea, and aching muscles. Within the next few hours, the body's airways (such as lungs) would become severely inflamed (swollen and hot), excess fluid would build up in the lungs, breathing would become even more difficult, and the skin might turn blue. Excess fluid in the lungs would be diagnosed by x-ray or by listening to the chest with a stethoscope.

- **Ingestion:** If someone swallows a significant amount of ricin, he or she would have internal bleeding of the stomach and intestines that would lead to vomiting and bloody diarrhea. Eventually, the person's liver, spleen, and kidneys might stop working, and the person could die.

* **Injection:** Injection of a lethal amount of ricin at first would cause the muscles and lymph nodes near the injection site to die. Eventually, the liver, kidney s, and spleen would stop working, and the person would have massive bleeding from the stomach and intestines. The person would die from multiple organ failure.

Death from ricin poisoning could take place within 36 to 48 hours of exposure, whether by injection, ingestion, or inhalation. If the person lives longer than 5 days without complications, he or she will probably not die.

How is ricin poisoning treated?

No antidote exists for ricin. Ricin poisoning is treated by giving the victim supportive medical care to minimize the effects of the poisoning. The types of supportive medical care would depend on several factors, such as the route by which the victim was poisoned (that is, by inhalation, ingestion, or injection). Care could include such measures as helping the victim breathe and giving him or her intravenous fluids and medications to treat swelling.

VX

VX is a human-made chemical warfare agent classified as a nerve agent. It was originally developed in the United Kingdom in the early 1950s. VX is odorless and tasteless; it is an oily liquid that is amber in color and very slow to evaporate. It evaporates about as slowly as motor oil. Because VX vapor is heavier than air, it will sink to low-lying areas and create a greater exposure hazard there.

How does VX work?

The extent of poisoning caused by VX depends on the amount of VX to which a person was exposed, how the person was exposed, and the length of time of the exposure. Symptoms will appear within a few seconds after exposure to the vapor form of VX, and within a few minutes to up to 18 hours after exposure to the liquid form.

VX is the most potent of all nerve agents. Compared with the nerve agent sarin (also known as GB), VX is considered to be much more toxic by entry through the skin and somewhat more toxic by inhalation. It is possible that any visible VX liquid contact on the skin, unless washed off immediately, would be lethal.

Because it evaporates so slowly, VX can be a long-term threat as well as a short-term threat. Surfaces contaminated with VX should therefore be considered a long-term hazard.

The immediate signs and symptoms of VX exposure are:

- People may not know they were exposed to VX because it has no odor.

- People exposed to a low or moderate dose of VX by inhalation, ingestion (swallowing), or skin absorption may experience some or all of the following symptoms within seconds to hours of exposure: runny nose; watery eyes; small, pinpoint pupils; eye pain; blurred vision; drooling and excessive sweating; cough; chest tightness; rapid breathing; diarrhea; increased urination; confusion; drowsiness; weakness; headache; nausea, vomiting, and/or abdominal pain; slow or fast heart rate; abnormally low or high blood pressure; even a tiny drop of nerve agent on the skin can cause sweating and muscle twitching where the agent touched the skin.

- Exposure to a large dose of VX by any route may result in these additional health effects: loss of consciousness; convulsions; paralysis; respiratory failure possibly leading to death.

- Showing these signs and symptoms does not necessarily mean that a person has been exposed to VX.

Mild or moderately exposed people usually recover completely. Severely exposed people are not likely to survive. Unlike some organophosphate pesticides, nerve agents have not been associated with neurological problems lasting more than 1 to 2 weeks after the exposure.

How can people protect themselves, and what should they do if they are exposed to VX?

Recovery from VX exposure is possible with treatment, but the antidotes available must be used quickly to be effective. Therefore, the best thing to do is avoid exposure:

- Leave the area where the VX was released and get to fresh air. Quickly moving to an area where fresh air is available is highly effective in reducing the possibility of death from exposure to VX vapor.

- If the VX release was outdoors, move away from the area where the VX was released. Go to the highest ground possible, because VX is heavier than air and will sink to low-lying areas.

- If the VX release was indoors, get out of the building.

- If people think they may have been exposed, they should remove their clothing, rapidly wash their entire body with soap and water, and get medical care as quickly as possible.

How is VX exposure treated?

Treatment consists of removing VX from the body as soon as possible and providing supportive medical care in a hospital setting. Antidotes are available for VX. They are most useful if given as soon as possible after exposure.

Part Six

Infectious Disease Research

Chapter 68

Infectious Disease
Milestones and Statistics

Top 10 Infectious Disease Events of the 20th Century

Vaccine—Eradication of smallpox in 1977: The total mortality attributed to smallpox in the 20th century is 300–500 million or 3–5 times the total of all world wars. The cost of the eradication program was $100 million. No Nobel prize was ever given for this feat which many authorities consider the most important medical accomplishment of the 20th century.

Antibiotic—Discovery of penicillin in 1927: Penicillin is the grandfather of antibiotics and has had an extraordinary impact on infectious diseases. In fact, some compare this development to the development of the steam engine in terms of impact on society. A 93% decline in mortality due to pneumonia in children was reported; this decrease is largely ascribed to penicillin [*NEJM* 2000;342:1399].

This chapter includes "Top 10 Infectious Disease Events of the 20th Century," "Ten Most Commonly Reported Nationally Notifiable Infectious Diseases in Adults 1992–94," "Ten Most Important Newly-Described Microbial Pathogens 1987–1998," "Top Ten Infectious Diseases—Globe: Frequency," "Top Ten Infectious Diseases—Globe: Mortality," "Top 10 Infectious Diseases That Cause Hospitalization," by John G. Bartlett, © 1997–2002 The Johns Hopkins University on behalf of its Division of Infectious Diseases, all rights reserved; reprinted with permission. For more information visit http://www.hopkins-id.edu. Information is also included from "FastStats: Infectious Disease," National Center for Health Statistics, Centers for Disease Control and Prevention, reviewed April 2003.

Epidemic—Influenza epidemic of 1918–19: This major epidemic had an attack rate of 28%, causing 675,000 deaths in the U.S., and a global toll of 20 million. This epidemic decreased life expectancy in the U.S. by 11 years.

Bacterium—Tuberculosis (century): Second to HIV as the major microbial cause of death on earth—1.8 million deaths/year, 7.8 million new cases/year, and 1.7 billion infected persons.

Virus—HIV 1981: It is currently estimated that there are 34 million people living with HIV, 2.6 million deaths/year, and 5.6 million new infections/year. HIV accounts for an anticipated 20–30 year decrease in life expectancy in much of Africa.

Controversy—H. pylori, 1983: Set the precedent for an infectious agent as the cause of chronic diseases that bear no features of infectious diseases. The debate regarding cause and effect persisted for nine years, from the time it was presented at the American Gastroenterological Association meeting by Barry Marshall in 1983 until David Grahan showed the dramatic impact of antibiotic treatment on ulcer recurrences [*Ann Int Med* 1992;116:705]. This experience has fostered the pursuit of infectious agents in coronary artery disease, rheumatologic diseases, diabetes and many enigmatic neurologic syndromes.

Anti-viral—AZT (Zidovudine), 1986: The antiviral agent of the century because it spawned the subsequent development of other antiretroviral agents that have had an enormous impact on HIV. The results of the initial trial were "spectacular" when announced in September 1986: 19 deaths in the placebo group and one death in the AZT group.

Public Health—Chlorination of water: This is probably the most significant of many public health activities that had a major impact on reducing infectious diseases prior to antibiotics, and at an incredibly low price.

Basic Science—Plasmids, 1970: There needs to be recognition of many very important basic science discoveries: the double helix, polymerase chain reaction (PCR), restriction enzymes, mechanism of cholera + EC toxins, cloning, etc. Plasmids were selected in recognition of bacteria's ability to evade antibiotics in creative and unpredictable ways.

Clinical Research—The controlled trial, 1945: Specifically, the study of streptomycin and TB gave credibility to claims of benefit at a time when medical management was largely based on anecdotes, hearsay, and folklore.

Table 68.1. Ten Most Commonly Reported Nationally Notifiable Infectious Diseases in Adults*

| Condition | No. Cases | Rate/100,000 | |
		Female	Male
Gonorrhoeae	875,817	122.0	205.2
AIDS	222,083	12.1	71.0
Syphilis	71,397	11.0	15.0
Tuberculosis	69,344	8.1	17.5
Salmonellosis	55,229	10.5	9.5
Hepatitis A	43,987	6.3	9.8
Hepatitis B	35,627	4.9	8.2
Shigellosis	22,328	5.0	3.1
Lyme disease	21,176	3.8	3.9
Hepatitis C	14,393	1.7	3.8

*Statistics for 1992–94 (*MMWR* 1997;46:637).

Table 68.2. Ten Most Important Newly Described Microbial Pathogens 1987–1998 (in order by year of publication)

Agent	Disease	Year of Discovery
Human herpes virus 6	Roseola-infantum	1988
Hepatitis E	Foodborne hepatitis	1988
Hepatitis C	Non A, non B hepatitis	1989
Bartonella henselae	Cat scratch disease	1990
Guanarito virus	Venezuelan hemorrhagic fever	1991
Vibrio cholera 0139	Cholera (new strain)	1992
T. whippelii	Whipple disease	1992
Si Nombre Virus	Hantavirus Pulmonary Syndrome	1993
Sabia virus	Brazilian hemorrhagic fever	1994
Human herpes virus 8	Kaposi's sarcoma	1995

Table 68.3. Top Ten Infectious Diseases, Global, by Frequency

Condition	Frequency (x 1000)
Diarrhea	4,000,000
Tuberculosis	1,900,000
Worms	1,400,000
Malaria	500,000
Hepatitis (HBV & HCV)	450,000
Pneumonia	395,000
Sexually transmitted diseases	330,000
Measles	42,000
Pertussis	40,000
HIV (new infections)	3,100
Meningococcal meningitis	350

Table 68.4. Top Ten Infectious Diseases, Global, Mortality

Condition	Frequency (x 1000)
Pneumonia	4,400
Diarrhea	3,100
Tuberculosis	3,100
Malaria	2,100
AIDS	1,500
Hepatitis B	1,100
Measles	1,000
Neonatal tetanus	460
Pertussis	350
Worms	135

Table 68.5. Top Infectious Diseases That Cause Hospitalization (Based on data from the National Hospital Discharge Survey for U.S. hospitals in 1994*)

Rank	Infectious Disease	Estimated No. Hospitalizations (#/100,000 population)	Increase or Decrease Compared to 1980
1	Lower respiratory tract infection	1,4480,600 (568)	+28,700
2	Urinary tract infection	470,200 (180)	+6,600
3	Cellulitus	335,300 (129)	+2,200
4	Septicemia	301,800 (116)	+18,300
5	Abdominal and rectal infections	282,600 (108)	-3,900
6	Upper respiratory tract infections	191,400 (73)	-38,700
7	Enteric infections	154,200 (59)	-900
8	Infections of prosthetic devices	73,500 (28)	+4,000
9	Postoperative infection	72,800 (28)	+2,300
10	Infections in pregnancy	56,000 (22)	+100
11	Osteomyelitis	48,100 (18)	+1,800
12	Pelvic inflammatory disease	40,000 (18)	-7,800
13	HIV/AIDS	41,700 (16)	+2,300
14	Mycosis	29,500 (11)	+900
15	Viral CNS infection	28,100 (11)	+400

*Adapted from Simonsen L, et al., *Arch Intern Med* 110;1923:1998.

Table 68.6. Infectious Diseases in the United States

Disease	Number of Cases (year reported)
Number of Hepatitis B Cases Annually:	8,036 (2000)
Number of Tuberculosis Cases Annually:	16,337 (2000)
Number of Syphilis Cases Annually:	31,575 (2000)
Number of Chlamydia Cases Annually:	702,093 (2000)
Number of Gonorrhea Cases Annually:	358,995 (2000)
Number of Salmonella Cases Annually:	39,574 (2000)

Source: *Health, United States: 2002*, National Center for Health Statistics, Centers for Disease Control and Prevention, Table 53.

Chapter 69

Addressing the
Problem of Infectious Disease
Transmission

Infectious diseases are a continuing menace to all segments of society, regardless of age, gender, lifestyle, ethnic background, and socioeconomic status. They cause suffering and death and impose an enormous financial burden on society. Because we do not know what new diseases will arise, we must always be prepared for the unexpected.

Foodborne and Waterborne Diseases

Foodborne and waterborne infections are major public health problems. Each year, millions of people in the United States are infected with foodborne diseases, and several thousand die. Hospitalization costs for these illnesses are estimated at over $3 billion a year, and costs from lost productivity are much higher. Waterborne diseases also contribute significantly to the U.S. disease burden. Many different pathogens can be foodborne or waterborne, and more are likely to be discovered. Preventing these diseases depends on understanding how food or water becomes contaminated and involves working with many partners to reduce or prevent contamination.

Foodborne pathogens are numerous and have many ways to enter the food chain, which makes disease prevention very complex. Some

Excerpted from "Preventing Emerging Infectious Diseases: A Strategy for the 21st Century," Centers for Disease Control and Prevention, 1998. Despite the date of this document, the issues and programs described will help the reader understand the concepts involved.

513

emerging foodborne pathogens are found in food animals, including cattle, poultry, fish, and shellfish. Although these animals may appear healthy, the meat, eggs, milk, or other products derived from them can be contaminated with *Escherichia coli* O157: H7, *Salmonella,* or other pathogens. Fresh produce is an important component of a healthy diet, but fruits and vegetables can also be sources of infection if they are contaminated in the field or after harvest. Moreover, some pathogens are spread from infected people who contaminate the food while preparing it. Safe food production and preparation practices applied throughout the food industry can reduce the risk of contamination. For some food products further safety may be ensured by pasteurization, irradiation, or similar processes.

New challenges due to foodborne pathogens are likely to emerge in the future. Wide commercial distribution of food products means that outbreaks can affect many people simultaneously over a large geographic area. Pathogens common in the developing world now cause illness in the United States because more of our food crosses international borders. In addition, the frequent use of antibiotics in food animals may select for antibiotic-resistant bacteria that can be transmitted to humans.

The problems posed by waterborne pathogens are also changing. In the past, most cases of waterborne diseases were due to bacterial contamination, which can be prevented by standard water disinfection treatments such as chlorination. In much of the developing world, however, this level of protection remains unachievable. In the United States and Europe, pathogens that are resistant to routine disinfection are now more commonly recognized as causes of waterborne diseases. These include Norwalk-like viruses and the parasite *Cryptosporidium,* which caused the largest single waterborne disease outbreak in the United States in 1993, affecting more than 400,000 people. Of the waterborne outbreaks reported to Centers for Disease Control and Prevention (CDC) during 1993 and 1994, more than half of those for which an infectious cause could be identified were due to contamination by chlorine-resistant microbes.

In partnership with other governmental agencies and international groups, the CDC is working toward effective global surveillance and control of foodborne and waterborne pathogens. The CDC is a major participant in the National Food Safety Initiative (NFSI), which was created in 1997 to address food safety problems in the United States. Through the NFSI, the CDC is improving surveillance and response to foodborne diseases, while the FDA, the USDA, and other agencies are expanding food safety inspection, research, training, and prevention activities. Similarly, the CDC is collaborating with the EPA and the drinking water industry to better estimate the risk of waterborne disease, develop better methods for detecting new pathogens in drinking water, and identify human and animal sources of water contamination.

Foodborne and Waterborne Pathogens

- *Campylobacter* is the most common contaminant of chicken.

- *Cryptosporidium* is a parasite that infects many wild and domestic animals and humans. It is highly resistant to disinfectants used to purify drinking water and can get through many types of water filters.

- *Cyclospora* is a parasite that has been traced to raspberries, basil in pesto sauces, and drinking water.

- *E. coli* O157: H7 is a bacterium found primarily in meats, in produce contaminated by manure in growing fields (e.g., sprouts), and in water. Although easily killed by water disinfectants, it has caused outbreaks in people in swimming pools not adequately chlorinated and in communities served by well water that was not disinfected.

- *Giardia* is one of the most common parasites implicated in waterborne outbreaks in the United States. It is moderately resistant to water disinfectants.

- *Listeria* is a contaminant of cold foods like soft cheeses and deli meats.

- *Salmonella enteritidis* is found in eggs.

- *Shigella* are bacteria that cause serious illness when water supplies are not adequately disinfected.

- Unpasteurized milk is a source of *Salmonella typhimurium* DT-104, an aggressive strain of *Salmonella* that is resistant to many antibiotics.

Bloodborne Diseases

Improvements in donor screening, serologic testing, and transfusion practices have made the U.S. blood supply one of the safest in the world, despite its size and complexity. Every year, 12 million units of blood are donated by volunteers and used to treat 4 million people.

An additional 13 million units of plasma are used to produce blood products such as immunoglobulins and clotting factors.

Because blood is a human tissue, it is a vehicle for transmission of infectious agents. During the 1970s and early 1980s, human immunodeficiency virus (HIV) was transmitted through transfusions of blood and clotting factors, and until the early 1990s, blood and blood products were contaminated with hepatitis C virus. Although research on artificial blood substitutes is underway, it is unlikely that such products will be available in the near future. Therefore, continued vigilance is required to safeguard our blood supply from recognized and emerging infectious disease threats.

Although the Food and Drug Administration (FDA) has regulatory responsibility for blood safety in the United States, CDC is responsible for detecting and assessing public health risks associated with blood and blood products. CDC and its partners are currently designing new strategies to prevent diseases from being transmitted by transfusions and ensure both the safety and availability of blood and blood products. Those strategies include devising and evaluating ways to screen donated blood, inactivating infectious agents in blood and blood products; finding new ways to ensure that people at risk of transmitting bloodborne infections do not donate blood; and identifying newly recognized pathogens that may be transmitted through blood transfusions.

Vectorborne and Zoonotic Diseases

A number of infectious diseases are "vectorborne," which in means that they are transmitted to animals and humans by blood-feeding arthropods, such as mosquitoes and ticks. Vectorborne diseases of public health importance include dengue fever, human ehrlichiosis, malaria, Lyme disease, and West Nile virus infection. As more people come in contact with previously undisturbed environments, their risk of infection with vectorborne diseases is increased. For example, residential building in the rural northeastern United States increased the risk for humans to come into contact with ticks that transmit Lyme disease.

Other infectious diseases are "zoonoses," which means that they are transmitted to humans by animals. Important zoonotic diseases include hantavirus pulmonary syndrome, influenza, leptospirosis, rabies, and salmonellosis, as well as most vectorborne diseases. The growing commercial pet trade is one way in which human risk of infection with zoonotic diseases is increased as these exotic animals may bring with them viruses, bacteria, and parasites new to North Americans.

The reemergence of certain vectorborne and zoonotic diseases may also be intensified by engineering projects such as land-clearing, dam-building, or creating irrigation systems, all of which bring humans into contact with animals and arthropods.

For example, when the Aswan Dam was built in Egypt during the 1950s, it created excellent breeding grounds for snails carrying parasites that cause schistosomiasis. While many vectorborne and zoonotic diseases are associated with the tropics or the developing world, some pathogens that cause diseases, such as Lyme disease, human ehrlichiosis, and hantavirus pulmonary syndrome, were first identified in North America. The emergence of Lyme disease in the United States was associated with the reversion of agricultural lands to secondary growth forest, the immigration of deer that carry infected ticks into these areas, and increasing urbanization.

West Nile virus encephalitis is another disease that has emerged in recent years in temperate regions of Europe and North America, presenting a threat to both people and animals. The public health implications of West Nile virus are serious. To prevent and control West Nile virus infection and other mosquito-borne diseases, the public health system must be fully equipped to conduct active surveillance, identify birds and animals that act as hosts, monitor human illness, and carry out mosquito control activities.

Travelers, Immigrants, and Refugees

People who cross international boundaries, such as travelers (tourists, businesspeople, and other workers), immigrants, and refugees, may be at increased risk of contracting infectious diseases, especially tourists or workers who have no immunity because the disease agents are uncommon in their native countries. Immigrants may come from nations where diseases like tuberculosis and malaria are endemic, and refugees may come from situations where crowding and malnutrition create ideal conditions for the spread of diseases like cholera, shigellosis, malaria, and measles.

From 1984 through 1994, the annual number of people traveling outside the United States doubled, from 20 million to 40 million, a substantial increase. Moreover, about half of those people visited tropical locations, putting them at risk for diseases they would not normally encounter. Travelers on commercial flights can reach most American cities from any part of the world within 36 hours, which is less time than the incubation period (the time between infection and the appearance of symptoms) for many infectious diseases. Thus, travelers who have been infected may not appear ill when they enter the United States through an airport or seaport or by crossing the border from Canada or Mexico. Travelers who become ill after they enter the United States must be identified through state and local surveillance efforts.

CDC operates eight quarantine stations which evaluate sick persons at United States ports of entry: Atlanta, Chicago, Honolulu, Los Angeles, Miami, New York, San Francisco, and Seattle. CDC also distributes health information to international travelers, provides guidelines and monitors the required medical assessment of immigrants and refugees. Other priorities include detecting and responding to diseases in travelers, refugees, and immigrants, and conducting studies to help prevent and control diseases in these populations. CDC also alerts local health departments and physicians about countries where outbreaks are occurring.

Chapter 70

Inside a Biosafety Level 4 (BSL-4) Laboratory

What Is a Biosafety Level 4 (BSL-4) Laboratory?

BSL-4 laboratories are designed to prevent infectious microbes from being released into the environment and to provide the highest possible level of safety to scientists carrying out experiments with infectious microbes. BSL-4 facilities may contain clinical components and/or those where animal experiments can be safely carried out.

BSL-4 uses several measures to ensure infectious agents are properly contained or destroyed. They include microfiltration of air, airlock buffer zones, "space suits" with positive-pressure air supply, chemical decontamination, and decontamination at high temperature for long periods of all materials produced in the facility.

Biosafety Lab Tour

In Biosafety Level 4 (BSL-4) laboratories, scientists study some of the world's potentially most dangerous microbes. These labs are designed to prevent microbes from being released into the environment and to provide maximum safety for the scientists. When a laboratory is designated BSL-4, that means the highest possible containment measures are in place.

This chapter includes "What is a Biosafety Level 4 (BSL-4) Laboratory?" from "An Integrated Research Facility at Rocky Mountain Laboratories," April 16, 2003, "Biosafety Lab Tour," undated, National Institutes of Health (NIH), National Institute of Allergy and Infectious Diseases (NIAID) Biodefense Research.

From the Outside

A Biosafety Level-4 (BSL-4) lab may look like an ordinary building from the outside, but these buildings are anything but ordinary. They are designed and constructed by experts so that nothing gets in or out that isn't supposed to, not even something as tiny as a bacterium or virus.

BSL-4 design features include the following:

Table 70.1. What do the Biosafety Level (BSL) numbers mean? (*continued on next page*)

BSL 1
Appropriate for: Educational Facilities

Types of biological agents: Strains of viable microorganisms not known to consistently cause disease in healthy adults

BSL-2
Appropriate for: Clinical or Diagnostic Facilities

Types of biological agents: Moderate-risk agents that are present in the community and can cause disease of varying severity (for example, testing blood or body fluids of unknown infectivity for hepatitis B or salmonella).

Safety considerations: Samples can be handled at the laboratory bench if the potential for producing splashes or aerosols is low. Scientists and technicians must wear splash shields, face protection, gowns, and gloves while using extra care with needles and glass, and they must decontaminate the work area and materials after each procedure. Biological Safety Cabinets (BSCs) are used to work with concentrated cultures or procedures that generate aerosols.

BSL-3
Appropriate for: Clinical, Research, or Production Facilities

Types of biological agents: Indigenous or exotic agents that may cause serious or potentially lethal infection and have potential for respiratory transmission by personnel exposure to infectious aerosols (for example, *Mycobacterium tuberculosis*, the cause of tuberculosis, and *Coxielli burnetii*, the cause of Q fever).
BSL-3 continued on next page

- All seams, joints, and doors are sealed to make the building airtight. You cannot open a window in a BSL-4 lab. Air does not flow in or out under the doors

- Air is pumped in and out of the building through a filtration system that catches even the tiniest microscopic particles, bacteria and viruses included

- All air ducts are welded stainless steel and tested to be airtight

Table 70.1. What do the Biosafety Level (BSL) numbers mean? (*continued from previous page*)

BSL-3 (continued)
Safety considerations: BSL-3 laboratories are required to include BSCs, controlled double-door laboratory access, and engineering controls, including maintaining negative air pressure relative to the surrounding rooms (so that all air flow is directed into the BSL-3 suites, not out into the surrounding rooms); microfiltration of air; and air-lock buffer zones. As necessary, before an individual can begin work in a BSL-3 laboratory, he or she will be required to undergo special training and receive preventive vaccines. Operational safeguards to ensure that infectious agents are properly contained or destroyed include long-time, high-temperature decontamination of all materials produced in a BSL-3 suite.

BSL-4
Appropriate for: Research

Types of biological agents: Dangerous or exotic agents that have a high risk of a life-threatening disease for which there is no available vaccine or therapy (for example, Ebola virus).

Safety Considerations: BSL-4 laboratories use all of the safety measures required for BSL-3. A BSL-4 facility also requires security measures to control access. Some BSL-4 laboratories may require personnel to use "space suits" with positive-pressure air supply. Decontamination is required of all materials produced in BSL-4 laboratories, either chemical decontamination or decontamination at high temperature for long periods.

Source: Excerpted from "An Integrated Research Facility at Fort Detrick, Maryland," National Institute of Allergy and Infectious Diseases, April 16, 2003.

- Inside many BSL-4 facilities, the laboratories are surrounded by buffer corridors that help protect the labs in the event of a bombing attack from outside

- Features such as airlocks, fumigation chambers, disinfectant "dunk tanks" and waste water treatment systems ensure that absolutely everything that leaves a BSL-4 lab is decontaminated

Outside Security

Security around a BSL-4 laboratory is tight. Only authorized personnel can pass through perimeter security.

Security measures here typically include combinations of the following:

- Perimeter fencing
- Security guards
- Closed-circuit TV surveillance
- Intrusion alarms
- Nighttime security lighting

Interior Security

Once past outside security, BSL-4 lab workers must pass an interior security station.

Measures here typically include combinations of the following:

- Extensive background checks prior to employment for everyone who works in the building

- Guards who check everyone's identification and credentials

- Special identification cards that are scanned to provide an electronic record of who goes in and out and when

- Identification devices such as retinal or fingerprint scanners

Scouring the Air

Once inside a BSL-4 lab, scientists breathe air filtered by a high-efficiency particulate air (HEPA) filter system. HEPA filters use ultra-fine fibers to remove microscopic particles 0.3 microns in size and smaller from the air with nearly 100 percent efficiency. (One micron is a millionth of a meter, about the length of a typical bacterium.)

Larger particles are of course removed more easily. HEPA filters can trap any bacteria or viruses that may be in the air. Exhaust air from the building always passes through two HEPA filters. The air pressure across these filters is monitored, and if a filter becomes clogged and the pressure drops, an alarm sounds. The filters are inspected regularly, and they are sterilized before being replaced.

Changing Room

Researchers must leave their clothes behind in a changing room, take a decontaminating shower, and put on laboratory clothes (even socks and underwear are provided) or a biocontainment suit before entering the lab.

Inside the Lab

Once past security and inside the lab, redundant safety systems, procedures, and equipment protect researchers and the environment. Safety features here include the following:

- Entries and exits have double-door airlocks

- Work surfaces are regularly decontaminated

- If a vaccine exists, researchers are vaccinated against the microbe they are studying

- All solid and liquid waste is decontaminated by heat sterilization, gaseous sterilization, or liquid disinfectant. Before it leaves the facility, this waste meets or exceeds the environmental standards of the community where the facility is built

Biocontainment Suits and Biosafety Cabinets

Researchers in biocontainment suits conjure up images of danger. However, highly trained laboratory personnel in suits such as these perform their research day in and day out without incident.

Some facts about laboratory safety measures and equipment:

- The airtight, pressurized suits have dedicated life-support systems that include redundant breathing air compressors, alarms and emergency backup air tanks, and a HEPA air filtration system

- Work stations called biosafety cabinets serve as additional barriers protecting the worker and the environment. With their own inward-directed and HEPA-filtered air systems, these cabinets are designed to prevent potentially dangerous microbes from escaping

Decontaminating Shower

Once their work is completed, researchers in biocontainment suits must shower with strong disinfectant before leaving the lab and removing the suit.

The Community and Environment

The multiple, redundant safety measures at BSL-4 facilities protect not only the people working in the laboratory, but the environment and the community in which the laboratory is located.

Chapter 71

Deciphering Pathogens: Blueprints for New Medical Tools

Understanding the Inner Workings of Disease-Causing Microbes

The human species has co-existed with microbes—tiny organisms like bacteria, viruses, fungi, and parasites—since we first appeared on Earth. During the hundreds of millennia since then, it has been a complex and sometimes uneasy relationship. Indeed, humans cannot live without certain microbes that help maintain proper physiological conditions inside our bodies, nourish our soil, or keep our environment in balance. At the same time, these tiny creatures have also swiftly devastated human populations around the world.

Scientists who study microbes that cause human illness, commonly called pathogens, have continually developed newer and better strategies to understand how the germs cause disease and how to stop them. That knowledge has led to the control of many diseases, like measles, diphtheria, tetanus, pertussis, mumps, and polio, and the complete eradication of natural disease from one-time killers like smallpox.

At the end of the 20th century, the new research approach known as "genomics" emerged as a powerful investigative tool for understanding biology. Now, investigators in every area of the life sciences use the vast and orderly collections of an organism's genetic information,

National Institute of Allergy and Infectious Diseases, National Institutes of Health (NIH), September 2002.

known as its "genome," to understand each and every process an organism carries out, all at once, as a complete system.

The Burden of Infectious Diseases

Probably nowhere in science is genomics making more inroads into understanding human diseases than in the field of microbiology—the study of microbes and their interactions with human beings and the environment. With the complete genomes of dozens of pathogenic microbes in hand—and many more on the way—scientists have begun a powerful new assault on some of humankind's oldest enemies. Illnesses caused by pathogenic microbes are today the second leading cause of death worldwide and third leading cause of death in the United States. Throughout the world, infectious diseases are also responsible for countless hospitalizations, sick days, missed work, and other lost opportunities. Those losses cost hundreds of billions of dollars each year.

Three infectious diseases alone—TB, malaria, and HIV/AIDS— illustrate the tremendous human toll taken by microbes each year. Though an ancient disease, TB remains a leading case of death worldwide, claiming 2 million lives every year. One-third of the world's population is infected with the TB bacterium, *Mycobacterium tuberculosis*, and someone is newly infected every second. Malaria, which is caused by a single-celled parasite spread to people by mosquitoes, kills up to 2.7 million people annually, most of them African children. Between 400 million and 900 million acute malaria cases occur each year in African children alone. HIV/AIDS first emerged in the early 1980s and

Table 71.1. The Leading Infectious Causes of Death Worldwide, 2000

Lower respiratory infections	3.9 million
HIV/AIDS	2.9 million
Diarrheal diseases	2.1 million
Tuberculosis	1.7 million
Malaria	1.1 million
Measles	777,000

Source: *World Health Report 2001*, World Health Organization, p. 144.

has since killed more than 20 million people around the world. As of the end of 2001, 40 million people were living with HIV/AIDS.

Those three diseases, however, are not the only threats to human health. Infectious diarrheal diseases kill almost as many people each year as HIV/AIDS, and respiratory infections kill far more. In the United States, pneumococcal pneumonia and influenza account for thousands of deaths during an ordinary year. That death toll surged to more than 20 million worldwide during the influenza pandemic that occurred during the 1918 flu season. While many important, infectious killers are held in check by vaccines and antibiotics, others cannot be stopped because there is currently no way to prevent or treat them. Other infections, such as West Nile fever, dengue, mad cow disease, and those caused by Ebola and hanta viruses, can emerge suddenly out of nowhere.

A Closer Look: Tuberculosis

Genomics Yield Clues for Vaccines, New Treatments for Tuberculosis

Tuberculosis (TB) is a contagious disease that has exacted a devastating toll throughout human history. TB kills two million people each year, and experts expect 500 million new infections to occur globally over the next decade. To make matters worse, worrisome new multidrug-resistant strains of the TB bacterium have emerged, making treatment more difficult.

NIAID and its collaborators sponsored the genomic analysis of the TB bacterium, *Mycobacterium tuberculosis*, as well as that of the closely related *Mycobacterium leprae*, which causes leprosy. Although leprosy is a much different disease, the two pathogens nonetheless have a great deal in common. For example, both are able to sidestep critical defensive responses of an infected person's immune system. Detailed comparisons of their genomes therefore will help researchers learn how they and other microbes can circumvent immune responses.

Researchers studying the *M. tuberculosis* genome are developing other noteworthy insights into the germ's biochemical makeup and disease-causing properties. For instance, about 10 percent of that pathogen's genes are devoted to making lipids—fatty substances used in its outer coat that enable it to withstand human immune responses and to ward off the actions of several antibiotics. In addition, both *M. tuberculosis* and *M. leprae* are missing genes that enable other microorganisms to grow more efficiently, which helps explain a frustrating feature of these microorganisms—they are extraordinarily difficult to grow in laboratories. That characteristic has repeatedly thwarted scientists and clinical microbiologists in their efforts to examine and learn more about these pathogens.

NIAID has also teamed with the National Institute of General Medical Sciences (NIGMS) to co-fund the *Mycobacterium tuberculosis* Structural Genomics Consortium. The consortium is a collaboration of scientists from 12 different countries who are analyzing the molecular structures of more than 400 proteins identified from the microbe's genome. Obtaining those structures should help researchers develop new or improved drugs and vaccines against tuberculosis.

A Closer Look: Malaria

Using Genomics to Solve the Complexities of a Notorious Killer

As many as 300 to 500 million new cases of malaria develop each year, and the disease is responsible for up to 2.7 million deaths yearly, many among young children. Although potent drugs and aggressive mosquito control measures once appeared to have malaria on the retreat in some areas of the world, widening drug resistance and concerns about unsafe uses of insecticides are among the reasons why malaria is now resurgent.

The parasites that cause malaria in humans, *Plasmodium falciparum* and three closely related species, are considerably more complex than bacteria. Not only does the parasite spend part of its life in a mosquito, but once it infects humans it undergoes distinct changes in form and size as it invades different cell types, including red blood cells and liver cells. As might be expected, the complex life cycle of *Plasmodium* species reflects its similarly complex underlying genetics. It's genome is nearly 10-times the size of a typical bacterium and is divided among several chromosomes. In the case of *P. falciparum*, 14 different chromosomes contain about 30 million base pairs of DNA.

During the mid-1990s, NIAID joined forces with other agencies and private foundations in the United States and United Kingdom to establish an international consortium for determining the genomic sequence of *P. falciparum*. Genomics experts working as part of that consortium have been steadily accelerating their efforts to determine the sequence of this parasite. By 1998, the DNA sequence for one of the 14 chromosomes had been completed, quickly leading to the identification of genes encoding a family of proteins that help this parasite elude the human immune system. The completed *P. falciparum* genome sequence was published in 2002, along with the genome of its mosquito host. Those sequences can now be combined with the recently completed human genome sequence to help paint a complete picture of the genetic mechanisms that control malaria infection, transmission, and immunity.

The accumulating genomic data have helped researchers determine how the parasite becomes resistant to malaria drugs and to identify promising targets for new antimalaria agents. For instance, a group of researchers in Germany scanned the public genome database to learn that the first fully sequenced *P. falciparum* chromosome contains genes encoding a relatively unusual means for making steroids. Further analysis suggested a point of vulnerability where drugs might inhibit some of this vital biochemical process within the parasite without affecting similar processes within infected people. Preliminary findings confirm that a drug called fosmidomycin and other closely related compounds are effective when used to treat malaria-like infections in mice—a sign that these drugs should be further evaluated for their safety and effectiveness in humans.

Understanding the Genomes of Microbes Will Provide New Insights into Health

By rigorously evaluating and funding laboratory, clinical, and field investigations that analyze the genomes of pathogenic microbes, the National Institute of Allergy and Infectious Diseases (NIAID), National Institutes of Health, a component of the U.S. Department of Health and Human Services, supports a diverse research program to define exactly how a microbe's genetic instructions drive it to make people sick. NIAID genomics research focuses on these areas

- Obtaining the complete genome sequence of organisms that are pathogenic to humans

- Analyzing pathogen genomes to understand how the microbe causes disease

- Using knowledge of microbe gene function to identify targets for new drugs or vaccines that can interrupt the infectious or disease-causing process

- Identifying mechanisms of drug resistance in microbes

- Studying the human genome to identify genetic variations that may protect or predispose people to infection or make resistant to the benefits of vaccines or antibiotics

- Making the data freely available for use by all researchers

Reading a Microbe's Genetic Language

In an earlier time, the vast range in size and complexity of microbes and their genetic instructions presented huge technical difficulties for scientists trying to parse out the molecular instructions that give germs the upper hand over human beings. Although researchers have long known a pathogen's sinister behaviors are encoded in the genetic language of DNA (deoxyribonucleic acid), or its related molecule, RNA (ribonucleic acid), deciphering the code in the laboratory once took months to years for even the smallest organisms. But now, thanks to the push to advance DNA sequencing of much larger genomes, newer automated technology allows researchers to read relatively small microbe genomes in days or even hours.

The instructions in a genome are contained in sets of DNA bases represented by the letters A, C, T, and G, and organized into genes. (Some virus genomes consist of RNA, a type of chemical photocopy of DNA.) The sequence of bases in DNA or RNA spells out the recipe for a pathogen's full set of biochemical ingredients—typically, anywhere from several hundred to several thousand kinds of proteins. Those proteins in turn are used to build cell structures and to carry out most of its activities. Using genome sequencing, scientists studying pathogenic microbes can for the first time look at complete collections of genes and the proteins they encode. Genomes therefore enable researchers to identify previously hidden molecules and biological processes that may give way to new drugs and vaccines aimed at interrupting them.

Since the first genomic sequence of a bacterial pathogen was completed in 1995, pathogen genome sequencing efforts have continued to accelerate at an astonishing rate. The genomes of several dozen microbes known to cause disease in humans have now been sequenced, with more soon to be reported. An up-to-date list of completed and ongoing genome sequencing projects can be found on the NIAID Web site at wwwniaid.nih.gov.

How a Genome Is Sequenced

Microbial genome projects start with laboratory procedures aimed at dividing large DNA molecules into smaller fragments for easier handling. Special enzymes are used to cut a microbe's single DNA-containing chromosome (or, in some cases, its several separate DNA molecules) randomly into hundreds of pieces, which are collected into separate entities, or "clones," for follow-up analytical procedures. The entire collection of clones from a particular microorganism often is referred to as a "library," symbolizing its role as a comprehensive and orderly collection of the organism's genetic information.

Typically, specialized instruments determine the base-pair sequence of DNA in each clone, and researchers repeat a sequencing analysis several times to ensure the information is accurate. That raw information is fed into computer programs that collect the sequences of the separate fragments, determine overlaps between fragments, and eventually reassemble them. The completed process catalogs each bit of formation in the exact order it was in the overall genome.

Even with a pathogen's full base-pair sequence in hand, the genome still contains many mysteries that remain to be ferreted out. Important follow-up efforts known as "annotation" involve a series of steps, many of them involving sophisticated computer analysis, to determine the identity and function of a microbe's full set of genes. So far, researchers studying microbial genomic sequences can identify and categorize perhaps one-third to one-half of the genes in a newly sequenced microbe. But many of the other gene sequences are yet to be identified.

Genomic Studies Explain How Microbes Cause Disease

Many of the genes within a microbial cell perform what scientists call "housekeeping" functions by providing energy, structural components, and other mundane but essential features to meet life's basic demands at the cellular level. However, some of those genes are peculiar to specific microbial pathogens, helping to set them apart from benign microorganisms and also from other pathogens. For instance, some pathogens infect the respiratory tract and may cause pneumonia, others infect the skin or soft tissues, and others infect the genital tract and are sexually transmitted. Still others may be foodborne and cause gastrointestinal disorders.

Genomic approaches are used to identify key similarities and differences among different microbes. Comparative genomics is a field of study that examines variation between genomes. By identifying genetic differences among different microbe species or strains, researchers can identify the genes that enable the microbes to behave as they do.

Comparative genomics can also identify common genetic features that can be targeted for new drugs, vaccines, or diagnostic tests.

For example, researchers have used genome sequencing to glean insights about two similar pathogens—*Vibrio cholerae* and *Escherichia coli*.

Both bacteria sometimes cause severe gastrointestinal diseases but at other times are benign.

V. cholerae is responsible for causing outbreaks of cholera, a severe diarrheal disease that kills thousands of people each year. During pandemics, which typically occur several times per century, global tolls rise sharply, causing high death rates particularly among vulnerable children living in developing countries where the bacteria are particularly common in water sources.

In 2001, a team of NIAID-supported cholera and genome-sequencing experts determined the full DNA sequence of the bacterium. Initial genomic analysis indicates that each comma-shaped *V. cholerae* bacterium contains two unevenly sized chromosomes that, taken together, comprise about 4 million DNA base pairs and encode nearly 4,000 genes. Information obtained from the bacterium's genomic sequence already is providing researchers with a better understanding of how this pathogen persists in open marine environments, often in a quiescent state while not causing harm to humans or wildlife between periods when it causes major cholera outbreaks.

Researchers have learned that most of *V. cholerae's* genes are much like those found in another more common bacteria, *E. coli*, which ordinarily is not nearly so harmful to humans. Despite the extensive genetic similarity between the two microbes, nearly 500 of the *V. cholerae* genes have no known counterpart in *E. coli*. Scientists are further analyzing the 500 "anonymous" *V. cholerae* genes to learn how they may play important roles in making it such a devastating pathogen.

Even different strains of the same microbe can carry different abilities to cause illness. *E. coli* O157:H7, for example, is a virulent strain that can cause bloody diarrhea, kidney troubles, and even death. Recognized since the early 1980s, this form of *E. coli* is responsible for nearly 75,000 cases of foodborne illness each year and as many as 60 deaths. Genomic sequence comparisons with benign strains of *E. coli* indicate that the two types share some 4,000 genes but the virulent *E. coli* O157:H7 strain carries 1,387 genes that the benign strain lacks.

This initial analysis immediately provides insights into genetic features that likely contribute to the virulence of O157:H7. Some of its additional genes apparently encode enzymes that help it survive the acidic conditions of the stomach while other genes encode proteins that enable this bacterium to adhere tenaciously to the intestinal walls of its host. The analysis also suggests many of these virulence traits were assembled into the O157:H7 genome relatively recently, indicating the strain's extraordinary virulence may have arisen through natural exchanges of genes among microorganisms.

Such genomics-based analyses are providing researchers with valuable clues into identifying potentially important targets for drug and vaccine research. With knowledge of different genes' functions, researchers can determine how those genes contribute to a microbe's life processes and learn how to shut those processes down.

Thus, genomics experts anticipate working closely with their colleagues engaged in applied research to explore new leads and accelerate efforts to develop safe and effective new products to treat or prevent deadly outbreaks. For example, some of the sequence-specific signatures identified through the genomic analysis of *E. coli* O157:H7 may prove useful for identifying and monitoring this pathogenic microorganism in various settings, such as on farms where it may associate with cattle without causing outward signs of disease, to prevent its entry into the food supply.

Lessons from the Human Genome Project

Applying the full force of genomic analysis to disease-causing microbes is a direct offshoot from the Human Genome Project, an ambitious international research effort to characterize the 3 billion base-pair genome of the human being. The completed draft sequence of the human genome was published in February 2001 and marked a watershed moment in biomedical research. The Project also encompasses DNA sequencing of other organisms important to human health research, such as common laboratory animals and several microbes used for studying the basic processes of cell biology. In addition, information obtained about human genes can be combined with microbial genetic information to paint a comprehensive picture of the myriad interactions between microbe and host. The Human Genome Project and microbial genomics research are also linked in other ways. Both rely on collaborations and partnerships with other government agencies, as well as with commercial and non-profit organizations in the United States and abroad. Microbial genomics also uses much of the technology developed for human genome sequencing.

A Closer Look: Sexually Transmitted Diseases

Seeking Common Threads Among Pathogens Causing STDs

The microbes that cause sexually transmitted diseases (STDs) are a disparate lot—viruses, bacteria, and several more complex organisms, including yeasts and protozoa, They also cause a disparate set of diseases, some short-lived and little more than annoying, others invisible but potentially serious, and still others unambiguously harmful and life threatening, According to the Institute of Medicine, some 12 million new cases of STDs occur each year in the United States, about one-fourth of them among teenagers. The annual costs associated with these diseases are estimated at $10 billion, or $17 billion if sexually transmitted HIV is included in the tabulation.

Despite the variety of microbes responsible for STDs, the germs that cause them share many similarities because of the specialized niche the pathogens occupy in their human hosts and because of the way in which most of them are transmitted.

To facilitate studies of STDs, NIAID began a collaborative effort with scientists at the Los Alamos National Laboratory in New Mexico to compile a special series of STD genomic databases. The initial focus of these efforts was the human papillomavirus (HPV), a virus that causes genital warts over the short term, and cervical and other cancers over the longer term. Because only certain genetic strains of HPV appear to cause disease, scientists developed an extensive genomic database to determine the genetic basis for the different strain properties.

The modest effort to catalog and track HPV grew into a broader effort to catalog and analyze a series of STD pathogens using genomic and other database information. Eventually, researchers gathered the genomic sequences of human herpes virus, some of which cause genital lesions, and at least a half-dozen bacterial pathogens responsible for a variety of well-known STDs, including syphilis, gonorrhea, and chlamydial infections that can lead to pelvic inflammatory disease and sterility.

Researchers have begun to comb the databases to look for common genes and gene products the pathogens require for infection and survival in people. To date they have discovered at least four different STD bacteria deploy essentially the same biochemical ingredients in the early stages of establishing an infection, This and other information coming from continuing genomic analysis should lead to new targets for drugs or vaccines.

A Closer Look: Microbes and Chronic Diseases

Chronic Chlamydia pneumoniae *Infections May Contribute to Heart Disease*

The bacterium *Chlamydia pneumoniae* causes respiratory tract infections and is a common cause of pneumonia, accounting for about 10 percent of cases in the United States. Infections can also occur with only mild or no symptoms, however, and many adults throughout the world carry antibodies to the bacterium, indicating prior exposure. Researchers are now focusing considerable attention on *C. pneumoniae* because of its possible link to another serious illness—heart disease. Although the story is far from complete, medical researchers have compiled persuasive circumstantial evidence linking *C. pneumoniae* with the blood vessel plaques that cause coronary heart disease. Studies suggest the persistent presence of these bacteria in blood vessels near the heart could provoke an exaggerated and damaging response of the host immune system.

If *C. pneumoniae* indeed is responsible for a substantial portion of coronary heart disease, it may be possible to reduce the incidence of that disease and save lives with a vaccine that can prevent chronic *C. pneumoniae* infections. Toward that end, researchers are now using the genomic sequence of *C. pneumoniae* and those of other closely related pathogens to identify specific genes whose products might be used in a vaccine to trigger a protective immune response. In addition, researchers are counting on genomic information to uncover other genes that enable the microbe to cause an array of damage in its human hosts.

Genomics Meets Bioinformatics

As genome sequences continue to become available, scientists must develop ways to efficiently deal with the accumulating data. Comprehensive data sets are currently released by investigators and widely shared among scientists, who now can access these vast databases by way of the Internet. The free availability of data about microbial genomes encourages important analytical comparisons with those of other pathogens, as well as with humans.

Because the genomes of each one of the microbes may contain upwards of several million base pairs of DNA and thousands of genes, analyzing information on this immense scale looms as a daunting task. Genomics provides far more data than can be interpreted using uncomplicated calculations jotted on the back of an envelope. Rather, such analysis requires the help of sophisticated computers and the use of innovative software.

To undertake such analysis, biologists now depend on the cooperation of a new class of scientists who are knowledgeable not only about the biological properties of the organisms they study but also in newer computer and "bioinformatics" skills essential for making the best use of the huge volume of data.

Some of these approaches will be aimed at developing new diagnostic procedures for rapidly identifying pathogens, including those carrying unique medically important traits such as antibiotic resistance. Someday, such information may enable physicians to more quickly diagnose an infection, identify the microbial culprit, and more closely tailor specific treatments to the disease. In other cases, rapid diagnostic procedures may indicate that a virus is responsible for causing a patient's problem, thereby avoiding antibiotic treatment and thus helping to curb the development of resistance through unwarranted uses of such drugs.

Proteomics

Knowing the complete set of genes within a microbe is just one step in understanding the biology of that organism. Proteins, which are encoded by the genes, do most of the actual work. Researchers therefore are beginning to use genomics in combination with other technologies to determine all of the proteins within an organism, a process dubbed proteomics. Scientists hope to identify each protein in a microbe, learn its functions, and decipher how all the proteins interact to help the organism survive. In the past, investigators have relied on specific biological properties of a microbe to hint at the possible presence of different proteins. In other cases, researchers have broken a virus or microbe into its chemical components to get a rough idea of the number and physical properties of its proteins. Scientists have then relied on laborious biochemical analyses to isolate and identify individual proteins and determine their function. Genomics greatly accelerates that process because it provides a starting list of genes, and by extension the proteins they encode.

Combining Pathogen and Human Genomics

Researchers are also exploring the details of host-pathogen interactions. For instance, some pathogens make their way into host cells on specific receptors. Once identified, those entry ports could provide researchers with new means for interfering with such pathogens. In addition, detailed knowledge about the bevy of molecules human cells produce in response to certain pathogens may enable scientists to better orchestrate host defenses. At an even more detailed level, such analysis eventually may explain why some individuals are susceptible to a particular infectious disease while others are resistant.

On the pathogen side, researchers are focusing on the genes needed to invade, colonize, and disrupt normal functions in a human host.

Cells and organ systems of the infected person also play important roles during such infections. Some cells serve as the target of the pathogen, while other cells and organs play an active role in a patient's immune response. Using powerful microarray analysis, researchers hope to identify the key features of human-pathogen interactions as another very promising way to tilt the contest in favor of humans.

For example, some researchers are studying how cells that are part of the host defense system respond during first encounters with pathogens. Initial experiments indicate that part of the first response appears to be the same regardless of the pathogen involved; several distinct groups of human genes switch on shortly after the cells are accosted by a variety of different types of microbial intruders. Other components of the immune system, however, respond to only one type of pathogen but not others.

Microarrays

Because of genomics, new technologies are being designed to assist basic and applied research on microbial pathogens. One of these technologies, called a DNA microarray, combines DNA and computer technology to rapidly scan the genetic activity of a given organism. In a microarray, scientists coat a small chip with hundreds or thousands of fragments of DNA; each one corresponds to a different gene within the cell being studied. Those fragments can be made to light up when they encounter their partner gene, an event that means the gene is actively being read by the cell. Microarrays therefore enable researchers to see which genes are being switched on and off under different conditions. Scientists can use microarrays to determine the underlying genetics behind how a microbe responds to drugs, infects different hosts, survives outside of its hosts, and responds to different environmental conditions.

Genomics and Biodefense

The possibility of a bioterrorist attack on U.S. soil has shed new light on the importance of infectious diseases research. In response to that threat, NIAID and other federal health agencies are accelerating basic microbial research and developing new ways to diagnose, prevent, or treat infections that may be caused by the intentional release of a pathogen.

Microbial genomics is a vital part of a comprehensive approach to biodefense. The genomes of several smallpox virus strains are already known, as are those for different hemorrhagic fever viruses. NIAID currently funds the genome sequencing of many other potential bioterrorism microbes and collaborates with the Defense Advanced Research Products Agency (DARPA) to sequence such potential agents of bioterror as the bacteria that cause brucellosis, Q fever, gangrene, and epidemic typhus. In 2002, the genome sequences of the anthrax and plague bacteria also were completed.

Rapid sequencing of microbial DNA quickly unveils many secrets of bioterrorism's most frightening pathogens. In the short term, scientists can use the information to develop gene-based diagnostic and sampling tests to quickly detect dangerous germs and assess their susceptibility to different types of treatment. Genomes also provide molecular fingerprints of different strains of a given microbe, thereby enabling investigators to better track future outbreaks to their source. In the longer term, the genetic blueprints revealed by genome sequencing will identify key genes required for microbes to infect people and thrive. The protein molecules encoded by some of those genes will be likely targets for new drugs and vaccines to protect the public from disease.

In 2002, NIAID released its "Biodefense Research Agenda for CDC Category A Agents." A key element to that agenda was comprehensive genomic analysis of the microbes considered the greatest bioterror threat. Those include the pathogens that cause anthrax, tularemia, smallpox, plague, botulism, and viral hemorrhagic fevers such as Ebola.

Anthrax

In 2001, a string of letters containing the anthrax bacterium were mailed to several destinations in the United States. The deadly bacterium, *Bacillus anthracis*, infected at least 18 people, killing eight. At the time the letters were mailed, researchers were well on their way to determining the genome sequence of the bacterium. After the mail attack, scientists used genome sequencing technology to determine the genetic blueprints of the strain isolated from one of the letters and compared it to the blueprints of other *B. anthracis* strains. As a result of that work, investigators gathered information on the potential source of the bioterror bacteria. In addition, the gene sequences provided researchers with the vital data required to quickly analyze the bacterium for potential vulnerabilities to new drugs and vaccines. Work on the *B. anthracis* genome continues as scientists sequence additional strains.

In Conclusion

As infectious diseases emerge, reemerge, and persist throughout the world, genomics research promises to be a valuable weapon in the fight to keep those diseases in check. By deciphering a pathogen's genetic blueprint, researchers can more quickly learn about the different genes and proteins required for that organism to survive, infect people, and cause disease. Some genes will point to unique biochemical processes that scientists can block with new drugs, thereby destroying a microbe without harming the people it infects. Other genes will identify key proteins on a pathogen that stimulate a person's immune response. Those proteins can then be used as the basis for new vaccines. Genome sequencing also can identify how microbes alter their makeup to avoid the effects of drugs or immune detection, enabling researchers to stay one step ahead by refining vaccines or medicines. Still other genes will provide potential targets for tests to rapidly diagnose an infection or identify the presence of harmful microbes in the field.

Pathogen genome sequencing therefore remains a high research priority at NIAID. Scientists continue to decipher the genetic secrets of infectious microbes and the organisms that transmit them to people. By understanding the underlying genes that make those microbes tick, researchers will continue to make advances in the diagnosis, prevention, and treatment of infectious diseases.

Chapter 72

Stress and Disease: New Perspectives

For thousands of years, people believed that stress made you sick. Up until the nineteenth century, the idea that the passions and emotions were intimately linked to disease held sway, and people were told by their doctors to go to spas or seaside resorts when they were ill. Gradually these ideas lost favor as more concrete causes and cures were found for illness after illness. But in the last decade, scientists like Dr. Esther Sternberg, director of the Integrative Neural Immune Program at NIH's (National Institutes of Health) National Institute of Mental Health (NIMH), have been rediscovering the links between the brain and the immune system.

The Immune System and the Brain

When you have an infection or something else that causes inflammation such as a burn or injury, many different kinds of cells from the immune system stream to the site. Dr. Sternberg likens them to soldiers moving into battle, each kind with its own specialized function. Some are like garbage collectors, ingesting invaders. Some make antibodies, the "bullets" to fight the infectious agents; others kill invaders directly. All these types of immune cells must coordinate their actions, and the way they do that is by sending each other signals in the form of molecules that they make in factories inside the cell.

"Stress and Disease: New Perspectives," by Harrison Wein, Ph.D., National Institutes of Health (NIH), October 2000.

"It turns out that these molecules have many more effects than just being the walkie-talkie communicators between different kinds of immune cells," Dr. Sternberg says. "They can also go through the blood-stream to signal the brain or activate nerves nearby that signal the brain."

These immune molecules, Dr. Sternberg explains, cause the brain to change its functions. "They can induce a whole set of behaviors that we call sickness behavior... You lose the desire or the ability to move, you lose your appetite, you lose interest in sex." Scientists can only speculate about the purpose of these sickness behaviors, but Dr. Sternberg suggests that they might help us conserve energy when we're sick so we can better use our energy to fight disease.

These signaling molecules from the immune system can also activate the part of the brain that controls the stress response, the hypothalamus. Through a cascade of hormones released from the pituitary and adrenal glands, the hypothalamus causes blood levels of the hormone cortisol to rise. Cortisol is the major steroid hormone produced by our bodies to help us get through stressful situations. The related compound known as cortisone is widely used as an anti-inflammatory drug in creams to treat rashes and in nasal sprays to treat sinusitis and asthma. But it wasn't until very recently that scientists realized the brain also uses cortisol to suppress the immune system and tone down inflammation within the body.

Stress and the Immune System

This complete communications cycle from the immune system to the brain and back again allows the immune system to talk to the brain, and the brain to then talk back and shut down the immune response when it's no longer needed.

"When you think about this cross-talk, this two-way street," Dr. Sternberg explains, "you can begin to understand the kinds of illnesses that might result if there is either too much or too little communication in either direction."

According to Dr. Sternberg, if you're chronically stressed, the part of the brain that controls the stress response is going to be constantly pumping out a lot of stress hormones. The immune cells are being bathed in molecules which are essentially telling them to stop fighting. And so in situations of chronic stress your immune cells are less able to respond to an invader like a bacteria or a virus.

This theory holds up in studies looking at high-levels of shorter term stress or chronic stress: in caregivers like those taking care of relatives with Alzheimer's, medical students undergoing exam stress, Army Rangers undergoing extremely grueling physical stress, and couples with marital stress. People in these situations, Dr. Sternberg says, show a prolonged healing time, a decreased ability of their immune systems to respond to vaccination, and an increased susceptibility to viral infections like the common cold.

Some Stress is Good

People tend to talk about stress as if it's all bad. It's not.

"Some stress is good for you," Dr. Sternberg says. "I have to get my stress response to a certain optimal level so I can perform in front of an audience when I give a talk." Otherwise, she may come across as lethargic and listless.

But while some stress is good, too much is not good. "If you're too stressed, your performance falls off," Dr. Sternberg says. "The objective should be not to get rid of stress completely because you can't get rid of stress—stress is life, life is stress. Rather, you need to be able to use your stress response optimally."

The key is to learn to move yourself to that optimal peak point so that you're not underperforming but you're also not so stressed that you're unable to perform. How much we're able to do that is the challenge, Dr. Sternberg admits. This may not be possible in all situations, or for all people, because just as with the animals Dr. Sternberg studies, some people may have a more sensitive stress response than others.

"But your goal should be to try to learn to control your stress to make it work for you," Dr. Sternberg says. "Don't just think of getting rid of your stress; think of turning it to your advantage."

Controlling the Immune Response

Problems between the brain and the immune system can go the other way, too. If for some reason you're unable to make enough of these brain stress hormones, you won't be able to turn off the immune cells once they're no longer needed.

"There has to be an exit strategy for these battles that are being fought by the immune system, and the brain provides the exit strategy through stress hormones," Dr. Sternberg says. "If your brain can't make enough of these hormones to turn the immune system off when it doesn't have to be active anymore, then it could go on unchecked and result in autoimmune diseases like rheumatoid arthritis, lupus, or other autoimmune diseases that people recognize as inflammation."

Dr. Sternberg says that there are several factors involved in these autoimmune conditions. There are many different effects that the brain and its nervous system can have on the immune system, depending on the kinds of nerve chemicals that are being made, where they're being made, what kind of nerves they come from, and whether they're in the bloodstream or not. Still, at least part of the problem in these diseases seems to involve the brain's hormonal stress response.

"So if you have too much stress hormone shutting down the immune response, you can't fight off infection and you're more susceptible to infection," Dr. Sternberg concludes. "Too little stress hormones and the immune response goes on unchecked and you could get an inflammatory disease."

Pinpointing the Problems

Why these miscommunications between the brain and the immune system come about is still largely unknown, and involves many genes and environmental factors. But by studying animals, scientists have finally been able to start understanding how the miscommunications occur.

Dr. Sternberg first started publishing work on the links between the brain and the immune system back in 1989 studying rats with immune problems. "In many of these cases it's very hard to show the mechanism in humans," Dr. Sternberg explains, "but you can show the mechanism in animals because you can manipulate all the different parts of the system and you can begin to understand which parts affect which other parts." It has taken "a good ten years" to gather enough evidence in human studies to show that the principles her lab uncovered in rats were also relevant to human beings.

Drugs that have been tested in rats to correct brain/immune system problems have had unpredictable effects. That is because nothing happens in isolation when it comes to the brain and the immune system. Dr. Sternberg points out that our bodies are amazing machines which at every moment of the day are constantly responding to a myriad of different kinds of stimuli—chemical, psychological, and physical. "These molecules act in many different ways in different parts of the system," she says. Understanding how the brain and the immune system work together in these different diseases should help scientists develop new kinds of drugs to treat them that would never have occurred to them before.

Taking Control Now

Dr. Sternberg thinks that one of the most hopeful aspects of this science is that it tells us it's not all in our genes. A growing number of studies show that, to some degree, you can use your mind to help treat your body. Support groups, stress relief, and meditation may, by altering stress hormone levels, all help the immune system. For example, women in support groups for their breast cancer have longer life spans than women without such psychological support.

There are several components of stress to think about, including its duration, how strong it is, and how long it lasts. Every stress has some effect on the body, and you have to take into account the total additive effect on the body of all stressors when considering how to reduce stress.

Perhaps the most productive way to think about stress is in terms of control. Dr. Sternberg shows a slide of an F-14 jet flying sideways by the deck of an aircraft carrier, its wings completely vertical. "The Navy Commander who flew that jet told me that he was the only one in the photo who was not stressed, and that's because he was the one in control. The officer sitting in the seat ten feet behind him was in the exact same physical situation but was not in control. Control is a very important part of whether or not we feel stressed.

So if you can learn to feel that you're in control or actually take control of certain aspects of the situation that you're in, you can reduce your stress response." Studies show that gaining a sense of control can help patients cope with their illness, if not help the illness itself.

Until science has more solid answers, it can't hurt to participate in support groups and seek ways to relieve stress, Dr. Sternberg says. But what you need to remember is if you do these things and you're not successful in correcting whatever the underlying problem is, it's not your fault because there's a biology to the system. "You need to know the benefits of the system," she says, "but its limitations as well." In other words, try not to get too stressed about being stressed.

Stress Control

First try to identify the things in your life that cause you stress: marital problems, conflict at work, a death or illness in the family. Once you identify and understand how these stressors affect you, you can begin to figure out ways to change your environment and manage them.

If there's a problem that can be solved, set about taking control and solving it. For example, you might decide to change jobs if problems at work are making you too stressed.

But some chronic stressors can't be changed. For those, support groups, relaxation, meditation, and exercise are all tools you can use to manage your stress. If nothing you do seems to work for you, seek a health professional who can help. Also seek professional help if you find that you worry excessively about the small things in life.

Keep in mind that chronic stress can be associated with mental conditions like depression and anxiety disorders as well as physical problems. Seek professional help if you have:

- Difficulty sleeping
- Changes in appetite
- Panic attacks
- Muscle tenseness and soreness
- Frequent headaches
- Gastrointestinal problems
- Prolonged feelings of sadness or worthlessness

Chapter 73

Food Irradiation: A Tool against Foodborne Pathogens

Facts about Food Irradiation

Like the pasteurization of milk and pressure cooking of canned foods, food irradiation can destroy bacteria and parasites that would otherwise cause foodborne disease. As was initially the case in the 19th century with the pasteurization of milk, food irradiation has raised public concerns about the safety of the process. The opposition stems from a variety of concerns—particularly a fear of anything "radioactive," fears about worker/environmental safety, and apprehension that food irradiation would serve as a substitute for sanitary and safe food handling.

While some consumers may have fears about irradiated foods, many do not realize that the same technology is already used and safely applied, e.g., it is used widely to sterilize surgical instruments and medical devices prior to use in patients. A highly relevant and little appreciated fact is that the food consumed by NASA astronauts is sterilized by irradiation to avoid foodborne illnesses during space travel.

The burden of illness due to foodborne disease in the United States has been substantially reduced during the past century because of improved food and water sanitation, food animal inspection, use of refrigeration, and safer food processing practices. Yet even with these improvements, 5,000 Americans die annually from infections caused by foodborne microbes while another 76 million are sickened, according to estimates from the Centers for Disease Control and Prevention (CDC). Newly emergent foodborne pathogens, consumer preferences for fresh or minimally processed foods and increases in groups of persons with increased susceptibility to enteric infection underscore the pressing need to push forward to improve food safety beyond the levels already achieved. For the 21st century, this will entail a comprehensive farm-to-table approach to minimize contamination during food production and, where necessary, the use of additional measures to control residual pathogens.

Infectious Diseases Society of America (IDSA) supports the use of irradiation, in conjunction with other food safety measures, for those foods for which irradiation is an effective means of decreasing residual pathogens. While IDSA supports measures that increase the acceptance and availability of this technology, IDSA recognizes that irradiation does not abrogate the need for other food safety measures.

In 1999, IDSA—along with a coalition of food industry groups, health care organizations and consumer groups—filed a petition with the Food and Drug Administration (FDA) urging the agency to expand the use of food irradiation to include a variety of ready-to-eat meat and poultry products as well as fruits and vegetables.

This information is intended to explain the current status of food irradiation in the United States and to answer the most commonly asked questions about its use.

Commonly Asked Questions and Answers about Food Irradiation

What is food irradiation?

Food irradiation is the process of exposing food to a carefully measured amount of ionizing radiant energy (e.g., electrons, gamma rays or x-rays), which travel through the food destroying pathogens such as *E. coli* O157:H7 without raising the temperature of the food. Food irradiation should complement, not supplant, other food safety practices. It is not intended as a substitute for scientifically sound safe food handling practices.

What are the benefits of food irradiation?

Food irradiation reduces the risk of foodborne illnesses by destroying pathogens such as *E. coli* O157:H7, *Campylobacter* and *Salmonella*.

Food irradiation also prolongs the shelf life of some foods, such as produce, thereby reducing spoilage and waste. Food irradiation generally destroys nearly all bacteria and parasites and many viruses. While viruses are more resistant to irradiation, any virus found in food is of human origin, so safe food handling procedures such as frequent hand washing to avoid contaminating food with human fecal matter will protect foods from contamination with viruses.

Is irradiated food safe?

Yes. Irradiated food does not become "radioactive." Based on a variety of scientific evidence (taking into account potential toxicity, nutritional adequacy and potential microbiological risk), FDA, the American Medical Association, the World Health Organization and many other organizations, including IDSA, have concluded that irradiated food products are safe to consume.

How does irradiation affect foods?

The nutritional value of irradiated foods is not changed in any significant way at the doses used. The nutritive values of the macronutrients in the diet (such as proteins, fats and carbohydrates) are not significantly altered by irradiation. Although the levels of certain vitamins may be reduced, the extent of the reduction depends upon the specific vitamin, the food type and conditions of irradiation. Levels of thiamine, for example, are slightly reduced, but the reduction is not enough to result in vitamin deficiency. Some foods may taste slightly different (just as pasteurized milk tastes slightly different from unpasteurized milk). If the food still has living cells, the cells will be damaged or destroyed just as the pathogens are. This effect can be useful in some cases and undesirable in others.

How much radiation is used to treat food?

During the irradiation process, food is exposed to the ionizing energy source in such a way that a precise and specific dose is absorbed. A dose is defined as the amount of radiation absorbed by the food, which is less than the level of energy transmitted from the radiation source. The absorbed dose is controlled by the intensity of the radiation source and the length of time the food is exposed. The unit used to measure the dose (or amount of absorbed radiation) is the gray (Gy). One gray is equal to 1 joule of absorbed energy per kilogram. (As a means of comparison, a 100 watt light bulb uses 100 joules of energy per second.)

- Low doses: Doses of 1 kGy or less are used on a variety of foods to eliminate insect pests as a replacement for fumigation with toxic chemicals. Low doses of irradiation can also inhibit the growth of molds, inhibit sprouting or prolong shelf life.

- High doses: Doses greater than 10 kGy are used on a variety of foods, such as meat, poultry, grains, many seafoods, fruits and vegetables, to eliminate parasites and bacteria that cause food-borne disease.

What is the regulatory status of food irradiation in the United States?

Irradiation was first approved in 1963 for use on wheat flour to control mold. For meats and poultry, the use of food irradiation needed the approval of both the FDA and the U.S. Department of Agriculture (USDA)—the latter responsible for developing procedures that govern food irradiation. Food irradiation is now approved in the United States for use on a variety of food products, including some produce, seeds, poultry and, as of last year, meat. While some specific grocery stores carry food products that have undergone irradiation, the practice is not widespread in the United States mainly because of consumer fears of irradiated foods.

Who ensures the safety of irradiation facilities?

The Nuclear Regulatory Commission regulates facilities that use radioactive sources. E-beam and x-ray sources are monitored by FDA and the same state authorities that regulate other medical, dental and industrial uses of these technologies. There has not been one fatal accident involving an irradiation facility in the United States.

Who ensures the safety of irradiated foods?

Irradiated foods are regulated as a food safety process by USDA and FDA. As is the case with all food products, state authorities also oversee food safety.

Will consumers need to prepare irradiated foods any differently?

No, but consumers should be reminded of the possibility of cross-contamination when handling and preparing all food. It is important to take appropriate precautions such as washing hands and preparation surfaces often. Thorough cooking, proper refrigeration and storage procedures must also be followed.

Will consumers be able to identify foods that have been irradiated?

FDA requires irradiated foods to have the international radura symbol (green petals in a broken circle) and the written statement: "Treated by irradiation" or "Treated with radiation" clearly displayed on the packaging.

Sources

1. "Food irradiation." National Food Processors Association, 1999.

2. "Food irradiation's hysteria industry," *Washington Times*, Feb. 19, 1999.

3. "Frequently asked questions about food irradiation." Division of Bacterial and Mycotic Diseases, Centers for Disease Control and Prevention, 1999.

4. Mead, P.S., et al. "Food-related illness and death in the United States." *Emerging Infectious Diseases*, Sept.-Oct. 1999.

5. Morehouse, K. M. "Food Irradiation: The treatment of foods with ionizing radiation." *Food Testing & Analysis*, June/July 1998.

6. Osterholm, M.T. and Potter, M.E. "Irradiation pasteurization of solid foods: taking food safety to the next level." *Emerging Infectious Diseases*, Oct.-Dec. 1997.

Chapter 74

Pressure Combined with Heat Reduces Prion Infectivity in Processed Meats

The combination of high temperature and very high pressure in the preparation of processed meats such as hot dogs and salami may effectively reduce the presence of infective prions while retaining the taste, texture, and look of these meats, according to a study in the May 5, 2003 *Proceedings of the National Academy of Sciences (PNAS) Early Edition*.

The study was led by Paul Brown, M.D., of the National Institute of Neurological Disorders and Stroke (NINDS), a component of the National Institutes of Health within the U.S. Department of Health and Human Services. Other collaborators on the study, which was conducted in Europe with partial funding provided by the Ministero della Salute, Italy, included Rich Meyer (Tacoma Farms, Washington State) and Franco Cardone and Maurizio Pocchiari (both with the Ministero della Salute).

Scientists believe that bovine spongiform encephalopathy, also known as "mad cow" disease, entered the human food chain through beef products containing abnormal, or folded, proteins called prions. The disease manifests itself in humans as variant Creutzfeldt-Jakob disease. Since 1995 more than 140 patients, mostly in the United Kingdom, have died as a probable result of eating contaminated meat products.

"Pressure Combined with Heat Reduces Prion Infectivity in Processed Meats," National Institute of Neurological Disorders and Stroke (NINDS), National Institutes of Health (NIH), May 5, 2003.

Scientists have been looking for strategies to inactivate any possible infectivity in meats, and although processes such as autoclaving and exposure to strong alkali or bleach are known to kill prions, they cannot be used successfully in food preparation.

Richard T. Johnson, M.D., former neurologist-in-chief at the Johns Hopkins University School of Medicine and a senior advisor to the National Institutes of Health on the transmissible spongiform encephalopathies, said, "The idea of using high pressure to decrease prion activity is interesting and unique and may lead to additional studies." Extensive surveillance by the U.S. Department of Agriculture has not detected bovine spongiform encephalopathy in the United States. The transmission of prion diseases through the food chain is a concern among public health officials.

To conduct the study, the scientists prepared a paste of scrapie prion-infected brain tissue mixed with hot dogs. They then exposed the paste to temperatures of 120–135 degrees Celsius (250–275 degrees Fahrenheit) and short bursts of ultra high pressure, in excess of 100,000 lbs. per square inch. The scientists found that they were able to retain the basic texture and flavor of the processed meat while reducing the prions to non-infective levels. This may have application in improving the safety of meat products.

The combination of temperature and high pressure has been used commercially for the past 15 years to reduce the amount of bacteria in foodstuffs and to preserve ham, chicken, salsa, and other foods. Dr. Brown said his team, "took the process one step further, to see if it would kill prions, which it did." He called the discovery a relatively inexpensive, practical step to potentially improve the safety of processed meats.

He added the approach may have implications for understanding the prion structure. "At a constant high temperature, we know that more and more prion inactivation occurs at higher and higher pressures. We hope that studying the structure of prions at increasing levels of pressure may allow us to better understand how the abnormal prion misshapes or unfolds," said Dr. Brown.

The NINDS is a component of the National Institutes of Health in Bethesda, Maryland, part of the U.S. Department of Health and Human Services, and is the nation's primary supporter of biomedical research on the brain and nervous system.

Chapter 75

Single Protein is Key in Response to Bacterial, Viral Infections

A single protein acts as a key switch point in frontline immune system reactions to both bacterial and viral infections, according to a report published online on July 20, 2003 in the journal *Nature*. In determining how this protein functions, a team of scientists supported by the National Institute of Allergy and Infectious Diseases (NIAID) can now explain why certain symptoms, such as fever, occur regardless of the cause of infection.

Bruce Beutler, M.D., of The Scripps Research Institute in La Jolla, CA, who led the team, says, "This protein, Trif, stands at a crossroads in the mouse innate immune system and, by inference, we believe in the human immune system as well." A clear understanding of Trif's role in sparking inflammation gives scientists an obvious target for drugs designed to combat the runaway inflammation characteristic of many infectious and immune-mediated diseases.

Mammals, including humans, employ a family of proteins (called toll-like receptors, or TLRs) in first-line defense against bacteria and viruses. One protein, TLR-3, is activated by viruses, while another, TLR-4, responds to molecules frequently contained in bacterial cell walls. The TLRs are an important part of the innate immune system, the all-purpose "first-responder" arm of the immune system. Once activated by invading pathogens, TLRs relay the alarm to other actors in the immune system. In short order, the innate immune system responds

"Single Protein is Key in Response to Bacterial, Viral Infections," National Institute of Allergy and Infectious Diseases (NIAID), National Institutes of Health (NIH), July 20, 2003.

with a surge of chemicals that together cause inflammation, fever, and other responses to infection or injury.

Defining the intervening steps in the signaling pathway from TLR activation to inflammatory response is an important objective of Dr. Beutler's research. Previously, scientists had discovered a "transducer" protein responsible for passing on the news of a bacterial attack. Mice lacking this protein could still fight bacterial infection, although not very well. There had to be at least one more transducer protein.

Dr. Beutler's team found this mystery protein through a technique called forward genetics. Genetic mutations are randomly introduced into strains of mice. A sensitive screening mechanism allows the researchers to pick out any mice that, by chance, show interesting characteristics, such as weakened responses to infection. In the latest research, Dr. Beutler and his colleagues identified a mouse whose immune system did not react to a substance called endotoxin, a component of bacterial cell walls. Subsequently, the team determined the consequence of the genetic error in these mice—they cannot produce working Trif protein.

Lack of Trif explained why the mutant mice could not respond adequately to endotoxin (which mimics bacterial infection). However, Dr. Beutler notes, the team also made the surprising observation that mice missing Trif are also unable to respond to the double-stranded RNA produced by most viruses and thus could not fight off viral infections.

The scientists inferred that both the bacteria-sensing TLR-4 pathway and the virus-sensing TLR-3 pathway are blocked when Trif is defective. This is the first innate immune system transducer protein discovered that mediates signals generated by both bacterial and viral infection.

"Scientists have been searching for the endotoxin signaling molecules of the innate immune system for more than four decades," says Daniel Rotrosen, M.D., director of NIAID's Division of Allergy, Immunology, and Transplantation. "We've witnessed an explosion of information on innate immunity in the past five years, catalyzed by the discovery of the TLR family of signaling molecules," he adds. "NIAID's grant to Scripps enables scientists from diverse disciplines spanning biology and informatics to tackle a wide variety of problems in innate immunity. This finding is the first of what we anticipate will be many discoveries made possible by forward genetics and other cutting-edge technologies supported through this grant."

Reference: K Hoebe et al. Identification of Lps2 as a key transducer of MyD88-independent TIR signaling. *Nature*. Published online July 20, 2003. DOI: 10.1038/nature01889.

Chapter 76

First Test for West Nile Virus

The Food and Drug Administration (FDA) cleared the first test for use as an aid in the clinical laboratory diagnosis of West Nile virus infection in July 2003. The West Nile Virus IgM Capture ELISA is intended for use in patients with clinical symptoms consistent with viral encephalitis/meningitis.

"Emerging infectious diseases such as West Nile virus present a challenge to the public health community," said Tommy G. Thompson, Secretary of Health and Human Services. "When industry and government collaborate closely to meet a public health need, the resulting new technology will strengthen our joint efforts to confront diseases earlier and should lower rates of infection."

The new test works by detecting the levels of a particular type of antibody, IgM, to the disease in a patient's serum. IgM antibodies can be detected within the first few days of the onset of illness and can assist in the diagnosis of these patients.

"The rapid review and approval of this blood test, which uses antibody levels to identify persons who were recently exposed to West Nile virus, reflects FDA's commitment to making safe and effective medical products available promptly," said FDA Commissioner Mark B. McClellan, M.D., Ph.D. "This test provides a useful tool to combat the important public health problem of West Nile virus infection, just in time for the start of the West Nile season."

"FDA Clears First Test for West Nile Virus," U.S. Food and Drug Administration (FDA), July 9, 2003.

The PanBio West Nile IgM assay was evaluated using over 1000 patient sera, which were tested at four different clinical sites. The test correctly identified antibody in up to 90 to 99% of West Nile virus disease cases. Because detection of antibody is not always specific in patients with acute viral infections, this test is considered presumptive and should be confirmed by more specific testing.

Although the PanBio test is a valuable aid in the diagnosis of West Nile virus encephalitis, due to similarities with other viruses in the same family, there is a need to confirm positive results by an additional test or by using the current CDC diagnostic guidelines for diagnosis of this disease.

West Nile virus is a mosquito-borne virus which first appeared in the United States in 1999. While the virus often presents as a mild infection that clears without further treatment, some patients develop severe infection resulting in neurological disease and even death.

The disease is most prevalent during the peak mosquito season which is expected to begin in July and end in October. Over the past several years, the geographic range of the virus as well as the number of new infections has expanded and now covers most of the continental United States.

Since September 2002, FDA has also worked very closely with industry to prepare for this upcoming West Nile virus season and has encouraged industry to develop blood donor screening tests. In mid June 2003, blood testing centers began testing the blood supply for West Nile virus, using experimental test kits that FDA has evaluated and permitted to be used. FDA also developed guidance to industry recommending procedures to assess donor suitability and to retrieve and quarantine potentially contaminated blood products. The investigational screening procedure has now successfully identified the first human West Nile virus infection in an asymptomatic blood donor.

The West Nile Virus IgM Capture ELISA is manufactured by PanBio Limited in Windsor, Australia.

Chapter 77

The Continuing Fight against Emerging Infectious Diseases

One fall day in 1996, a little girl experienced diarrhea and stomach cramps and, within days, was in the hospital, kidneys failing, fighting futilely for her life. Laboratory tests showed that the cause was a deadly toxin-armed bacterium known as *Escherichia coli*, or *E. coli*, O157:H7—the same microbe that killed four children in 1993 and sickened hundreds of others after they ate undercooked hamburger from a fast-food chain. Since this virulent strain of *E. coli* was first identified in 1982, it has become one of the most feared food-related threats to the health of the American public.

With the little girl's death, health officials asked many questions: Where did the *E. coli* come from? Are others sick? Who will be sick tomorrow? Summoned to investigate, medical detectives from the state health department and the Centers for Disease Control and Prevention (CDC) questioned relatives and friends, pored over medical records, and investigated possible sources. They traced the child's infection to unpasteurized apple juice, a brand touted for its natural freshness.

Some might view a toddler's death from *E. coli*-contaminated apple juice as a disturbing but isolated incident. In reality; though, it is part of an ongoing life-and-death struggle in an invisible biological war. The enemy is a growing list of disease-causing microorganisms that

Excerpted from "Preventing Emerging Infectious Diseases: A Strategy for the 21st Century," Centers for Disease Control and Prevention (CDC), 1998. Despite the date of this document, the issues and programs described will help the reader understand the concepts involved.

are emerging or rebounding all over the world, some are appearing in new forms armed with new methods of attack. *E. coli* O157:H7 continues to strike in communities around the United States. For example, in June 1998 it infected 26 small children who played in a contaminated wading pool at a large water park in Georgia.

The Continuing Microbial Threat

Only a few decades ago, a grateful public trusted that science had triumphed over infectious diseases by building a fortress of health protections. Antibiotics, vaccines, and aggressive public health campaigns had yielded a string of victories over old enemies like pneumonia, polio, and smallpox, and Americans were lulled into believing that microbial threats were a thing of the past. But the global spread of acquired immunodeficiency syndrome (AIDS), the resurgence of tuberculosis, and the appearance of new enemies like hantaviruses, Ebola virus, and deadly *E. coli* strains are reminders of the resilience and adaptability of our microbial adversaries. Within the last few years,

- A "bird flu" virus that had never before attacked humans began to kill people in Hong Kong.

- A new variant of a fatal brain disease, Creutzfeldt-Jakob disease, was identified in the United Kingdom, apparently transmitted by beef from animals with "mad cow disease."

- *Staphylococcus* bacteria with reduced susceptibility to vancomycin, long the antibiotic of last resort, were seen for the first time.

- The country has been hit with several major multistate foodborne outbreaks, including those caused by parasites on raspberries, viruses on strawberries, and bacteria in produce, ground beef, cold cuts, and breakfast cereal.

- A new strain of tuberculosis that is resistant to many drugs, and occurs most often in people infected with human immunodeficiency virus (HIV), persists in New York City and some other large cities.

The emergence and reemergence of these and other disease agents have been fueled by

- Unprecedented worldwide population growth
- Increased international travel

- Increasing worldwide transport of animals and food products

- Changes in food processing and handling

- Changes in human behavior

- Human encroachment on wilderness habitats that are reservoirs for insects and animals that harbor infectious agents

- Microbial evolution and the development of resistance to antibiotics and other antimicrobial drugs

Whatever the cause, the resurgence of diseases attributed to newly emerging microbes poses a continuing challenge for the nation's public health and health-care systems. As pathogens strengthen their hold, broaden their reach, and pierce our defenses, our vulnerability is extending to the most mundane activities. Questions arise such as—Is my tap water safe to drink? Is the food I ordered in a restaurant safe to eat? Are my children likely to be bitten by disease-carrying insects or ticks while playing in the yard? Does my sex partner have an infection that might be passed on to me? Is it safe to vacation in a tropical country? Is the coughing person next to me on the subway or airplane spreading a deadly strain of influenza or tuberculosis?

CDC's Plan for the New Millenium

The battle lines are drawn: new diseases are emerging and old diseases are regaining a foothold. This is happening not just in a faraway locale, but also in our own neighborhoods and homes. The enemy is invisible, furtive, and gaining in strength and numbers. As we approach the new millennium, we must be prepared for the unexpected today and for prolonged conflict tomorrow.

- We must enhance our watchfulness worldwide.

- We must prepare to fight diseases that we have never heard of while we learn to cope again with those we thought we had vanquished.

- We must keep our food, water, and blood supplies safe from contamination.

- We must develop new antibiotics and vaccines.

- We must combat drug-resistant illnesses.

- We must ensure that diseases carried by animals do not spread to people.

- We must protect the most vulnerable among us—children, pregnant women, the sick, the elderly, people without easy access to health care.

- We must be ready to act decisively in the event of a deliberate release of infectious microbes by terrorists or rogue nations.

In short, we must redouble our efforts to be vigilant, increase our understanding of microbes new and old, develop better weapons, and be prepared to respond with decisive action when needed.

CDC—the nation's disease prevention agency—is dedicated to this mission. CDC's vision for the 21st century is of individuals, communities, and nations joined in a common effort to combat today's emerging infectious diseases and to prevent those of tomorrow. To realize this vision, CDC scientists have designed a plan to respond to microbial emergence and resurgence in the new millennium—*Preventing Emerging Infectious Diseases: A Strategy for the 21st Century.*

This plan is the second phase of an effort launched in 1994 with the publication of CDC's *Addressing Emerging Infectious Disease Threats: A Prevention Strategy for the United States.* The implementation of the 1994 strategy is well underway, and results are already evident. However, fulfilling CDC's vision of a safer world requires a long-term commitment and sustained effort. *Preventing Emerging Infectious Diseases: A Strategy for the 21st Century* describes CDC's next steps in the battle to prevent and control emerging infections. It takes into account the discoveries and challenges of the past few years and builds on new experiences, successes, and knowledge. Like the initial strategy, the plan is organized around four interdependent goals:

- Surveillance and Response,
- Applied Research,
- Infrastructure and
- Training, and Prevention and Control.

How Disease Prevention Works

Surveillance systems at the state and national levels monitor emerging infections and detect outbreaks of disease. When surveillance data or other information uncovers a change in the occurrence or distribution of a disease, or when a new strain of a microbe becomes a health threat, specially trained public health workers investigate, assess the potential public health implications, and mount a rapid response. Through applied research, scientists ask and answer questions about the disease's causes, transmission, diagnosis, prevention, and control. A specialized infrastructure supports and equips public health workers and laboratories and links them in national and global communications networks. Training the next generation to fight emerging infectious diseases is a crucial component of public health. All of these efforts are ultimately directed toward disease prevention and control—the application of the most effective tools and technologies to strengthen personal and national defenses against infectious diseases.

Surveillance and Response

In 1997, U.S. public health authorities received the long-dreaded alert: strains of the common, but potentially deadly, microbe *Staphylococcus aureus* had acquired the ability to partially withstand vancomycin, the antibiotic used when all other licensed drugs are ineffective. The discovery of the drug-resistant *Staphylococcus* strain in patients in Michigan and New Jersey came just 3 months after a similar resistant strain was found in an infant in Japan. Although the newly identified bacteria are not fully resistant to vancomycin, the possibility of a widespread untreatable infection marks a turn for the worse in the fight against infectious diseases and underscores the need for renewed attention to disease surveillance.

Surveillance means watchfulness: What is the threat? What caused it? Where is it appearing? How is it moving? Surveillance detects changes in disease occurrence and sounds the alarm for action. It provides the basis for timely public health decisions and timely responses.

Many of our most visible disease control successes have their basis in effective surveillance and response: tracing contaminated foods and prompting national warnings and recalls, identifying the most prevalent influenza virus strains to make the best possible vaccine, monitoring the blood supply to keep it safe, tracking the proliferation of drug-resistant infections and instituting controls. To maintain these successes and to heighten our watchfulness to detect new threats, the country's surveillance and response systems—and the essential laboratory services on which they depend—need support and resources from all levels of government and the full cooperation of health-care networks and providers nationwide.

Throughout the United States, surveillance for foodborne diseases is a high priority. In the past, outbreaks of foodborne illness tended to be local events that were easily recognized. Now, however, outbreaks are often scattered over a wide geographic area—the consequence of regional or national distribution of food products. As part of the 1997 National Food Safety Initiative, the federal government is boosting its ability to track foodborne illnesses from coast to coast. In mid-1998, officials unveiled a new early warning system called PulseNet—a national network of laboratories that rapidly perform DNA "finger-printing" on bacteria samples from sick people and contaminated food. The network permits speedy comparison of fingerprint patterns through an electronic database at CDC. When patterns submitted from different sites are very similar, the computer alerts health agencies to a possible widespread outbreak so that further illnesses and deaths can be prevented.

Applied Research

A sustained, forward-thinking applied research program enables scientists to uncover the weak links in the armor of emerging microbes, create novel ways to identify and fight microbial foes, and evaluate the preventive power of new approaches. For example, a growing body of evidence shows that emerging pathogens do more than cause acute infectious diseases. They can also be major contributors to chronic diseases traditionally associated with lifestyle and environment. Many stomach and duodenal ulcers—long thought to be due to stress and spicy food—are now known to result from infection with the bacterium *Helicobacter pylori.* Another bacterium, *Chlamydia pneumoniae,* may play a role in heart disease. Cancer of the cervix has been linked to infection with some types of human papillomavirus, and chronic liver disease and liver cancer are associated with chronic infection with hepatitis B and C viruses. Thus, some of the leading causes of death and disability may turn out to be to some degree infectious, and common infection-fighting drugs may help bring them under control.

Research is also a crucial part of the response to new and reemerging diseases. In 1976, when a horrific tropical fever appeared out of nowhere in Sudan and Zaire (now the Democratic Republic of the Congo), no one knew what caused it, how it was spread, or how to control it. Researchers hurried to identify the cause of the epidemic, pinpoint its source, and halt its spread. The disease became known as Ebola hemorrhagic fever—"Ebola" after a nearby river and "hemorrhagic" because of the massive internal bleeding it often causes.

Because of the research conducted during and after this first outbreak, investigators were better prepared in 1995 when a major Ebola outbreak struck Zaire, in and around the city of Kikwit. By then, scientists knew that Ebola is caused by a virus spread by contact with body fluids. International teams of disease detectives used epidemiologic methods and laboratory tools to determine that the outbreak had been in progress at least 4 months before health authorities were alerted. Much of the ongoing transmission was occurring in hospitals, and the number of new cases dropped sharply after CDC, WHO, and their partners encouraged the use of barrier precautions, supplied protective clothing and disposable syringes, and disinfected healthcare facilities.

While the 1995 outbreak was still going on, a research pathologist at CDC noticed that people who died of Ebola hemorrhagic fever had virus particles in their skin. Building on this finding, he and his colleagues developed a surveillance kit that lets health teams safely take diagnostic skin samples from people who have died from what appears to be Ebola. The samples can then be sent to laboratories for testing. CDC has provided kits to healthcare facilities in the Kikwit area and has trained local staff to identify and test people with suspected Ebola. Prompt diagnosis of Ebola hemorrhagic fever will help provide early identification of outbreaks and allow control measures to be instituted as quickly as possible.

Infrastructure and Training

Public health infrastructure and training support public health actions. Nations, states, and communities need strong infrastructures to sustain disease surveillance, research, and prevention activities and to prepare for the unexpected. They need modern laboratories that are equipped to recognize stealthy microbial agents like hepatitis C virus and *E. coli* O157:H7. They need people, equipment, and know-how to perform jobs as diverse as disease reporting, microbe identification, restaurant inspections, water-supply tests, vaccination campaigns, and public education. They need communications technologies to link scientists in national and global networks. They need training to teach laboratory researchers how to perform diagnostic tests and safely process deadly specimens, to instruct workers about new tools and techniques, and to prepare the next generation of scientists to confront emerging disease challenges.

The U.S. experience with rubella shows the importance of a strong public health infrastructure. Rubella (German measles) is an acute viral infection that is spread from person to person. Although the disease is usually mild, when a pregnant women gets this infection, her baby can be born with severe birth defects, including heart defects, deafness, and mental retardation, and other outcomes of the condition known as congenital rubella syndrome (CRS).

Since a rubella vaccine was licensed in 1969, no major epidemics of rubella have occurred in the United States, and rubella infections have sharply decreased. Over the past few years, however, the epidemiology of rubella has changed, and it now occurs mainly in adults, rather than in children. Many of the affected adults come from countries without rubella vaccination programs. This shift puts susceptible pregnant women and their fetuses at risk.

Since 1994, CDC has provided grants to all states to bolster the infrastructure for fighting vaccine-preventable diseases like rubella. North Carolina used its grant to strengthen disease monitoring and control. Thus, when an outbreak of rubella hit nine North Carolina counties in 1997, a rubella surveillance system was already in place. The outbreak was detected early, and control measures were initiated without delay. No cases of CRS were reported in the months that followed.

Achievements like North Carolina's triumph over rubella are certainly impressive, but many health departments remain inadequately prepared for the fight against the new public health threats. Strengthening the public health infrastructure requires an ongoing and sizable investment in modernization and training to boost local, state, national, and global disease-monitoring capacity and to augment outbreak-response expertise. Making these improvements is the only way to guarantee that the United States, and the world, are prepared with trained experts, well equipped laboratories, and cutting-edge technology to combat emerging and reemerging microbes in the decades to come.

Prevention and Control

The culmination of all of these efforts is the prevention and control of infectious diseases. Disease prevention alerts people to the threats of new and reemerging diseases and teaches them how to protect themselves and their families. Disease control applies the most effective tools and technologies to combat infectious microbes.

The crusade against group B streptococcal infection illustrates the power of effective prevention and control. Scientists have known for a long time that 1 woman in 5 carries group B streptococcus bacteria in her body. The bacteria usually cause no symptoms. However, when transmitted from an infected pregnant woman to her newborn during childbirth, the bacteria can kill the baby—or leave a tiny survivor cruelly handicapped.

Until recently, most parents-to-be never learned about the possibility of this infection during their prenatal visits to the doctor's office. Unsuspecting new parents would typically be told about the disease only after delivery, when faced with a critically ill newborn. Although studies in the 1980s showed that giving antibiotics during childbirth to women at high risk can prevent group B streptococcus infection in newborns, antibiotics were not routinely given, and thousands of U.S. babies continued to be stricken each year.

Why were these deadly but preventable infections still occurring? Surveys found that doctors were confused about recommendations to prevent group B streptococcal disease. CDC responded to this problem by joining with several partner organizations to develop and distribute new recommendations for disease prevention. As obstetricians adopted the new policies, the number of cases in newborns dropped— by more than 50% in some places—and the action saved thousands of babies from permanent disability, shielded thousands of parents from heartbreak, and saved the nation millions in medical costs. CDC is now working with community groups, health departments, and professional organizations to bring standardized prevention protocols to a wider audience.

These actions exemplify CDC's approach to disease prevention and control and the success that comes from translating the results of surveillance and research into practice. The nation can build on the strengths gained by investments in surveillance, research, infrastructure building, and training and apply them systematically to reducing illnesses and deaths from infectious diseases.

Fighting Emerging Infections around the World

Infectious diseases remain the number one cause of death around the world, and the global upswing in new and reemerging microbes increases the danger to us all. The reality of that threat was dramatized recently by worldwide concern that a 1997 outbreak of avian influenza ("bird flu") in Hong Kong might be the start of the next global pandemic.

Influenza is a wily adversary that routinely taxes the skills and resources of the public health community. Influenza is not caused by a single organism but by a group of related viruses that are constantly changing. Because the viruses vary so much from year to year, a new vaccine must be developed for each winter season.

Looming over the yearly routine of preparing for each flu season is the threat that a pandemic strain might emerge—a virulent new type of flu that can span the globe in months and decimate the world's population—the kind that killed more than 20 million people in 1918–1919. Such a lethal virus can sweep the world without warning.

The recent influenza scare raised the specter of a possible global pandemic and jolted the world from any renewed complacency about infectious diseases. It also reminded us of the value and urgency of a strategy of national and international watchfulness, knowledge, preparedness, and action.

Scientists have done their best to build a sturdy defense against influenza. A worldwide detection system tracks the yearly changes in flu viruses. Timely global watchfulness pays off by giving manufacturers the lead time to prepare each year's vaccine. The surveillance system worked well enough in 1997 to detect the new flu strain in Hong Kong that many feared might be the next worldwide killer.

Each year, scientists need to characterize the circulating flu strains early enough for vaccine to be created. They study thousands of virus samples from dozens of laboratories around the world to predict which types are likely to dominate the next flu season. From that knowledge, manufacturers can develop an appropriate vaccine. Laboratory research makes it possible to understand a new virus at its most basic level, develop tests to detect infected persons, and produce large quantities of effective vaccine quickly and safely.

Delivering influenza vaccine to people at high risk is a yearly public health priority. In the case of a potential pandemic, inoculating hundreds of millions of Americans would be a dizzying logistical feat—but possible within the parameters of state and national influenza preparedness plans. The challenge is to be ready.

Once a new strain actually strikes, the public health community is set into action—informing the public, educating medical workers, and vaccinating millions to meet the threat of an emerging influenza strain.

Pandemic flu is not the only threat facing us in the next millennium. An equivalent level of commitment and action is needed to thwart the full assemblage of emerging infectious diseases. The groundwork has already been laid, new tools are expanding our arsenal, and the challenges and opportunities of a new century await.

Partners in Disease Prevention and Control

Realizing CDC's vision of a safer world requires the sustained and coordinated work of many people and groups, from the highest levels of government and most respected research institutions to individual health-care providers, businesses, communities, and families.

In the national government, CDC has responsibility for disease surveillance and investigation of emerging threats. Other federal agencies share responsibilities for conducting research and activating control measures. State and local public health departments lead the effort to detect, prevent, and control emerging infectious diseases in their jurisdictions.

The campaign against infectious diseases also extends beyond public agencies. Laboratories test human samples for infectious agents and report results to health departments. Universities and research groups find and promote treatments, cures, and new methods for preventing infections. Health-care providers report notifiable diseases to public health authorities, take actions to check the spread of illness, and instruct patients on how to avoid infection. Pharmaceutical companies develop vaccines and antibiotics. Schools and child-care centers enforce immunization requirements and teach good health practices. Advocacy groups educate the public about diseases that threaten their neighborhoods and communities.

These groups often come together to tackle problems that require people and expertise beyond the resources of any one entity. One such challenge was to halt the nationwide increase in babies born infected with HIV, the virus that causes AIDS. Before preventive treatments were available, 1,000 to 2,000 U.S. infants were born with HIV infection each year. In 1994, clinical trials sponsored by the National Institutes of Health (NIH) found that the anti-HIV drug zidovudine, given to HIV-infected mothers prenatally and at delivery and to their babies immediately after birth, could reduce the risk of mother-to-child (perinatal) HIV transmission by more than two-thirds. Zidovudine (also known as AZT or ZDV) was developed by industry scientists who built on the findings of researchers supported by NIH and private foundations. The drug was first licensed by the Food and Drug Administration (FDA) in 1987.

Based on the results of the clinical trials, the U.S. Public Health Service (PHS) issued guidelines in 1995 recommending HIV counseling and voluntary testing for all pregnant women and zidovudine therapy for those infected. A consortium of federal, state, and local health officials, AIDS service providers, and private physicians and researchers wrote the PHS guidelines. Putting them into action required the teamwork of public agencies, private institutions, and nonprofit organizations. Community representatives worked with health departments to meet local needs and link patients, doctors, counselors, scientists, activists, and public health workers. Public and private clinics, medical centers, and nonprofit sites provided counseling, testing, and treatment.

From 1992 through 1997, the number of babies in the United States with HIV/AIDS fell dramatically, by more than 40%. The public/private partnerships continue today and have expanded to include international groups, such as the Joint United Nations Programme on AIDS (UNAIDS).

Entering the 21st Century

Despite our best efforts to stop the onslaught of new and resurgent infections, infectious diseases probably will never be wholly subdued. Microbial pathogens are unpredictable, ever-changing, endlessly adaptable, and ready to ambush us any time our defenses falter. Therefore, we must be ready for whatever new threats arise.

CDC's publication, *Preventing Emerging Infectious Diseases: A strategy for the 21st Century*, lays out the battle plan. The challenge for the nation is to respond with the resources and commitment needed to

- Maintain our watchfulness through surveillance

- Invigorate our knowledge through research

- Heighten our preparedness by strengthening public health systems

- Arm our communities, our nation, and the world for decisive preventive action against emerging and resurgent infectious diseases.

Part Seven

Additional Help
and Information

Chapter 78

Glossary of Terms Related to Infectious Diseases

antibiotic: Type of antimicrobial agent made from a mold or a bacterium that kills, or slows the growth of other microbes, specifically bacteria. Examples include penicillin and streptomycin.

antibody: A protein molecule (also called an immunoglobulin) produced by B cells in response to an antigen. When an antibody attaches to an antigen, it destroys the antigen.

antigen: A substance or molecule that is recognized by the immune system. The molecule can be from a foreign material such as bacteria or viruses.

antimicrobial agents: A general term for the drugs, chemicals, or other substances that either kill or slow the growth of microbes. Among the antimicrobial agents in use today are antibacterial drugs (which kill bacteria), antiviral agents (which kill viruses), antifungal agents (which kill fungi), and antiparasitic drugs (which kill parasites).

antimicrobial resistance: Antimicrobial resistance is the result of microbes changing in ways that reduce or eliminate the effectiveness of drugs, chemicals, or other agents to cure or prevent infections.

This glossary contains terms excerpted from "Antimicrobial Resistance: Glossary," July 2000, and "Rocky Mountain Spotted Fever," August 2000, National Center for Infectious Diseases, with additional terms from "Malaria," September 2002, and "Primary Immune Deficiency," March 2003, National Institute of Allergy and Infectious Diseases.

attenuated: Treated in such a way as to weaken the infection or disease.

B cells: Small white blood cells crucial to the immune defenses. Also known as B lymphocytes, they come from bone marrow and develop into blood cells called plasma cells, which are the source of antibodies.

bacteria: Microscopic organisms composed of a single cell and lacking a defined nucleus and membrane-enclosed internal compartment. Bacteria live in and around us. They may be helpful, but in certain conditions may cause illnesses such as strep throat, most ear infections, and bacterial pneumonia.

bacterium: The singular form of bacteria.

bronchi: Airways in the lungs

carriers: Apparently healthy people who harbor disease-causing microbes in the body and who can infect others by passing the microbes on to them.

cell: The smallest unit of life; the basic living unit that makes up tissues, organs, systems, and bloodstream of the body.

chromosome: Physical structure in a cell that houses genes. Almost every human cell has 23 pairs of chromosomes (egg and sperm cells have half).

complement: A series of blood proteins whose action "complements" the work of antibodies. Complement destroys bacteria, produces inflammation, and regulates immune reactions.

disease: A state in which a function or part of the body is no longer in a healthy condition.

DNA (deoxyribonucleic acid): A complex molecule found in the cell nucleus which contains an organism's genetic information.

drug resistance: Drug resistance is the result of microbes changing in ways that reduce or eliminate the effectiveness of drugs, chemicals, or other agents to cure or prevent infections.

endemic: Constantly present.

epidemic: A disease outbreak that affects many people in a region at the same time.

epidemiology: The study of the spread of diseases. Epidemiologists are often sent to investigate outbreaks.

fungi: Single-celled or multicellular organisms. Fungi can be either opportunistic pathogens (such as aspergillosis, candidiasis, and cryptococcosis) that cause infections in immunocompromised persons (including cancer patients, transplant recipients, and persons with AIDS) or pathogens (such as the endemic mycoses, histoplasmosis and coccidioidomycosis, and superficial mycoses) that cause infections in healthy people. Fungi are also used for the development of antibiotics, antitoxins, and other drugs used to control various human diseases.

gametes: Reproductive elements, male and female.

gene: A unit of genetic material that is inherited from a parent. A gene carries the directions a cell uses to perform a specific function, like making proteins. Genes are made of DNA, the basic chemical unit of life.

genes: Units of genetic material (DNA) that carry the directions a cell uses to perform a specific function.

genus: A category of organisms.

granulocyte: A cell filled with potent chemicals that destroy germs and reduce inflammation.

hemoglobin: The oxygen-carrying part of the red blood cell.

IgA (immunoglobulin A): A type of antibody concentrated in mucous membranes and body fluids like tears, saliva, and secretions of the respiratory and gastrointestinal tract.

IgG (immunoglobulin G): The major antibody found in the blood that can enter tissues. It coats germs, helping other cells to seek and destroy them.

IgM (immunoglobulin M): An antibody that remains in the bloodstream where it can kill bacteria that enter the blood stream.

immune response: Reactions of the immune system to foreign substances.

immune system: A complex network of specialized cells, tissues, and organs that defends the body against attacks by disease-causing microbes.

immunity: The protection generated by the body's immune system in response to invasion by "foreign" invaders, including bacteria and viruses as well as parasites.

immunization: The process or procedure by which a subject (person, animal, or plant) is rendered immune, or resistant to a specific disease. This term is often used interchangeably with vaccination or inoculation, although the act of inoculation does not always result in immunity.

immunoglobulins: A large family of proteins, also known as antibodies. There are five classes of immunoglobulins: IgA, IgM, IgG, IgD, and IgE. Only IgA, IgG, and IgM are further classified into specific subclasses, denoted by a numeric suffix (for example, IgG2).

infection: A state in which disease-causing microbes have invaded or multiplied in body tissues.

infectious diseases: Diseases caused by microbes that can be passed to or among humans by several methods.

inflammation: An immune system process that stops the progression of disease-causing microbes, often seen at the site of an injury like a cut. Signs include redness, swelling, pain, and heat.

larvae: An immature stage that differs from the adult form; in insects such as mosquitos, an immature wingless form.

latent: Present but not seen. A latent viral infection is one in which no virus can be found in the blood cells but in which those virus-infected cells can produce virus under certain circumstances.

lymph nodes: Small bean-shaped organs of the immune system, distributed widely throughout the body. They are fortresses of B, T, and other immune cells.

lymphocytes: Small white blood cells (B and T cells) that are the major players in immune defense.

meningitis: Inflammation of the meninges, the membranes that surround the brain and spinal cord.

microbes: Organisms so small that a microscope is required to see them. Microbes are also called microorganisms.

microorganisms: Microscopic organisms, including bacteria, viruses, fungi, plants, and animals.

microscopic: Too small to be seen with the naked eye.

molecules: The smallest physical units of a substance that still retain the chemical properties of that chemical substance; molecules are the building blocks of a cell. Some examples are proteins, fats, carbohydrates, and nucleic acids.

mucous membrane: The moist lining of certain body cavities such as the mouth.

mutation: A change in a cell's DNA that may cause the cell to produce an abnormal protein.

neutrophils: An important white blood cell that is both a phagocyte and a granulocyte abundant in the blood.

nosocomial: Referring to an infection acquired by a patient while in a hospital.

oocyst: A parasite stage within the mosquito, produced by the union of male and female gametes.

opportunistic infections: Infections caused by microbes that usually do not cause disease in healthy individuals, but which can result in overwhelming and widespread infection in people with immune deficiency.

organism: Any living thing. Organisms include humans, animals, plants, bacteria, protozoa, and fungi.

pandemics: Diseases that affect many people in different regions around the world.

parasite: An animal (or plant) that must live on or in an organism of another species, from which it draws its nourishment, without benefiting the host organism; commonly refers to pathogens, most commonly in reference to protozoans and helminths.

paroxysm: An attack of a disease that is likely to recur at periodic intervals.

pathogens: Disease-causing organisms, such as bacteria, viruses, parasites, or fungi.

phagocytes: Large white blood cells that contribute to immune defense by engulfing microbes, such as bacteria and fungi, or other cells and foreign particles.

relapse: The recurrence of disease some time after it has been apparently cured.

resistance: The ability of an organism to develop strains that are impervious to specific threats to their existence.

RNA (ribonucleic acid): A complex molecule that is found in the cell cytoplasm and nucleus. One function of RNA is to direct the building of proteins.

rotavirus: A group of viruses that can cause digestive problems and diarrhea in young children.

species: Organisms in the same genus that have similar characteristics.

strain: A genetic variant within a species.

surveillance systems: The ongoing systematic collection and analysis of data. The data may lead to actions taken to prevent and control an infectious disease.

T cells (T lymphocytes): White blood cells that either orchestrate the immune response (regulatory T cells) or directly attack infected or malignant cells (cytotoxic T cells).

tissues: Groups of similar cells joined to perform the same function.

toxins: Agents produced by plants and bacteria, normally very damaging to human cells.

vaccine: Substance that contains parts of antigens from an infectious microbe. By stimulating an immune response (but not disease), it protects the body against subsequent infection by that organism.

vector: The organism, typically an insect, that transmits an infectious agent to its alternate host, typically a vertebrate. For example, in human malaria, the vector of the parasite are mosquitoes; the "carriers" or "hosts" are humans.

virulent: Characterized by rapid, severe, and malignant course.

virus: A strand of DNA or RNA in a protein coat that must get inside a living cell to grow and reproduce. Viruses cause many types of illness; for example, varicella virus causes chickenpox, and the human immunodeficiency virus (HIV) causes the acquired immune deficiency syndrome, or AIDS.

Chapter 79

Resources for Information about Infectious Diseases

Centers for Disease Control and Prevention

Centers for Disease Control and Prevention
1600 Clifton Road
Atlanta, GA 30333
Toll-Free: 800-311-3435
Website: http://www.cdc.gov

Division of Bacterial and Mycotic Diseases
Website: http://www.cdc.gov/ncidod/dbmd

Division of Global Migration and Quarantine
Website: http://www.cdc.gov/ncidod/dq

Division of Healthcare Quality Promotion
Website: http://www.cdc.gov/ncidod/hip

Division of Parasitic Diseases
Website: http://www.cdc.gov/ncidod/dpd

Division of Vector-Borne Infectious Diseases
Website: http://www.cdc.gov/ncidod/dvbid

Division of Viral and Rickettsial Diseases
Website: http://www.cdc.gov/ncidod/dvrd

Healthy Swimming
Website: http://www.cdc.gov/healthyswimming
E-mail: healthyswimming@cdc.gov

Information in this chapter was compiled from many sources deemed accurate. All contact information was updated and verified in January 2004. Inclusion does not constitute endorsement.

National Center for Infectious
Diseases
Office of Health Communication
Centers for Disease Control and
Prevention
1600 Clifton Road
Mailstop C-14
Atlanta, GA 30333
Phone: 404-639-3401
Website: http://www.cdc.gov/
ncidod
E-mail: ncid@cdc.gov

*National Immunization
Information Program*
Toll Free: 800-232-2522
Toll Free Fax: 888-232-3299
Spanish: 800-232-0233
Website: http://www.cdc.gov/nip
E-mail: NIPINFO@cdc.gov

*Public Health Emergency
Preparedness and Response*
Toll Free Hotline: 888-246-2675
Spanish: 888-246-2857
TTY: 866-874-2646
Website: http://www.bt.cdc.gov

Select Agent Program
Phone: 404-498-2255
Fax: 404-498-2265
Website: http://www.cdc.gov/od/
sap
E-mail: lrsat@cdc.gov

Special Pathogens Branch
Phone: 404-639-1510
Fax: 404-639-1509
Website: http://www.cdc.gov/
ncidod/dvrd/spb
E-mail: dvd1spath@cdc.gov

Traveler's Health
Toll Free: 877-FYI-TRIP
Toll Free Fax: 888-232-3299
Website: http://www.cdc.gov/
travel

Other Resources

Agricultural Research Service
U.S. Department of Agriculture
5601 Sunnyside Avenue
Beltsville, MD 20705-5134
Phone: 301-504-6078
Website: http://www.ars.usda
.gov
E-mail: info@ars.udsa.gov

American Academy of Family Physicians
11400 Tomahawk Creek Parkway
Leawood, KS 66211-2672
Toll Free: 800-274-2237
Phone: 913-906-6000
Website: http://
www.familydoctor.org
E-mail: email@familydoctor.org

American Lyme Disease Foundation, Inc.
Mill Pond Offices
293 Route 100
Somers, NY 10589
Phone: 914-277-6970
Fax: 914-277-6974
Website: http://www.aldf.com
E-mail: inquire@aldf.com

American Society for Microbiology
1752 N Street, NW
Washington, DC 20036-2904
Phone: 202-942-9297
Fax: 202-942-9367
Website: http://www.asm.org
E-mail: communications@
asmusa.org

Association for Professionals in Infection Control and Epidemiology, Inc.
1275 K Street, NW, Suite 1000
Washington, DC 20005-4006
Phone: 202-789-1890
Fax: 202-789-1899
Website: http://www.apic.org
E-mail: APICinfo@apic.org

Association of State and Territorial Directors of Health Promotion and Public Health Education
1101 15th Street, NW, Suite 601
Washington, DC 20005
Phone: 202-689-2230
Fax: 202-659-2339
Website: http://www.dhpe.org

Bureau of Infectious Diseases
Health Canada
A.L. 0900C2
Ottawa, Canada K1A 0K9
Phone: 613-957-2991
Fax 613-941-5366
Toll Free TTY: 800-267-1245
Website: http://www.hc-sc.gc.ca/
pphb-dgspsp/bid-bmi
E-mail: pphb_web_mail@hc-
sc.gc.ca

Center for Biosecurity
University of Pittsburgh Medical
Center
200 Lothrop St.
Pittsburgh, PA 15213
Phone: 443-573-3304
Fax: 443-573-3305
Website: http://www.upmc-
biosecurity.org

Center for Food Safety and Applied Nutrition
U.S. Food and Drug Admin.
5100 Paint Branch Parkway
College Park, MD 20740-3825
Toll Free: 888-SAFEFOOD (888-
723-3366)
Website: http://www.cfsan.fda.gov

Center for Infectious Disease Research and Policy
University of Minnesota
Academic Health Center
420 Delaware Street, SE
MMC 263
Minneapolis, MN 55455
Phone: 612-626-6770
Fax: 612-626-6783
Website: http://www.cidrap.umn
.edu
E-mail: cidrap@umn.edu

Florida Infectious Diseases Society
James A. Haley Veterans'
Hospital
13000 Bruce B. Downs Blvd.
Tampa, FL 33612
Phone: 813-972-1000 ext. 6184
Website: http://www.geocities
.com/~fids
E-mail: idfla@yahoo.com

Food Safety and Inspection Service
U.S. Department of Agriculture
Washington, DC 20250-3700
Toll Free: 800-535-4555
Toll Free TTY: 800-256-7072
Website: http://www.fsis.usda .gov
E-mail: MPHotline.fsis@usda .gov

Infectious Diseases Society of America
66 Canal Center Plaza
Suite 600
Alexandria, VA 22314
Phone: 703-299-0200
Fax: 703-299-0204
Website: http://www.idsociety.org
E-mail: info@idsociety.org

International Society for Infectious Diseases
181 Longwood Avenue
Boston, MA 02115
Phone: 617-277-0551
Fax: 617-731-1541
Website: http://www.isid.org
E-mail: info@isid.org

Johns Hopkins University
Division of Infectious Diseases
Baltimore, MD 21287
Phone: 410-614-8976
Fax: 410-955-7889
Website: http://www.hopkins-id.edu
E-mail: feedback@hopkins-aids.edu

National Foundation for Infectious Diseases
4733 Bethesda Avenue
Suite 750
Bethesda, MD 20814
Phone: 301-656-0003
Fax: 301-907-0878
Website: http://www.nfid.org
E-mail: info@nfid.org

National Institute of Allergy and Infectious Diseases
Building 31, Room 7A50
31 Center Drive, MSC 2520
Bethesda, MD 20892-2520
Phone: 301-496-5717
Website: http://www.niaid.nih.gov

National Institute of Diabetes and Digestive and Kidney Diseases
Center Drive, MSC 2560
Building 31, Room 9A04
Bethesda, MD 20892
Toll Free: 877-946-4627
Website: http://www.niddk.nih.gov

National Institute of Neurological Disorders and Stroke
NIH Neurological Institute
P.O. Box 5801
Bethesda, MD 20824
Toll Free: 800-352-9424
Phone: 301-496-5751
TTY: 301-468-5981
Website: http://www.ninds.nih .gov

National Institutes of Health
9000 Rockville Pike
Bethesda, MD 20892
Phone: 301-496-4000
Website: http://www.nih.gov

National Library of Medicine
8600 Rockville Pike
Bethesda, MD 20894
Toll Free: 888-346-3656
Phone: 301-594-5983
Fax: 301-402-1384
Website: http://www.nlm.nih.gov

Nemours Center for Children's Health
12735 West Gran Bay Parkway
Jacksonville, FL 32258
Toll Free: 866-390-3610
Website: http://www.KidsHealth
.org

Office of Ground Water and Drinking Water
U.S. Environmental Protection Agency
Ariel Rios Building
1200 Pennsylvania Avenue, NW
Washington, DC 20460-0003
Toll Free: 800-426-4791
Phone: 202-564-3750
Fax: 202-564-3751
Website: http://www.epa.gov/
safewater
E-mail: sdwa@epa.gov

Pediatric Infectious Disease Society (PIDS)
66 Canal Center Plaza
Suite 600
Alexandria, VA 22314
Phone: 703-299-6764
Fax: 703-299-0473
Website: http://www.pids.org
E-mail: pids@idsociety.org

U.S. Department of Homeland Security
Washington, DC 20528
Toll Free: 800-BE-READY
Website: http://www.ready.gov

U.S. Food and Drug Administration
5600 Fishers Lane
Rockville, MD 20857-0001
Toll-Free: 888-INFO-FDA (888-463-6332)
Website: http://www.fda.gov

World Health Organization
Avenue Appia 20
1211 Geneva 27
Switzerland
Phone: (011 + 41 22) 791 21 11
Fax: (011 + 41 22) 791 3111
Website: http://www.who.int
E-mail: info@who.int

Chapter 80

Additional Reading on Infectious Diseases

Magazine and Journal Articles

Brachman, Philip S. "Bioterrorism: An Update with a Focus on Anthrax," *American Journal of Epidemiology*, vol. 155, no. 11 (06/01/2002) p. 981-7.

Cox, Nadine. "Infant Botulism," *American Family Physician*, vol. 65, no. 7 (04/01/2002) p. 1388-92.

Craun, Gunther F. "Outbreaks in Drinking-Water Systems, 1991-1998," *Journal of Environmental Health*, vol. 65, no. 1 (07–08/2002) p. 16-23.

Daniels, Anthony. "Germs against Man. Bioterror: A Brief History," *National Review* vol. 53, no. 23 (12/03/2001) p. 42-4.

Gammons, Matthew, "Tick Removal," *American Family Physician*, vol. 66, no. 4 (08/15/2002) p. 643-6.

Hall, Stephen S. "On The Trail of the West Nile Virus," *Smithsonian*, vol. 34, no. 4 (07/2003) p. 88-94, 96, 98-102.

Harder, B. "A Safe Solution," *Science News*, vol. 163, no. 9 (03/01/2003) p. 136-8.

The resources listed in this chapter provide a starting point for further research. They were selected to provide a diverse sampling of the many types of resources available. Inclusion does not constitute endorsement. All websites were verified in January 2004.

Hawaleshka, Danylo, "Zapping the Germs," *Maclean's* vol. 115, no. 49 (Dec. 9 2002) p. 66.

Hawaleshka, Danylo. "Worries over Water: *E. coli* in Canadian Drinking Water," *Maclean's*, vol. 113, no. 23 (06/05/2000) p. 37.

Hingley, Audrey. "Campylobacter: Low-Profile Bug Is Food Poisoning Leader," *FDA Consumer*, vol. 33, no. 5 (09–10/1999) p. 14-17.

Jaroff, Leon. "The New Antiseptics," *Time*, vol. 156, no. 4 (07/24/2000) p. 47.

Katz, J.R. and Hirsch, A.M. "When Global Health Is Local Health. Infectious Diseases Travel Easily," *American Journal of Nursing*, vol. 103, no. 12 (12/2003) p. 75-9.

Kuiken, T., Fouchier, R., Rimmelzwaan, G., and Osterhaus, A. "Emerging Viral Infections in a Rapidly Changing World," *Current Opinions in Biotechnology*, vol. 14, no. 6 (12/2003) p. 641-6.

Kurowski, Rene. "Overview of Histoplasmosis," *American Family Physician*, vol. 66, no. 12 (12/15/2002) p. 2247-52.

O'Brien, Karen K. "Recognition and Management of Bioterrorism Infections," *American Family Physician*, vol. 67, no. 9 (05/01/2003) p. 1927-34.

Prüss, Annette, "Estimating the Burden of Disease from Water, Sanitation, and Hygiene at a Global Level," *Environmental Health Perspectives*, vol. 110, no. 5 (05/2002) p. 537-42.

Rajan, T. V. "The Worm and the Parasite," *Natural History*, vol. 112, no. 1 (02/2003) p. 32-5.

Seppa, N. "Gene Variants [of *Helicobacter pylori*] Implicated in Stomach Cancer," *Science News*, vol. 162, no. 22 (11/30/2002) p. 341-2.

Swerdlow, Joel L. "Living with Microbes," *The Wilson Quarterly*, vol. 26 no. 2 (Spring 2002) p. 42-59.

"Top Food Safety Mistakes," *Restaurants & Institutions*, vol. 113, no. 4 (02/15/2003 suppl.) p. 8-10, 12.

Waldvogel F.A. "Infectious Diseases in the 21st Century: Old Challenges and New Opportunities," *International Journal of Infectious Diseases*, vol. 8, no. 1 (01/0004) p. 5-12.

Walling, Anne D. "Women Frequently Misdiagnose Vulvovaginal Infections," *American Family Physician*, vol. 65, no. 11 (06/01/2002) p. 2349-54.

Weinhold B. "Infectious Disease: The Human Costs of Our Environmental Errors," *Environmental Health Perspectives*, vol. 112, no. 1 (01/2004) p. A32-9.

Weiss, Peter. "Ultrasound Fizz Kills Microbes under Pressure," *Science News*, vol. 162, no. 23 (12/07/2002) p. 358.

Books

Armies of Pestilence: The Impact of Disease on History
A hardcover book by R. S. Bray
Published by Barnes & Noble Books, February 2000
ISBN: 076071908X

Infectious Diseases
A medical reference edited by Sherwood Gorbach, John G. Bartlett, and Neil R. Blacklow
Published by Lippincott Williams & Wilkins, November 2003
ISBN: 0781733715

Infectious Diseases: Principles and Practice, Fifth Edition
A medical reference by Gerald L. Mandell, R. Gordon Douglas, Raphael Dolin, and John E. Bennett
Published by Churchill Livingstone, Inc., September 1998
ISBN: 044307693X

Medical Microbiology, Fourth Edition
A textbook by Patrick R. Murray, George S. Kobayashi, Michael A. Pfaller, and Kenneth S. Rosenthal
Published by Elsevier Science, January 2001
ISBN: 0323012132

Microbe Hunters
A paperback book by Paul de Kruif
Published by Harcourt, October 2002
ISBN: 0156027771

Robbins Pathologic Basis of Disease, Sixth Edition
A textbook by Ramzi S. Cotran, Tucker Collins, Vinay Kumar
Published by Elsevier Science, November 1998
ISBN: 072167335X

Secret Agents: The Menace of Emerging Infections
A paperback book by Madeline Drexler
Published by Penguin, February 2003
ISBN: 0142002615

The Secret Life of Germs: Observations and Lessons of a Microbe Hunter
A hardcover book by Philip M. Tierno
Published by Simon & Schuster, October 2001
ISBN: 0743421876

Information Available on the Internet

Emerging Infectious Diseases
A journal produced by the Centers for Disease Control and Prevention
http://www.cdc.gov/ncidod/eid

Epidemic: The World of Infectious Diseases
An online exhibit of the American Museum of Natural History
http://amnh.org/exhibitions/epidemic

Fight Bac! Keep Food Safe From Bacteria
Online information for educators, consumers, and the media, produced by the Partnership for Food Safety Education
http://www.fightbac.org

Foodborne Pathogenic Microorganisms and Natural Toxins Handbook (the "Bad Bug Book")
A book produced by the U.S. Food and Drug Administration's Center for Food Safety and Applied Nutrition
http://www.cfsan.fda.gov/~mow/intro.html

Health Information for International Travel (the "Yellow Book")
An annual book produced by the Centers for Disease Control and Prevention
http://www.cdc.gov/travel/yb/index.htm

Infectious Diseases
A list of links to documents of interest, compiled by the National Library of Medicine
http://www.nlm.nih.gov/medlineplus/infectiousdiseases.html

Infectious Diseases / Bacterial Diseases / Microbiology
A list of links to documents of interest, compiled by the Hardin Library
for the Health Sciences at the University of Iowa
http://www.lib.uiowa.edu/hardin/md/micro.html

Infectious Diseases in Children
An online newsletter produced by Slack Inc.
http://idinchildren.com

Infectious Disease News
An online newsletter produced by Slack Inc.
http://infectiousdiseasenews.com

"Infectious Disorders," *The Merck Manual of Diagnosis and Therapy*
Section 13 (Chapters 150–164) from a book produced by Merck &
Co., Inc.
http://www.merck.com/mrkshared/mmanual/section13/sec13.jsp

Microbe World
An online educational site, developed by the American Society for
Microbiology
http://www.microbeworld.org

Microbe Library
A collection of online resources for educators, developed by the
American Society for Microbiology
http://www.microbelibrary.org

Microbes: Invisible Invaders... Amazing Allies
An online exhibit, produced by the Natural History Museum of
Los Angeles County Foundation
http://www.nhm.org/microbes/main.html

Scaling Up the Response to Infectious Diseases
A publication of the World Health Organization
http://www.who.int/infectious-disease-report/2002

Stalking the Mysterious Microbe
An online resource for kids, developed by the American Society for
Microbiology
http://www.microbe.org

Virtual Museum of Bacteria
An online exhibit sponsored by the Foundation of Bacteriology
http://www.bacteriamuseum.org

Index

Index

Page numbers followed by 'n' indicate a footnote. Page numbers in *italics* indicate a table or illustration.

diatoms 24–25
dinoflagellates, described 24
diphenoxylate 123
Dipylidium caninum 153–54
direct fluorescent antibody test 273
"Dirty Bombs" (CDC) 485n
dirty bombs, described 488–90
disease
    defined 574
    versus infection 9
disseminated histoplasmosis 387
Division of Bacterial and Mycotic Dis-
    eases (CDC), Web site address 579
Division of Global Migration and
    Quarantine (CDC), Web site ad-
    dress 579
Division of Healthcare Quality Pro-
    motion (CDC), Web site address 579
Division of Parasitic Diseases (CDC),
    Web site address 579
Division of Viral and Rickettsial Dis-
    eases, Web site address 579
Divison of Vector-Borne Diseases
    (CDC), Web site address 579
DNA *see* deoxyribonucleic acid
doctors *see* physicians
dog tapeworm, described 153–54
doxycycline 46, 57–58, 177, 214, 305,
    329, 433
drug resistance
    defined 574
    described 11

E

E. coli see Escherichia coli
eastern equine encephalitis 160–62
"Eastern Equine Encephalitis" (CDC)
    159n
ebola hemorrhagic fever 336–38
"Ebola Hemorrhagic Fever" (CDC)
    331n
Ehrlichia chaffeensis 175–76
ehrlichiosis
    described 293
    overview 175–79
elephantiasis, lymphatic filariasis
    222

emerging diseases, described 4
encephalitis
    overview 159–74
    West Nile virus 13, 345
"Encephalitis and Meningitis Infor-
    mation Page" (NINDS) 159n
endemic, defined 574
endocarditis 46, 375, 459
epidemic, defined 574
epidemic typhus 292
epidemiology, defined 575
Eppes, Stephen 149n
erythema migrans 210
erythromycin 399
Escherichia coli
    overview 75–78
    statistics 14
    transmission 7, 514, 515
    travelers' diarrhea 122
    urinary tract infections 430
esomeprazole *99*
eukaryotes, described 21
euryarchaeota, described 22
extremophiles, described 21

F

"Facts about Sarin" (CDC) 497n
"Facts about Sulfur Mustard" (CDC)
    497n
"Facts about Tetanus for Adults"
    (NFID) 423n
"Facts about Tetanus for Children"
    (KidsHealth) 423n
"Facts about VX" (CDC) 497n
"Fact Sheet: St. Louis Encephalitis"
    (CDC) 159n
famotidine *99*
"FastStats: Infectious Disease" (CDC)
    507n
fatal familial insomnia 225
FDA *see* US Food and Drug Adminis-
    tration
"FDA Clears First Test for West Nile
    Virus" (FDA) 557n
Federal Trade Commission
    (FTC), biothreats publication
    441n

I

J

K

L

Health Reference Series
COMPLETE CATALOG

Adolescent Health Sourcebook

Basic Consumer Health Information about Common Medical, Mental, and Emotional Concerns in Adolescents, Including Facts about Acne, Body Piercing, Mononucleosis, Nutrition, Eating Disorders, Stress, Depression, Behavior Problems, Peer Pressure, Violence, Gangs, Drug Use, Puberty, Sexuality, Pregnancy, Learning Disabilities, and More

Along with a Glossary of Terms and Other Resources for Further Help and Information

Edited by Chad T. Kimball. 658 pages. 2002. 0-7808-0248-9. $78.

"It is written in clear, nontechnical language aimed at general readers. . . . Recommended for public libraries, community colleges, and other agencies serving health care consumers."
— *American Reference Books Annual, 2003*

"Recommended for school and public libraries. Parents and professionals dealing with teens will appreciate the easy-to-follow format and the clearly written text. This could become a 'must have' for every high school teacher." — *E-Streams, Jan '03*

"A good starting point for information related to common medical, mental, and emotional concerns of adolescents." — *School Library Journal, Nov '02*

"This book provides accurate information in an easy to access format. It addresses topics that parents and caregivers might not be aware of and provides practical, useable information." — *Doody's Health Sciences Book Review Journal, Sep-Oct '02*

"Recommended reference source."
— *Booklist, American Library Association, Sep '02*

AIDS Sourcebook, 3rd Edition

Basic Consumer Health Information about Acquired Immune Deficiency Syndrome (AIDS) and Human Immunodeficiency Virus (HIV) Infection, Including Facts about Transmission, Prevention, Diagnosis, Treatment, Opportunistic Infections, and Other Complications, with a Section for Women and Children, Including Details about Associated Gynecological Concerns, Pregnancy, and Pediatric Care

Along with Updated Statistical Information, Reports on Current Research Initiatives, a Glossary, and Directories of Internet, Hotline, and Other Resources

Edited by Dawn D. Matthews. 664 pages. 2003. 0-7808-0631-X. $78.

ALSO AVAILABLE: *AIDS Sourcebook, 1st Edition.* Edited by Karen Bellenir and Peter D. Dresser. 831 pages. 1995. 0-7808-0031-1. $78.

AIDS Sourcebook, 2nd Edition. Edited by Karen Bellenir. 751 pages. 1999. 0-7808-0225-X. $78.

"Highly recommended."
— *American Reference Books Annual, 2000*

"Excellent sourcebook. This continues to be a highly recommended book. There is no other book that provides as much information as this book provides."
— *AIDS Book Review Journal, Dec-Jan 2000*

"Recommended reference source."
— *Booklist, American Library Association, Dec '99*

"A solid text for college-level health libraries."
— *The Bookwatch, Aug '99*

Cited in *Reference Sources for Small and Medium-Sized Libraries, American Library Association, 1999*

Alcoholism Sourcebook

Basic Consumer Health Information about the Physical and Mental Consequences of Alcohol Abuse, Including Liver Disease, Pancreatitis, Wernicke-Korsakoff Syndrome (Alcoholic Dementia), Fetal Alcohol Syndrome, Heart Disease, Kidney Disorders, Gastrointestinal Problems, and Immune System Compromise and Featuring Facts about Addiction, Detoxification, Alcohol Withdrawal, Recovery, and the Maintenance of Sobriety

Along with a Glossary and Directories of Resources for Further Help and Information

Edited by Karen Bellenir. 613 pages. 2000. 0-7808-0325-6. $78.

"This title is one of the few reference works on alcoholism for general readers. For some readers this will be a welcome complement to the many self-help books on the market. Recommended for collections serving general readers and consumer health collections."
— *E-Streams, Mar '01*

"This book is an excellent choice for public and academic libraries."
— *American Reference Books Annual, 2001*

"Recommended reference source."
— *Booklist, American Library Association, Dec '00*

"Presents a wealth of information on alcohol use and abuse and its effects on the body and mind, treatment, and prevention." — *SciTech Book News, Dec '00*

"Important new health guide which packs in the latest consumer information about the problems of alcoholism." — *Reviewer's Bookwatch, Nov '00*

SEE ALSO *Drug Abuse Sourcebook, Substance Abuse Sourcebook*

Allergies Sourcebook, 2nd Edition

Basic Consumer Health Information about Allergic Disorders, Triggers, Reactions, and Related Symptoms, Including Anaphylaxis, Rhinitis, Sinusitis, Asthma, Dermatitis, Conjunctivitis, and Multiple Chemical Sensitivity

Along with Tips on Diagnosis, Prevention, and Treatment, Statistical Data, a Glossary, and a Directory of Sources for Further Help and Information

Edited by Annemarie S. Muth. 598 pages. 2002. 0-7808-0376-0. $78.

ALSO AVAILABLE: *Allergies Sourcebook, 1st Edition.* Edited by Allan R. Cook. 611 pages. 1997. 0-7808-0036-2. $78.

"This book brings a great deal of useful material together. . . . This is an excellent addition to public and consumer health library collections."
— *American Reference Books Annual, 2003*

"This second edition would be useful to laypersons with little or advanced knowledge of the subject matter. This book would also serve as a resource for nursing and other health care professions students. It would be useful in public, academic, and hospital libraries with consumer health collections." — *E-Streams, Jul '02*

■

Alternative Medicine Sourcebook, 2nd Edition

Basic Consumer Health Information about Alternative and Complementary Medical Practices, Including Acupuncture, Chiropractic, Herbal Medicine, Homeopathy, Naturopathic Medicine, Mind-Body Interventions, Ayurveda, and Other Non-Western Medical Traditions

Along with Facts about such Specific Therapies as Massage Therapy, Aromatherapy, Qigong, Hypnosis, Prayer, Dance, and Art Therapies, a Glossary, and Resources for Further Information

Edited by Dawn D. Matthews. 618 pages. 2002. 0-7808-0605-0. $78.

ALSO AVAILABLE: *Alternative Medicine Sourcebook, 1st Edition.* Edited by Allan R. Cook. 737 pages. 1999. 0-7808-0200-4. $78.

"Recommended for public, high school, and academic libraries that have consumer health collections. Hospital libraries that also serve the public will find this to be a useful resource." — *E-Streams, Feb '03*

"Recommended reference source."
—*Booklist, American Library Association, Jan '03*

"An important alternate health reference."
— *MBR Bookwatch, Oct '02*

"A great addition to the reference collection of every type of library." — *American Reference Books Annual, 2000*

Alzheimer's Disease Sourcebook, 3rd Edition

Basic Consumer Health Information about Alzheimer's Disease, Other Dementias, and Related Disorders, Including Multi-Infarct Dementia, AIDS Dementia Complex, Dementia with Lewy Bodies, Huntington's Disease, Wernicke-Korsakoff Syndrome (Alcohol-Reated Dementia), Delirium, and Confusional States

Along with Information for People Newly Diagnosed with Alzheimer's Disease and Caregivers, Reports Detailing Current Research Efforts in Prevention, Diagnosis, and Treatment, Facts about Long-Term Care Issues, and Listings of Sources for Additional Information

Edited by Karen Bellenir. 645 pages. 2003. 0-7808-0666-2. $78.

ALSO AVAILABLE: *Alzheimer's, Stroke & 29 Other Neurological Disorders Sourcebook, 1st Edition.* Edited by Frank E. Bair. 579 pages. 1993. 1-55888-748-2. $78.

ALSO AVAILABLE: *Alzheimer's Disease Sourcebook, 2nd Edition.* Edited by Karen Bellenir. 524 pages. 1999. 0-7808-0223-3. $78.

"Provides a wealth of useful information not otherwise available in one place. This resource is recommended for all types of libraries."
—*American Reference Books Annual, 2000*

"Recommended reference source."
— *Booklist, American Library Association, Oct '99*

SEE ALSO Brain Disorders Sourcebook

■

Arthritis Sourcebook

Basic Consumer Health Information about Specific Forms of Arthritis and Related Disorders, Including Rheumatoid Arthritis, Osteoarthritis, Gout, Polymyalgia Rheumatica, Psoriatic Arthritis, Spondyloarthropathies, Juvenile Rheumatoid Arthritis, and Juvenile Ankylosing Spondylitis

Along with Information about Medical, Surgical, and Alternative Treatment Options, and Including Strategies for Coping with Pain, Fatigue, and Stress

Edited by Allan R. Cook. 550 pages. 1998. 0-7808-0201-2. $78.

". . . accessible to the layperson."
—*Reference and Research Book News, Feb '99*

■

Asthma Sourcebook

Basic Consumer Health Information about Asthma, Including Symptoms, Traditional and Nontraditional Remedies, Treatment Advances, Quality-of-Life Aids, Medical Research Updates, and the Role of Allergies, Exercise, Age, the Environment, and Genetics in the Development of Asthma

Along with Statistical Data, a Glossary, and Directories of Support Groups, and Other Resources for Further Information

Edited by Annemarie S. Muth. 628 pages. 2000. 0-7808-0381-7. $78.

"A worthwhile reference acquisition for public libraries and academic medical libraries whose readers desire a quick introduction to the wide range of asthma information." — *Choice, Association of College & Research Libraries, Jun '01*

"Recommended reference source."
— *Booklist, American Library Association, Feb '01*

"Highly recommended." — *The Bookwatch, Jan '01*

"There is much good information for patients and their families who deal with asthma daily."
— *American Medical Writers Association Journal, Winter '01*

"This informative text is recommended for consumer health collections in public, secondary school, and community college libraries and the libraries of universities with a large undergraduate population."
— *American Reference Books Annual, 2001*

■

Attention Deficit Disorder Sourcebook

Basic Consumer Health Information about Attention Deficit/Hyperactivity Disorder in Children and Adults, Including Facts about Causes, Symptoms, Diagnostic Criteria, and Treatment Options Such as Medications, Behavior Therapy, Coaching, and Homeopathy

Along with Reports on Current Research Initiatives, Legal Issues, and Government Regulations, and Featuring a Glossary of Related Terms, Internet Resources, and a List of Additional Reading Material

Edited by Dawn D. Matthews. 470 pages. 2002. 0-7808-0624-7. $78.

"Recommended reference source."
— *Booklist, American Library Association, Jan '03*

"This book is recommended for all school libraries and the reference or consumer health sections of public libraries." — *American Reference Books Annual, 2003*

■

Back & Neck Disorders Sourcebook

Basic Information about Disorders and Injuries of the Spinal Cord and Vertebrae, Including Facts on Chiropractic Treatment, Surgical Interventions, Paralysis, and Rehabilitation

Along with Advice for Preventing Back Trouble

Edited by Karen Bellenir. 548 pages. 1997. 0-7808-0202-0. $78.

"The strength of this work is its basic, easy-to-read format. Recommended."
— *Reference and User Services Quarterly, American Library Association, Winter '97*

Blood & Circulatory Disorders Sourcebook

Basic Information about Blood and Its Components, Anemias, Leukemias, Bleeding Disorders, and Circulatory Disorders, Including Aplastic Anemia, Thalassemia, Sickle-Cell Disease, Hemochromatosis, Hemophilia, Von Willebrand Disease, and Vascular Diseases

Along with a Special Section on Blood Transfusions and Blood Supply Safety, a Glossary, and Source Listings for Further Help and Information

Edited by Karen Bellenir and Linda M. Shin. 554 pages. 1998. 0-7808-0203-9. $78.

"Recommended reference source."
— *Booklist, American Library Association, Feb '99*

"An important reference sourcebook written in simple language for everyday, non-technical users. "
— *Reviewer's Bookwatch, Jan '99*

■

Brain Disorders Sourcebook

Basic Consumer Health Information about Strokes, Epilepsy, Amyotrophic Lateral Sclerosis (ALS/Lou Gehrig's Disease), Parkinson's Disease, Brain Tumors, Cerebral Palsy, Headache, Tourette Syndrome, and More

Along with Statistical Data, Treatment and Rehabilitation Options, Coping Strategies, Reports on Current Research Initiatives, a Glossary, and Resource Listings for Additional Help and Information

Edited by Karen Bellenir. 481 pages. 1999. 0-7808-0229-2. $78.

"Belongs on the shelves of any library with a consumer health collection." — *E-Streams, Mar '00*

"Recommended reference source."
— *Booklist, American Library Association, Oct '99*

SEE ALSO *Alzheimer's Disease Sourcebook*

■

Breast Cancer Sourcebook

Basic Consumer Health Information about Breast Cancer, Including Diagnostic Methods, Treatment Options, Alternative Therapies, Self-Help Information, Related Health Concerns, Statistical and Demographic Data, and Facts for Men with Breast Cancer

Along with Reports on Current Research Initiatives, a Glossary of Related Medical Terms, and a Directory of Sources for Further Help and Information

Edited by Edward J. Prucha and Karen Bellenir. 580 pages. 2001. 0-7808-0244-6. $78.

"It would be a useful reference book in a library or on loan to women in a support group."
— *Cancer Forum, Mar '03*

"Recommended reference source."
— *Booklist, American Library Association, Jan '02*

"This reference source is highly recommended. It is quite informative, comprehensive and detailed in nature, and yet it offers practical advice in easy-to-read language. It could be thought of as the 'bible' of breast cancer for the consumer." — *E-Streams, Jan '02*

"The broad range of topics covered in lay language make the *Breast Cancer Sourcebook* an excellent addition to public and consumer health library collections." — *American Reference Books Annual 2002*

"From the pros and cons of different screening methods and results to treatment options, *Breast Cancer Sourcebook* provides the latest information on the subject." — *Library Bookwatch, Dec '01*

"This thoroughgoing, very readable reference covers all aspects of breast health and cancer. . . . Readers will find much to consider here. Recommended for all public and patient health collections." — *Library Journal, Sep '01*

SEE ALSO *Cancer Sourcebook for Women, Women's Health Concerns Sourcebook*

■

Breastfeeding Sourcebook

Basic Consumer Health Information about the Benefits of Breastmilk, Preparing to Breastfeed, Breastfeeding as a Baby Grows, Nutrition, and More, Including Information on Special Situations and Concerns Such as Mastitis, Illness, Medications, Allergies, Multiple Births, Prematurity, Special Needs, and Adoption

Along with a Glossary and Resources for Additional Help and Information

Edited by Jenni Lynn Colson. 388 pages. 2002. 0-7808-0332-9. $78.

SEE ALSO *Pregnancy & Birth Sourcebook*

"Particularly useful is the information about professional lactation services and chapters on breastfeeding when returning to work. . . . *Breastfeeding Sourcebook* will be useful for public libraries, consumer health libraries, and technical schools offering nurse assistant training, especially in areas where Internet access is problematic." — *American Reference Books Annual, 2003*

■

Burns Sourcebook

Basic Consumer Health Information about Various Types of Burns and Scalds, Including Flame, Heat, Cold, Electrical, Chemical, and Sun Burns

Along with Information on Short-Term and Long-Term Treatments, Tissue Reconstruction, Plastic Surgery, Prevention Suggestions, and First Aid

Edited by Allan R. Cook. 604 pages. 1999. 0-7808-0204-7. $78.

"This is an exceptional addition to the series and is highly recommended for all consumer health collections, hospital libraries, and academic medical centers." — *E-Streams, Mar '00*

"This key reference guide is an invaluable addition to all health care and public libraries in confronting this ongoing health issue." — *American Reference Books Annual, 2000*

"Recommended reference source." — *Booklist, American Library Association, Dec '99*

SEE ALSO *Skin Disorders Sourcebook*

■

Cancer Sourcebook, 4th Edition

Basic Consumer Health Information about Major Forms and Stages of Cancer, Featuring Facts about Head and Neck Cancers, Lung Cancers, Gastrointestinal Cancers, Genitourinary Cancers, Lymphomas, Blood Cell Cancers, Endocrine Cancers, Skin Cancers, Bone Cancers, Sarcomas, and Others, and Including Information about Cancer Treatments and Therapies, Identifying and Reducing Cancer Risks, and Strategies for Coping with Cancer and the Side Effects of Treatment

Along with a Cancer Glossary, Statistical and Demographic Data, and a Directory of Sources for Additional Help and Information

Edited by Karen Bellenir. 1,119 pages. 2003. 0-7808-0633-6. $78.

ALSO AVAILABLE: *Cancer Sourcebook, 1st Edition.* Edited by Frank E. Bair. 932 pages. 1990. 1-55888-888-8. $78.

New Cancer Sourcebook, 2nd Edition. Edited by Allan R. Cook. 1,313 pages. 1996. 0-7808-0041-9. $78.

Cancer Sourcebook, 3rd Edition. Edited by Edward J. Prucha. 1,069 pages. 2000. 0-7808-0227-6. $78.

"This title is recommended for health sciences and public libraries with consumer health collections." — *E-Streams, Feb '01*

". . . can be effectively used by cancer patients and their families who are looking for answers in a language they can understand. Public and hospital libraries should have it on their shelves." — *American Reference Books Annual, 2001*

"Recommended reference source." — *Booklist, American Library Association, Dec '00*

Cited in *Reference Sources for Small and Medium-Sized Libraries, American Library Association, 1999*

"The amount of factual and useful information is extensive. The writing is very clear, geared to general readers. Recommended for all levels." — *Choice, Association of College & Research Libraries, Jan '97*

SEE ALSO *Breast Cancer Sourcebook, Cancer Sourcebook for Women, Pediatric Cancer Sourcebook, Prostate Cancer Sourcebook*

Cancer Sourcebook for Women, 2nd Edition

Basic Consumer Health Information about Gynecologic Cancers and Related Concerns, Including Cervical Cancer, Endometrial Cancer, Gestational Trophoblastic Tumor, Ovarian Cancer, Uterine Cancer, Vaginal Cancer, Vulvar Cancer, Breast Cancer, and Common Non-Cancerous Uterine Conditions, with Facts about Cancer Risk Factors, Screening and Prevention, Treatment Options, and Reports on Current Research Initiatives

Along with a Glossary of Cancer Terms and a Directory of Resources for Additional Help and Information

Edited by Karen Bellenir. 604 pages. 2002. 0-7808-0226-8. $78.

ALSO AVAILABLE: *Cancer Sourcebook for Women, 1st Edition.* Edited by Allan R. Cook and Peter D. Dresser. 524 pages. 1996. 0-7808-0076-1. $78.

"An excellent addition to collections in public, consumer health, and women's health libraries."
— *American Reference Books Annual, 2003*

"Overall, the information is excellent, and complex topics are clearly explained. As a reference book for the consumer it is a valuable resource to assist them to make informed decisions about cancer and its treatments." — *Cancer Forum, Nov '02*

"Highly recommended for academic and medical reference collections." — *Library Bookwatch, Sep '02*

"This is a highly recommended book for any public or consumer library, being reader friendly and containing accurate and helpful information."
— *E-Streams, Aug '02*

"Recommended reference source."
— *Booklist, American Library Association, Jul '02*

SEE ALSO *Breast Cancer Sourcebook, Women's Health Concerns Sourcebook*

Cardiovascular Diseases & Disorders Sourcebook, 1st Edition

SEE *Heart Diseases & Disorders Sourcebook, 2nd Edition*

Caregiving Sourcebook

Basic Consumer Health Information for Caregivers, Including a Profile of Caregivers, Caregiving Responsibilities and Concerns, Tips for Specific Conditions, Care Environments, and the Effects of Caregiving

Along with Facts about Legal Issues, Financial Information, and Future Planning, a Glossary, and a Listing of Additional Resources

Edited by Joyce Brennfleck Shannon. 600 pages. 2001. 0-7808-0331-0. $78.

"Essential for most collections."
— *Library Journal, Apr 1, 2002*

"An ideal addition to the reference collection of any public library. Health sciences information professionals may also want to acquire the *Caregiving Sourcebook* for their hospital or academic library for use as a ready reference tool by health care workers interested in aging and caregiving." — *E-Streams, Jan '02*

"Recommended reference source."
— *Booklist, American Library Association, Oct '01*

Child Abuse Sourcebook

Basic Consumer Health Information about the Physical, Sexual, and Emotional Abuse of Children, with Additional Facts about Neglect, Munchausen Syndrome by Proxy (MSBP), Shaken Baby Syndrome, and Controversial Issues Related to Child Abuse, Such as Withholding Medical Care, Corporal Punishment, and Child Maltreatment in Youth Sports, and Featuring Facts about Child Protective Services, Foster Care, Adoption, Parenting Challenges, and Other Abuse Prevention Efforts

Along with a Glossary of Related Terms and Resources for Additional Help and Information

Edited by Dawn D. Matthews. 625 pages. 2004. 0-7808-0705-7. $78.

Childhood Diseases & Disorders Sourcebook

Basic Consumer Health Information about Medical Problems Often Encountered in Pre-Adolescent Children, Including Respiratory Tract Ailments, Ear Infections, Sore Throats, Disorders of the Skin and Scalp, Digestive and Genitourinary Diseases, Infectious Diseases, Inflammatory Disorders, Chronic Physical and Developmental Disorders, Allergies, and More

Along with Information about Diagnostic Tests, Common Childhood Surgeries, and Frequently Used Medications, with a Glossary of Important Terms and Resource Directory

Edited by Chad T. Kimball. 662 pages. 2003. 0-7808-0458-9. $78.

Colds, Flu & Other Common Ailments Sourcebook

Basic Consumer Health Information about Common Ailments and Injuries, Including Colds, Coughs, the Flu, Sinus Problems, Headaches, Fever, Nausea and Vomiting, Menstrual Cramps, Diarrhea, Constipation, Hemorrhoids, Back Pain, Dandruff, Dry and Itchy Skin, Cuts, Scrapes, Sprains, Bruises, and More

Along with Information about Prevention, Self-Care, Choosing a Doctor, Over-the-Counter Medications, Folk Remedies, and Alternative Therapies, and Including a Glossary of Important Terms and a Directory of Resources for Further Help and Information

Edited by Chad T. Kimball. 638 pages. 2001. 0-7808-0435-X. $78.

"A good starting point for research on common illnesses. It will be a useful addition to public and consumer health library collections."
— American Reference Books Annual 2002

"Will prove valuable to any library seeking to maintain a current, comprehensive reference collection of health resources. . . . Excellent reference."
— The Bookwatch, Aug '01

"Recommended reference source."
— Booklist, American Library Association, July '01

■

Communication Disorders Sourcebook

Basic Information about Deafness and Hearing Loss, Speech and Language Disorders, Voice Disorders, Balance and Vestibular Disorders, and Disorders of Smell, Taste, and Touch

Edited by Linda M. Ross. 533 pages. 1996. 0-7808-0077-X. $78.

"This is skillfully edited and is a welcome resource for the layperson. It should be found in every public and medical library." — Booklist Health Sciences Supplement, American Library Association, Oct '97

■

Congenital Disorders Sourcebook

Basic Information about Disorders Acquired during Gestation, Including Spina Bifida, Hydrocephalus, Cerebral Palsy, Heart Defects, Craniofacial Abnormalities, Fetal Alcohol Syndrome, and More

Along with Current Treatment Options and Statistical Data

Edited by Karen Bellenir. 607 pages. 1997. 0-7808-0205-5. $78.

"Recommended reference source."
— Booklist, American Library Association, Oct '97

SEE ALSO Pregnancy & Birth Sourcebook

■

Consumer Issues in Health Care Sourcebook

Basic Information about Health Care Fundamentals and Related Consumer Issues, Including Exams and Screening Tests, Physician Specialties, Choosing a Doctor, Using Prescription and Over-the-Counter Medications Safely, Avoiding Health Scams, Managing Common Health Risks in the Home, Care Options for Chronically or Terminally Ill Patients, and a List of Resources for Obtaining Help and Further Information

Edited by Karen Bellenir. 618 pages. 1998. 0-7808-0221-7. $78.

"Both public and academic libraries will want to have a copy in their collection for readers who are interested in self-education on health issues."
— American Reference Books Annual, 2000

"The editor has researched the literature from government agencies and others, saving readers the time and effort of having to do the research themselves. Recommended for public libraries."
— Reference and User Services Quarterly, American Library Association, Spring '99

"Recommended reference source."
— Booklist, American Library Association, Dec '98

■

Contagious & Non-Contagious Infectious Diseases Sourcebook

Basic Information about Contagious Diseases like Measles, Polio, Hepatitis B, and Infectious Mononucleosis, and Non-Contagious Infectious Diseases like Tetanus and Toxic Shock Syndrome, and Diseases Occurring as Secondary Infections Such as Shingles and Reye Syndrome

Along with Vaccination, Prevention, and Treatment Information, and a Section Describing Emerging Infectious Disease Threats

Edited by Karen Bellenir and Peter D. Dresser. 566 pages. 1996. 0-7808-0075-3. $78.

■

Death & Dying Sourcebook

Basic Consumer Health Information for the Layperson about End-of-Life Care and Related Ethical and Legal Issues, Including Chief Causes of Death, Autopsies, Pain Management for the Terminally Ill, Life Support Systems, Insurance, Euthanasia, Assisted Suicide, Hospice Programs, Living Wills, Funeral Planning, Counseling, Mourning, Organ Donation, and Physician Training

Along with Statistical Data, a Glossary, and Listings of Sources for Further Help and Information

Edited by Annemarie S. Muth. 641 pages. 1999. 0-7808-0230-6. $78.

"Public libraries, medical libraries, and academic libraries will all find this sourcebook a useful addition to their collections."
— American Reference Books Annual, 2001

"An extremely useful resource for those concerned with death and dying in the United States."
— Respiratory Care, Nov '00

"Recommended reference source."
— Booklist, American Library Association, Aug '00

"This book is a definite must for all those involved in end-of-life care." — Doody's Review Service, 2000

■

Dental Care & Oral Health Sourcebook, 2nd Edition

Basic Consumer Health Information about Dental Care, Including Oral Hygiene, Dental Visits, Pain Management, Cavities, Crowns, Bridges, Dental Implants, and Fillings, and Other Oral Health Concerns, Such as Gum Disease, Bad Breath, Dry Mouth, Genetic and Developmental Abnormalities, Oral Cancers, Orthodontics, and Temporomandibular Disorders

Along with Updates on Current Research in Oral Health, a Glossary, a Directory of Dental and Oral Health Organizations, and Resources for People with Dental and Oral Health Disorders

Edited by Amy L. Sutton. 609 pages. 2003. 0-7808-0634-4. $78.

ALSO AVAILABLE: Oral Health Sourcebook, 1st Edition. Edited by Allan R. Cook. 558 pages. 1997. 0-7808-0082-6. $78.

"Unique source which will fill a gap in dental sources for patients and the lay public. A valuable reference tool even in a library with thousands of books on dentistry. Comprehensive, clear, inexpensive, and easy to read and use. It fills an enormous gap in the health care literature." — Reference and User Services Quarterly, American Library Association, Summer '98

"Recommended reference source." — Booklist, American Library Association, Dec '97

Depression Sourcebook

Basic Consumer Health Information about Unipolar Depression, Bipolar Disorder, Postpartum Depression, Seasonal Affective Disorder, and Other Types of Depression in Children, Adolescents, Women, Men, the Elderly, and Other Selected Populations

Along with Facts about Causes, Risk Factors, Diagnostic Criteria, Treatment Options, Coping Strategies, Suicide Prevention, a Glossary, and a Directory of Sources for Additional Help and Information

Edited by Karen Belleni. 602 pages. 2002. 0-7808-0611-5. $78.

"Invaluable reference for public and school library collections alike." — Library Bookwatch, Apr '03

"Recommended for purchase." — American Reference Books Annual, 2003

Diabetes Sourcebook, 3rd Edition

Basic Consumer Health Information about Type 1 Diabetes (Insulin-Dependent or Juvenile-Onset Diabetes), Type 2 Diabetes (Noninsulin-Dependent or Adult-Onset Diabetes), Gestational Diabetes, Impaired Glucose Tolerance (IGT), and Related Complications, Such as Amputation, Eye Disease, Gum Disease, Nerve Damage, and End-Stage Renal Disease, Including Facts about Insulin, Oral Diabetes Medications, Blood Sugar Testing, and the Role of Exercise and Nutrition in the Control of Diabetes

Along with a Glossary and Resources for Further Help and Information

Edited by Dawn D. Matthews. 622 pages. 2003. 0-7808-0629-8. $78.

ALSO AVAILABLE: Diabetes Sourcebook, 1st Edition. Edited by Karen Bellenir and Peter D. Dresser. 827 pages. 1994. 1-55888-751-2. $78.

Diabetes Sourcebook, 2nd Edition. Edited by Karen Bellenir. 688 pages. 1998. 0-7808-0224-1. $78.

"An invaluable reference." — Library Journal, May '00

Selected as one of the 250 "Best Health Sciences Books of 1999." — Doody's Rating Service, Mar-Apr 2000

"This comprehensive book is an excellent addition for high school, academic, medical, and public libraries. This volume is highly recommended." — American Reference Books Annual, 2000

"Provides useful information for the general public." — Healthlines, University of Michigan Health Management Research Center, Sep/Oct '99

". . . provides reliable mainstream medical information . . . belongs on the shelves of any library with a consumer health collection." — E-Streams, Sep '99

"Recommended reference source." — Booklist, American Library Association, Feb '99

Diet & Nutrition Sourcebook, 2nd Edition

Basic Consumer Health Information about Dietary Guidelines, Recommended Daily Intake Values, Vitamins, Minerals, Fiber, Fat, Weight Control, Dietary Supplements, and Food Additives

Along with Special Sections on Nutrition Needs throughout Life and Nutrition for People with Such Specific Medical Concerns as Allergies, High Blood Cholesterol, Hypertension, Diabetes, Celiac Disease, Seizure Disorders, Phenylketonuria (PKU), Cancer, and Eating Disorders, and Including Reports on Current Nutrition Research and Source Listings for Additional Help and Information

Edited by Karen Bellenir. 650 pages. 1999. 0-7808-0228-4. $78.

ALSO AVAILABLE: Diet & Nutrition Sourcebook, 1st Edition. Edited by Dan R. Harris. 662 pages. 1996. 0-7808-0084-2. $78.

"This book is an excellent source of basic diet and nutrition information." — Booklist Health Sciences Supplement, American Library Association, Dec '00

"This reference document should be in any public library, but it would be a very good guide for beginning students in the health sciences. If the other books in this publisher's series are as good as this, they should all be in the health sciences collections." — American Reference Books Annual, 2000

"This book is an excellent general nutrition reference for consumers who desire to take an active role in their health care for prevention. Consumers of all ages who select this book can feel confident they are receiving current and accurate information." — Journal of Nutrition for the Elderly, Vol. 19, No. 4, '00

"Recommended reference source." — Booklist, American Library Association, Dec '99

SEE ALSO Digestive Diseases & Disorders Sourcebook, Eating Disorders Sourcebook, Gastrointestinal Diseases & Disorders Sourcebook, Vegetarian Sourcebook

Digestive Diseases & Disorders Sourcebook

Basic Consumer Health Information about Diseases and Disorders that Impact the Upper and Lower Digestive System, Including Celiac Disease, Constipation, Crohn's Disease, Cyclic Vomiting Syndrome, Diarrhea, Diverticulosis and Diverticulitis, Gallstones, Heartburn, Hemorrhoids, Hernias, Indigestion (Dyspepsia), Irritable Bowel Syndrome, Lactose Intolerance, Ulcers, and More

Along with Information about Medications and Other Treatments, Tips for Maintaining a Healthy Digestive Tract, a Glossary, and Directory of Digestive Diseases Organizations

Edited by Karen Bellenir. 335 pages. 2000. 0-7808-0327-2. $78.

"This title would be an excellent addition to all public or patient-research libraries."
—*American Reference Books Annual, 2001*

"This title is recommended for public, hospital, and health sciences libraries with consumer health collections." —*E-Streams, Jul-Aug '00*

"Recommended reference source."
—*Booklist, American Library Association, May '00*

SEE ALSO *Diet & Nutrition Sourcebook, Eating Disorders Sourcebook, Gastrointestinal Diseases & Disorders Sourcebook*

■

Disabilities Sourcebook

Basic Consumer Health Information about Physical and Psychiatric Disabilities, Including Descriptions of Major Causes of Disability, Assistive and Adaptive Aids, Workplace Issues, and Accessibility Concerns

Along with Information about the Americans with Disabilities Act, a Glossary, and Resources for Additional Help and Information

Edited by Dawn D. Matthews. 616 pages. 2000. 0-7808-0389-2. $78.

"It is a must for libraries with a consumer health section." —*American Reference Books Annual 2002*

"A much needed addition to the Omnigraphics *Health Reference Series*. A current reference work to provide people with disabilities, their families, caregivers or those who work with them, a broad range of information in one volume, has not been available until now. . . . It is recommended for all public and academic library reference collections." —*E-Streams, May '01*

"An excellent source book in easy-to-read format covering many current topics; highly recommended for all libraries." —*Choice, Association of College and Research Libraries, Jan '01*

"Recommended reference source."
—*Booklist, American Library Association, Jul '00*

Domestic Violence Sourcebook, 2nd Edition

Basic Consumer Health Information about the Causes and Consequences of Abusive Relationships, Including Physical Violence, Sexual Assault, Battery, Stalking, and Emotional Abuse, and Facts about the Effects of Violence on Women, Men, Young Adults, and the Elderly, with Reports about Domestic Violence in Selected Populations, and Featuring Facts about Medical Care, Victim Assistance and Protection, Prevention Strategies, Mental Health Services, and Legal Issues

Along with a Glossary of Related Terms and Resources for Additional Help and Information

Edited by Dawn D. Matthews. 628 pages. 2004. 0-7808-0669-7. $78.

ALSO AVAILABLE: *Domestic Violence & Child Abuse Sourcebook, 1st Edition.* Edited by Helene Henderson. 1,064 pages. 2001. 0-7808-0235-7. $78.

"Interested lay persons should find the book extremely beneficial. . . . A copy of *Domestic Violence and Child Abuse Sourcebook* should be in every public library in the United States."
—*Social Science & Medicine, No. 56, 2003*

"This is important information. The Web has many resources but this sourcebook fills an important societal need. I am not aware of any other resources of this type." —*Doody's Review Service, Sep '01*

"Recommended for all libraries, scholars, and practitioners." —*Choice, Association of College & Research Libraries, Jul '01*

"Recommended reference source."
—*Booklist, American Library Association, Apr '01*

"Important pick for college-level health reference libraries." —*The Bookwatch, Mar '01*

"Because this problem is so widespread and because this book includes a lot of issues within one volume, this work is recommended for all public libraries."
—*American Reference Books Annual, 2001*

■

Drug Abuse Sourcebook

Basic Consumer Health Information about Illicit Substances of Abuse and the Diversion of Prescription Medications, Including Depressants, Hallucinogens, Inhalants, Marijuana, Narcotics, Stimulants, and Anabolic Steroids

Along with Facts about Related Health Risks, Treatment Issues, and Substance Abuse Prevention Programs, a Glossary of Terms, Statistical Data, and Directories of Hotline Services, Self-Help Groups, and Organizations Able to Provide Further Information

Edited by Karen Bellenir. 629 pages. 2000. 0-7808-0242-X. $78.

"Containing a wealth of information . . . . This resource belongs in libraries that serve a lower-division undergraduate or community college clientele as well as the general public." —*Choice, Association of College and Research Libraries, Jun '01*

SEE ALSO Alcoholism Sourcebook, Substance Abuse Sourcebook

Ear, Nose & Throat Disorders Sourcebook

Basic Information about Disorders of the Ears, Nose, Sinus Cavities, Pharynx, and Larynx, Including Ear Infections, Tinnitus, Vestibular Disorders, Allergic and Non-Allergic Rhinitis, Sore Throats, Tonsillitis, and Cancers That Affect the Ears, Nose, Sinuses, and Throat

Along with Reports on Current Research Initiatives, a Glossary of Related Medical Terms, and a Directory of Sources for Further Help and Information

Edited by Karen Bellenir and Linda M. Shin. 576 pages. 1998. 0-7808-0206-3. $78.

Eating Disorders Sourcebook

Basic Consumer Health Information about Eating Disorders, Including Information about Anorexia Nervosa, Bulimia Nervosa, Binge Eating, Body Dysmorphic Disorder, Pica, Laxative Abuse, and Night Eating Syndrome

Along with Information about Causes, Adverse Effects, and Treatment and Prevention Issues, and Featuring a Section on Concerns Specific to Children and Adolescents, a Glossary, and Resources for Further Help and Information

Edited by Dawn D. Matthews. 322 pages. 2001. 0-7808-0335-3. $78.

SEE ALSO Diet & Nutrition Sourcebook, Digestive Diseases & Disorders Sourcebook, Gastrointestinal Diseases & Disorders Sourcebook

Emergency Medical Services Sourcebook

Basic Consumer Health Information about Preventing, Preparing for, and Managing Emergency Situations, When and Who to Call for Help, What to Expect in the Emergency Room, the Emergency Medical Team, Patient Issues, and Current Topics in Emergency Medicine

Along with Statistical Data, a Glossary, and Sources of Additional Help and Information

Edited by Jenni Lynn Colson. 494 pages. 2002. 0-7808-0420-1. $78.

Endocrine & Metabolic Disorders Sourcebook

Basic Information for the Layperson about Pancreatic and Insulin-Related Disorders Such as Pancreatitis, Diabetes, and Hypoglycemia; Adrenal Gland Disorders Such as Cushing's Syndrome, Addison's Disease, and Congenital Adrenal Hyperplasia; Pituitary Gland Disorders Such as Growth Hormone Deficiency, Acromegaly, and Pituitary Tumors; Thyroid Disorders Such as Hypothyroidism, Graves' Disease, Hashimoto's Disease, and Goiter; Hyperparathyroidism; and Other Diseases and Syndromes of Hormone Imbalance or Metabolic Dysfunction

Along with Reports on Current Research Initiatives

Edited by Linda M. Shin. 574 pages. 1998. 0-7808-0207-1. $78.

Environmental Health Sourcebook, 2nd Edition

Basic Consumer Health Information about the Environment and Its Effect on Human Health, Including the Effects of Air Pollution, Water Pollution, Hazardous Chemicals, Food Hazards, Radiation Hazards, Biological Agents, Household Hazards, Such as Radon, Asbestos, Carbon Monoxide, and Mold, and Information about Associated Diseases and Disorders, Including Cancer, Allergies, Respiratory Problems, and Skin Disorders

Along with Information about Environmental Concerns for Specific Populations, a Glossary of Related Terms, and Resources for Further Help and Information

Edited by Dawn D. Matthews. 673 pages. 2003. 0-7808-0632-8. $78.

ALSO AVAILABLE: Environmentally Induced Disorders Sourcebook, 1st Edition. Edited by Allan R. Cook. 620 pages. 1997. 0-7808-0083-4. $78.

"Recommended reference source."
— *Booklist, American Library Association, Sep '98*

"This book will be a useful addition to anyone's library." — *Choice Health Sciences Supplement, Association of College and Research Libraries, May '98*

". . . a good survey of numerous environmentally induced physical disorders . . . a useful addition to anyone's library."
— *Doody's Health Sciences Book Reviews, Jan '98*

". . . provide[s] introductory information from the best authorities around. Since this volume covers topics that potentially affect everyone, it will surely be one of the most frequently consulted volumes in the *Health Reference Series.*" — *Rettig on Reference, Nov '97*

■

Environmentally Induced Disorders Sourcebook, 1st Edition

SEE Environmental Health Sourcebook, 2nd Edition

■

Ethnic Diseases Sourcebook

Basic Consumer Health Information for Ethnic and Racial Minority Groups in the United States, Including General Health Indicators and Behaviors, Ethnic Diseases, Genetic Testing, the Impact of Chronic Diseases, Women's Health, Mental Health Issues, and Preventive Health Care Services

Along with a Glossary and a Listing of Additional Resources

Edited by Joyce Brennfleck Shannon. 664 pages. 2001. 0-7808-0336-1. $78.

"Recommended for health sciences libraries where public health programs are a priority."
— *E-Streams, Jan '02*

"Not many books have been written on this topic to date, and the *Ethnic Diseases Sourcebook* is a strong addition to the list. It will be an important introductory resource for health consumers, students, health care personnel, and social scientists. It is recommended for public, academic, and large hospital libraries."
— *American Reference Books Annual 2002*

"Recommended reference source."
— *Booklist, American Library Association, Oct '01*

"Will prove valuable to any library seeking to maintain a current, comprehensive reference collection of health resources. . . . An excellent source of health information about genetic disorders which affect particular ethnic and racial minorities in the U.S."
— *The Bookwatch, Aug '01*

Eye Care Sourcebook, 2nd Edition

Basic Consumer Health Information about Eye Care and Eye Disorders, Including Facts about the Diagnosis, Prevention, and Treatment of Common Refractive Problems Such as Myopia, Hyperopia, Astigmatism, and Presbyopia, and Eye Diseases, Including Glaucoma, Cataract, Age-Related Macular Degeneration, and Diabetic Retinopathy

Along with a Section on Vision Correction and Refractive Surgeries, Including LASIK and LASEK, a Glossary, and Directories of Resources for Additional Help and Information

Edited by Amy L. Sutton. 543 pages. 2003. 0-7808-0635-2. $78.

ALSO AVAILABLE: Ophthalmic Disorders Sourcebook, 1st Edition. Edited by Linda M. Ross. 631 pages. 1996. 0-7808-0081-8. $78.

■

Family Planning Sourcebook

Basic Consumer Health Information about Planning for Pregnancy and Contraception, Including Traditional Methods, Barrier Methods, Hormonal Methods, Permanent Methods, Future Methods, Emergency Contraception, and Birth Control Choices for Women at Each Stage of Life

Along with Statistics, a Glossary, and Sources of Additional Information

Edited by Amy Marcaccio Keyzer. 520 pages. 2001. 0-7808-0379-5. $78.

"Recommended for public, health, and undergraduate libraries as part of the circulating collection."
— *E-Streams, Mar '02*

"Information is presented in an unbiased, readable manner, and the sourcebook will certainly be a necessary addition to those public and high school libraries where Internet access is restricted or otherwise problematic." — *American Reference Books Annual 2002*

"Recommended reference source."
— *Booklist, American Library Association, Oct '01*

"Will prove valuable to any library seeking to maintain a current, comprehensive reference collection of health resources. . . . Excellent reference."
— *The Bookwatch, Aug '01*

SEE ALSO Pregnancy & Birth Sourcebook

■

Fitness & Exercise Sourcebook, 2nd Edition

Basic Consumer Health Information about the Fundamentals of Fitness and Exercise, Including How to Begin and Maintain a Fitness Program, Fitness as a Lifestyle, the Link between Fitness and Diet, Advice for Specific Groups of People, Exercise as It Relates to Specific Medical Conditions, and Recent Research in Fitness and Exercise

Along with a Glossary of Important Terms and Resources for Additional Help and Information

Edited by Kristen M. Gledhill. 646 pages. 2001. 0-7808-0334-5. $78.

ALSO AVAILABLE: Fitness & Exercise Sourcebook, 1st Edition. Edited by Dan R. Harris. 663 pages. 1996. 0-7808-0186-5. $78.

"This work is recommended for all general reference collections."
— American Reference Books Annual 2002

"Highly recommended for public, consumer, and school grades fourth through college."
—E-Streams, Nov '01

"Recommended reference source." — Booklist, American Library Association, Oct '01

"The information appears quite comprehensive and is considered reliable. . . . This second edition is a welcomed addition to the series."
—Doody's Review Service, Sep '01

"This reference is a valuable choice for those who desire a broad source of information on exercise, fitness, and chronic-disease prevention through a healthy lifestyle." —American Medical Writers Association Journal, Fall '01

"Will prove valuable to any library seeking to maintain a current, comprehensive reference collection of health resources. . . . Excellent reference."
— The Bookwatch, Aug '01

Food & Animal Borne Diseases Sourcebook

Basic Information about Diseases That Can Be Spread to Humans through the Ingestion of Contaminated Food or Water or by Contact with Infected Animals and Insects, Such as Botulism, E. Coli, Hepatitis A, Trichinosis, Lyme Disease, and Rabies

Along with Information Regarding Prevention and Treatment Methods, and Including a Special Section for International Travelers Describing Diseases Such as Cholera, Malaria, Travelers' Diarrhea, and Yellow Fever, and Offering Recommendations for Avoiding Illness

Edited by Karen Bellenir and Peter D. Dresser. 535 pages. 1995. 0-7808-0033-8. $78.

"Targeting general readers and providing them with a single, comprehensive source of information on selected topics, this book continues, with the excellent caliber of its predecessors, to catalog topical information on health matters of general interest. Readable and thorough, this valuable resource is highly recommended for all libraries."
— Academic Library Book Review, Summer '96

"A comprehensive collection of authoritative information." — Emergency Medical Services, Oct '95

Food Safety Sourcebook

Basic Consumer Health Information about the Safe Handling of Meat, Poultry, Seafood, Eggs, Fruit Juices, and Other Food Items, and Facts about Pesticides, Drinking Water, Food Safety Overseas, and the Onset, Duration, and Symptoms of Foodborne Illnesses, Including Types of Pathogenic Bacteria, Parasitic Protozoa, Worms, Viruses, and Natural Toxins

Along with the Role of the Consumer, the Food Handler, and the Government in Food Safety; a Glossary, and Resources for Additional Help and Information

Edited by Dawn D. Matthews. 339 pages. 1999. 0-7808-0326-4. $78.

"This book is recommended for public libraries and universities with home economic and food science programs." — E-Streams, Nov '00

"Recommended reference source."
—Booklist, American Library Association, May '00

"This book takes the complex issues of food safety and foodborne pathogens and presents them in an easily understood manner. [It does] an excellent job of covering a large and often confusing topic."
—American Reference Books Annual, 2000

Forensic Medicine Sourcebook

Basic Consumer Information for the Layperson about Forensic Medicine, Including Crime Scene Investigation, Evidence Collection and Analysis, Expert Testimony, Computer-Aided Criminal Identification, Digital Imaging in the Courtroom, DNA Profiling, Accident Reconstruction, Autopsies, Ballistics, Drugs and Explosives Detection, Latent Fingerprints, Product Tampering, and Questioned Document Examination

Along with Statistical Data, a Glossary of Forensics Terminology, and Listings of Sources for Further Help and Information

Edited by Annemarie S. Muth. 574 pages. 1999. 0-7808-0232-2. $78.

"Given the expected widespread interest in its content and its easy to read style, this book is recommended for most public and all college and university libraries."
—E-Streams, Feb '01

"Recommended for public libraries."
—Reference & User Services Quarterly, American Library Association, Spring 2000

"Recommended reference source."
—Booklist, American Library Association, Feb '00

"A wealth of information, useful statistics, references are up-to-date and extremely complete. This wonderful collection of data will help students who are interested in a career in any type of forensic field. It is a great resource for attorneys who need information about types of expert witnesses needed in a particular case. It also offers useful information for fiction and nonfiction writers whose work involves a crime. A fascinating compilation. All levels." — Choice, Association of College and Research Libraries, Jan 2000

"There are several items that make this book attractive to consumers who are seeking certain forensic data.... This is a useful current source for those seeking general forensic medical answers."

—American Reference Books Annual, 2000

■

Gastrointestinal Diseases & Disorders Sourcebook

Basic Information about Gastroesophageal Reflux Disease (Heartburn), Ulcers, Diverticulosis, Irritable Bowel Syndrome, Crohn's Disease, Ulcerative Colitis, Diarrhea, Constipation, Lactose Intolerance, Hemorrhoids, Hepatitis, Cirrhosis, and Other Digestive Problems, Featuring Statistics, Descriptions of Symptoms, and Current Treatment Methods of Interest for Persons Living with Upper and Lower Gastrointestinal Maladies

Edited by Linda M. Ross. 413 pages. 1996. 0-7808-0078-8. $78.

". . . very readable form. The successful editorial work that brought this material together into a useful and understandable reference makes accessible to all readers information that can help them more effectively understand and obtain help for digestive tract problems."

— Choice, Association of College & Research Libraries, Feb '97

SEE ALSO *Diet & Nutrition Sourcebook, Digestive Diseases & Disorders, Eating Disorders Sourcebook*

■

Genetic Disorders Sourcebook, 2nd Edition

Basic Consumer Health Information about Hereditary Diseases and Disorders, Including Cystic Fibrosis, Down Syndrome, Hemophilia, Huntington's Disease, Sickle Cell Anemia, and More; Facts about Genes, Gene Research and Therapy, Genetic Screening, Ethics of Gene Testing, Genetic Counseling, and Advice on Coping and Caring

Along with a Glossary of Genetic Terminology and a Resource List for Help, Support, and Further Information

Edited by Kathy Massimini. 768 pages. 2001. 0-7808-0241-1. $78.

ALSO AVAILABLE: Genetic Disorders Sourcebook, 1st Edition. Edited by Karen Bellenir. 642 pages. 1996. 0-7808-0034-6. $78.

"Recommended for public libraries and medical and hospital libraries with consumer health collections."

—E-Streams, May '01

"Recommended reference source."

— Booklist, American Library Association, Apr '01

"Important pick for college-level health reference libraries." *— The Bookwatch, Mar '01*

"Provides essential medical information to both the general public and those diagnosed with a serious or fatal genetic disease or disorder." *—Choice, Association of College and Research Libraries, Jan '97*

Head Trauma Sourcebook

Basic Information for the Layperson about Open-Head and Closed-Head Injuries, Treatment Advances, Recovery, and Rehabilitation

Along with Reports on Current Research Initiatives

Edited by Karen Bellenir. 414 pages. 1997. 0-7808-0208-X. $78.

■

Headache Sourcebook

Basic Consumer Health Information about Migraine, Tension, Cluster, Rebound and Other Types of Headaches, with Facts about the Cause and Prevention of Headaches, the Effects of Stress and the Environment, Headaches during Pregnancy and Menopause, and Childhood Headaches

Along with a Glossary and Other Resources for Additional Help and Information

Edited by Dawn D. Matthews. 362 pages. 2002. 0-7808-0337-X. $78.

"Highly recommended for academic and medical reference collections." *— Library Bookwatch, Sep '02*

■

Health Insurance Sourcebook

Basic Information about Managed Care Organizations, Traditional Fee-for-Service Insurance, Insurance Portability and Pre-Existing Conditions Clauses, Medicare, Medicaid, Social Security, and Military Health Care

Along with Information about Insurance Fraud

Edited by Wendy Wilcox. 530 pages. 1997. 0-7808-0222-5. $78.

"Particularly useful because it brings much of this information together in one volume. This book will be a handy reference source in the health sciences library, hospital library, college and university library, and medium to large public library."

— Medical Reference Services Quarterly, Fall '98

Awarded "Books of the Year Award"

— American Journal of Nursing, 1997

"The layout of the book is particularly helpful as it provides easy access to reference material. A most useful addition to the vast amount of information about health insurance. The use of data from U.S. government agencies is most commendable. Useful in a library or learning center for healthcare professional students."

— Doody's Health Sciences Book Reviews, Nov '97

■

Health Reference Series Cumulative Index 1999

A Comprehensive Index to the Individual Volumes of the Health Reference Series, Including a Subject Index, Name Index, Organization Index, and Publication Index

Along with a Master List of Acronyms and Abbreviations

Edited by Edward J. Prucha, Anne Holmes, and Robert Rudnick. 990 pages. 2000. 0-7808-0382-5. $78.

"This volume will be most helpful in libraries that have a relatively complete collection of the Health Reference Series." —American Reference Books Annual, 2001

"Essential for collections that hold any of the numerous *Health Reference Series* titles." —Choice, Association of College and Research Libraries, Nov '00

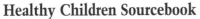

Healthy Aging Sourcebook

Basic Consumer Health Information about Maintaining Health through the Aging Process, Including Advice on Nutrition, Exercise, and Sleep, Help in Making Decisions about Midlife Issues and Retirement, and Guidance Concerning Practical and Informed Choices in Health Consumerism

Along with Data Concerning the Theories of Aging, Different Experiences in Aging by Minority Groups, and Facts about Aging Now and Aging in the Future; and Featuring a Glossary, a Guide to Consumer Help, Additional Suggested Reading, and Practical Resource Directory

Edited by Jenifer Swanson. 536 pages. 1999. 0-7808-0390-6. $78.

"Recommended reference source." —Booklist, American Library Association, Feb '00

SEE ALSO *Physical & Mental Issues in Aging Sourcebook*

Healthy Children Sourcebook

Basic Consumer Health Information about the Physical and Mental Development of Children between the Ages of 3 and 12, Including Routine Health Care, Preventative Health Services, Safety and First Aid, Healthy Sleep, Dental Care, Nutrition, and Fitness, and Featuring Parenting Tips on Such Topics as Bedwetting, Choosing Day Care, Monitoring TV and Other Media, and Establishing a Foundation for Substance Abuse Prevention

Along with a Glossary of Commonly Used Pediatric Terms and Resources for Additional Help and Information.

Edited by Chad T. Kimball. 647 pages. 2003. 0-7808-0247-0. $78.

Healthy Heart Sourcebook for Women

Basic Consumer Health Information about Cardiac Issues Specific to Women, Including Facts about Major Risk Factors and Prevention, Treatment and Control Strategies, and Important Dietary Issues

Along with a Special Section Regarding the Pros and Cons of Hormone Replacement Therapy and Its Impact on Heart Health, and Additional Help, Including Recipes, a Glossary, and a Directory of Resources

Edited by Dawn D. Matthews. 336 pages. 2000. 0-7808-0329-9. $78.

"A good reference source and recommended for all public, academic, medical, and hospital libraries." —Medical Reference Services Quarterly, Summer '01

"Because of the lack of information specific to women on this topic, this book is recommended for public libraries and consumer libraries." —American Reference Books Annual, 2001

"Contains very important information about coronary artery disease that all women should know. The information is current and presented in an easy-to-read format. The book will make a good addition to any library." —American Medical Writers Association Journal, Summer '00

"Important, basic reference." —Reviewer's Bookwatch, Jul '00

SEE ALSO *Heart Diseases & Disorders Sourcebook, Women's Health Concerns Sourcebook*

Heart Diseases & Disorders Sourcebook, 2nd Edition

Basic Consumer Health Information about Heart Attacks, Angina, Rhythm Disorders, Heart Failure, Valve Disease, Congenital Heart Disorders, and More, Including Descriptions of Surgical Procedures and Other Interventions, Medications, Cardiac Rehabilitation, Risk Identification, and Prevention Tips

Along with Statistical Data, Reports on Current Research Initiatives, a Glossary of Cardiovascular Terms, and Resource Directory

Edited by Karen Bellenir. 612 pages. 2000. 0-7808-0238-1. $78.

ALSO AVAILABLE: *Cardiovascular Diseases & Disorders Sourcebook, 1st Edition.* Edited by Karen Bellenir and Peter D. Dresser. 683 pages. 1995. 0-7808-0032-X. $78.

"This work stands out as an imminently accessible resource for the general public. It is recommended for the reference and circulating shelves of school, public, and academic libraries." —American Reference Books Annual, 2001

"Recommended reference source." —Booklist, American Library Association, Dec '00

"Provides comprehensive coverage of matters related to the heart. This title is recommended for health sciences and public libraries with consumer health collections." —E-Streams, Oct '00

SEE ALSO *Healthy Heart Sourcebook for Women*

Household Safety Sourcebook

Basic Consumer Health Information about Household Safety, Including Information about Poisons, Chemicals, Fire, and Water Hazards in the Home

Along with Advice about the Safe Use of Home Maintenance Equipment, Choosing Toys and Nursery Furni-

ture, Holiday and Recreation Safety, a Glossary, and Resources for Further Help and Information

Edited by Dawn D. Matthews. 606 pages. 2002. 0-7808-0338-8. $78.

"This work will be useful in public libraries with large consumer health and wellness departments."
— American Reference Books Annual, 2003

"As a sourcebook on household safety this book meets its mark. It is encyclopedic in scope and covers a wide range of safety issues that are commonly seen in the home." *— E-Streams, Jul '02*

Immune System Disorders Sourcebook

Basic Information about Lupus, Multiple Sclerosis, Guillain-Barré Syndrome, Chronic Granulomatous Disease, and More

Along with Statistical and Demographic Data and Reports on Current Research Initiatives

Edited by Allan R. Cook. 608 pages. 1997. 0-7808-0209-8. $78.

Infant & Toddler Health Sourcebook

Basic Consumer Health Information about the Physical and Mental Development of Newborns, Infants, and Toddlers, Including Neonatal Concerns, Nutrition Recommendations, Immunization Schedules, Common Pediatric Disorders, Assessments and Milestones, Safety Tips, and Advice for Parents and Other Caregivers

Along with a Glossary of Terms and Resource Listings for Additional Help

Edited by Jenifer Swanson. 585 pages. 2000. 0-7808-0246-2. $78.

"As a reference for the general public, this would be useful in any library." *— E-Streams, May '01*

"Recommended reference source."
— Booklist, American Library Association, Feb '01

"This is a good source for general use."
—American Reference Books Annual, 2001

Infectious Diseases Sourcebook

Basic Consumer Health Information about Non-Contagious Bacterial, Viral, Prion, Fungal, and Parasitic Diseases Spread by Food and Water, Insects and Animals, or Environmental Contact, Including Botulism, E. Coli, Encephalitis, Legionnaires' Disease, Lyme Disease, Malaria, Plague, Rabies, Salmonella, Tetanus, and Others, and Facts about Newly Emerging Diseases, Such as Hantavirus, Mad Cow Disease, Monkeypox, and West Nile Virus

Along with Information about Preventing Disease Transmission, the Threat of Bioterrorism, and Current

Research Initiatives, with a Glossary and Directory of Resources for More Information

Edited by Karen Bellenir. 634 pages. 2004. 0-7808-0675-1. $78.

Injury & Trauma Sourcebook

Basic Consumer Health Information about the Impact of Injury, the Diagnosis and Treatment of Common and Traumatic Injuries, Emergency Care, and Specific Injuries Related to Home, Community, Workplace, Transportation, and Recreation

Along with Guidelines for Injury Prevention, a Glossary, and a Directory of Additional Resources

Edited by Joyce Brennfleck Shannon. 696 pages. 2002. 0-7808-0421-X. $78.

"This publication is the most comprehensive work of its kind about injury and trauma."
— American Reference Books Annual, 2003

"This sourcebook provides concise, easily readable, basic health information about injuries. . . . This book is well organized and an easy to use reference resource suitable for hospital, health sciences and public libraries with consumer health collections."
— E-Streams, Nov '02

"Practitioners should be aware of guides such as this in order to facilitate their use by patients and their families." *—Doody's Health Sciences Book Review Journal, Sep-Oct '02*

"Recommended reference source."
—Booklist, American Library Association, Sep '02

"Highly recommended for academic and medical reference collections." *—Library Bookwatch, Sep '02*

Kidney & Urinary Tract Diseases & Disorders Sourcebook

Basic Information about Kidney Stones, Urinary Incontinence, Bladder Disease, End Stage Renal Disease, Dialysis, and More

Along with Statistical and Demographic Data and Reports on Current Research Initiatives

Edited by Linda M. Ross. 602 pages. 1997. 0-7808-0079-6. $78.

Learning Disabilities Sourcebook, 2nd Edition

Basic Consumer Health Information about Learning Disabilities, Including Dyslexia, Developmental Speech and Language Disabilities, Non-Verbal Learning Disorders, Developmental Arithmetic Disorder, Developmental Writing Disorder, and Other Conditions That Impede Learning Such as Attention Deficit/ Hyperactivity Disorder, Brain Injury, Hearing Impairment, Klinefelter Syndrome, Dyspraxia, and Tourette Syndrome

Along with Facts about Educational Issues and Assistive Technology, Coping Strategies, a Glossary of Re-

lated Terms, and Resources for Further Help and Information

Edited by Dawn D. Matthews. 621 pages. 2003. 0-7808-0626 3. $78.

ALSO AVAILABLE: *Learning Disabilities Sourcebook, 1st Edition.* Edited by Linda M. Shin. 579 pages. 1998. 0-7808-0210-1. $78.

"Teachers as well as consumers will find this an essential guide to understanding various syndromes and their latest treatments. [An] invaluable reference for public and school library collections alike."
— *Library Bookwatch, Apr '03*

Named **"Outstanding Reference Book of 1999."**
— *New York Public Library, Feb 2000*

"An excellent candidate for inclusion in a public library reference section. It's a great source of information. Teachers will also find the book useful. Definitely worth reading."
— *Journal of Adolescent & Adult Literacy, Feb 2000*

"Readable . . . provides a solid base of information regarding successful techniques used with individuals who have learning disabilities, as well as practical suggestions for educators and family members. Clear language, concise descriptions, and pertinent information for contacting multiple resources add to the strength of this book as a useful tool." — *Choice, Association of College and Research Libraries, Feb '99*

"Recommended reference source."
— *Booklist, American Library Association, Sep '98*

"A useful resource for libraries and for those who don't have the time to identify and locate the individual publications." — *Disability Resources Monthly, Sep '98*

Leukemia Sourcebook

Basic Consumer Health Information about Adult and Childhood Leukemias, Including Acute Lymphocytic Leukemia (ALL), Chronic Lymphocytic Leukemia (CLL), Acute Myelogenous Leukemia (AML), Chronic Myelogenous Leukemia (CML), and Hairy Cell Leukemia, and Treatments Such as Chemotherapy, Radiation Therapy, Peripheral Blood Stem Cell and Marrow Transplantation, and Immunotherapy

Along with Tips for Life During and After Treatment, a Glossary, and Directories of Additional Resources

Edited by Joyce Brennfleck Shannon. 587 pages. 2003. 0-7808-0627-1. $78.

Liver Disorders Sourcebook

Basic Consumer Health Information about the Liver and How It Works; Liver Diseases, Including Cancer, Cirrhosis, Hepatitis, and Toxic and Drug Related Diseases; Tips for Maintaining a Healthy Liver; Laboratory Tests, Radiology Tests, and Facts about Liver Transplantation

Along with a Section on Support Groups, a Glossary, and Resource Listings

Edited by Joyce Brennfleck Shannon. 591 pages. 2000. 0-7808-0383-3. $78.

"A valuable resource."
— *American Reference Books Annual, 2001*

"This title is recommended for health sciences and public libraries with consumer health collections."
— *E-Streams, Oct '00*

"Recommended reference source."
— *Booklist, American Library Association, Jun '00*

Lung Disorders Sourcebook

Basic Consumer Health Information about Emphysema, Pneumonia, Tuberculosis, Asthma, Cystic Fibrosis, and Other Lung Disorders, Including Facts about Diagnostic Procedures, Treatment Strategies, Disease Prevention Efforts, and Such Risk Factors as Smoking, Air Pollution, and Exposure to Asbestos, Radon, and Other Agents

Along with a Glossary and Resources for Additional Help and Information

Edited by Dawn D. Matthews. 678 pages. 2002. 0-7808-0339-6. $78.

"This title is a great addition for public and school libraries because it provides concise health information on the lungs."
— *American Reference Books Annual, 2003*

"Highly recommended for academic and medical reference collections." — *Library Bookwatch, Sep '02*

Medical Tests Sourcebook, 2nd Edition

Basic Consumer Health Information about Medical Tests, Including Age-Specific Health Tests, Important Health Screenings and Exams, Home-Use Tests, Blood and Specimen Tests, Electrical Tests, Scope Tests, Genetic Testing, and Imaging Tests, Such as X-Rays, Ultrasound, Computed Tomography, Magnetic Resonance Imaging, Angiography, and Nuclear Medicine

Along with a Glossary and Directory of Additional Resources

Edited by Joyce Brennfleck Shannon. 654 pages. 2004. 0-7808-0670-0. $78.

ALSO AVAILABLE: *Medical Tests, 1st Edition.* Edited by Joyce Brennfleck Shannon. 691 pages. 1999. 0-7808-0243-8. $78.

"Recommended for hospital and health sciences libraries with consumer health collections."
— *E-Streams, Mar '00*

"This is an overall excellent reference with a wealth of general knowledge that may aid those who are reluctant to get vital tests performed."
— *Today's Librarian, Jan 2000*

"A valuable reference guide."
— *American Reference Books Annual, 2000*

Men's Health Concerns Sourcebook, 2nd Edition

Basic Consumer Health Information about the Medical and Mental Concerns of Men, Including Theories about the Shorter Male Lifespan, the Leading Causes of Death and Disability, Physical Concerns of Special Significance to Men, Reproductive and Sexual Concerns, Sexually Transmitted Diseases, Men's Mental and Emotional Health, and Lifestyle Choices That Affect Wellness, Such as Nutrition, Fitness, and Substance Use

Along with a Glossary of Related Terms and a Directory of Organizational Resources in Men's Health

Edited by Robert Aquinas McNally. 644 pages. 2004. 0-7808-0671-9. $78.

ALSO AVAILABLE: *Men's Health Concerns Sourcebook, 1st Edition.* Edited by Allan R. Cook. 738 pages. 1998. 0-7808-0212-8. $78.

"This comprehensive resource and the series are highly recommended."
—*American Reference Books Annual, 2000*

"Recommended reference source."
— *Booklist, American Library Association, Dec '98*

■

Mental Health Disorders Sourcebook, 2nd Edition

Basic Consumer Health Information about Anxiety Disorders, Depression and Other Mood Disorders, Eating Disorders, Personality Disorders, Schizophrenia, and More, Including Disease Descriptions, Treatment Options, and Reports on Current Research Initiatives

Along with Statistical Data, Tips for Maintaining Mental Health, a Glossary, and Directory of Sources for Additional Help and Information

Edited by Karen Bellenir. 605 pages. 2000. 0-7808-0240-3. $78.

ALSO AVAILABLE: *Mental Health Disorders Sourcebook, 1st Edition.* Edited by Karen Bellenir. 548 pages. 1995. 0-7808-0040-0. $78.

"Well organized and well written."
—*American Reference Books Annual, 2001*

"Recommended reference source."
—*Booklist, American Library Association, Jun '00*

■

Mental Retardation Sourcebook

Basic Consumer Health Information about Mental Retardation and Its Causes, Including Down Syndrome, Fetal Alcohol Syndrome, Fragile X Syndrome, Genetic Conditions, Injury, and Environmental Sources

Along with Preventive Strategies, Parenting Issues, Educational Implications, Health Care Needs, Employment and Economic Matters, Legal Issues, a Glossary, and a Resource Listing for Additional Help and Information

Edited by Joyce Brennfleck Shannon. 642 pages. 2000. 0-7808-0377-9. $78.

"Public libraries will find the book useful for reference and as a beginning research point for students, parents, and caregivers."
—*American Reference Books Annual, 2001*

"The strength of this work is that it compiles many basic fact sheets and addresses for further information in one volume. It is intended and suitable for the general public. This sourcebook is relevant to any collection providing health information to the general public."
—*E-Streams, Nov '00*

"From preventing retardation to parenting and family challenges, this covers health, social and legal issues and will prove an invaluable overview."
—*Reviewer's Bookwatch, Jul '00*

■

Movement Disorders Sourcebook

Basic Consumer Health Information about Neurological Movement Disorders, Including Essential Tremor, Parkinson's Disease, Dystonia, Cerebral Palsy, Huntington's Disease, Myasthenia Gravis, Multiple Sclerosis, and Other Early-Onset and Adult-Onset Movement Disorders, Their Symptoms and Causes, Diagnostic Tests, and Treatments

Along with Mobility and Assistive Technology Information, a Glossary, and a Directory of Additional Resources

Edited by Joyce Brennfleck Shannon. 655 pages. 2003. 0-7808-0628-X. $78.

■

Obesity Sourcebook

Basic Consumer Health Information about Diseases and Other Problems Associated with Obesity, and Including Facts about Risk Factors, Prevention Issues, and Management Approaches

Along with Statistical and Demographic Data, Information about Special Populations, Research Updates, a Glossary, and Source Listings for Further Help and Information

Edited by Wilma Caldwell and Chad T. Kimball. 376 pages. 2001. 0-7808-0333-7. $78.

"The book synthesizes the reliable medical literature on obesity into one easy-to-read and useful resource for the general public."
— *American Reference Books Annual 2002*

"This is a very useful resource book for the lay public."
—*Doody's Review Service, Nov '01*

"Well suited for the health reference collection of a public library or an academic health science library that serves the general population." —*E-Streams, Sep '01*

"Recommended reference source."
—*Booklist, American Library Association, Apr '01*

" Recommended pick both for specialty health library collections and any general consumer health reference collection." — *The Bookwatch, Apr '01*

Ophthalmic Disorders Sourcebook, 1st Edition

SEE Eye Care Sourcebook, 2nd Edition

Oral Health Sourcebook

SEE Dental Care & Oral Health Sourcebook, 2nd Ed.

Osteoporosis Sourcebook

Basic Consumer Health Information about Primary and Secondary Osteoporosis and Juvenile Osteoporosis and Related Conditions, Including Fibrous Dysplasia, Gaucher Disease, Hyperthyroidism, Hypophosphatasia, Myeloma, Osteopetrosis, Osteogenesis Imperfecta, and Paget's Disease

Along with Information about Risk Factors, Treatments, Traditional and Non-Traditional Pain Management, a Glossary of Related Terms, and a Directory of Resources

Edited by Allan R. Cook. 584 pages. 2001. 0-7808-0239-X. $78.

"This would be a book to be kept in a staff or patient library. The targeted audience is the layperson, but the therapist who needs a quick bit of information on a particular topic will also find the book useful."
— Physical Therapy, Jan '02

"This resource is recommended as a great reference source for public, health, and academic libraries, and is another triumph for the editors of Omnigraphics."
— American Reference Books Annual 2002

"Recommended for all public libraries and general health collections, especially those supporting patient education or consumer health programs."
— E-Streams, Nov '01

"Will prove valuable to any library seeking to maintain a current, comprehensive reference collection of health resources. . . . From prevention to treatment and associated conditions, this provides an excellent survey."
— The Bookwatch, Aug '01

"Recommended reference source."
— Booklist, American Library Association, July '01

SEE ALSO Women's Health Concerns Sourcebook

Pain Sourcebook, 2nd Edition

Basic Consumer Health Information about Specific Forms of Acute and Chronic Pain, Including Muscle and Skeletal Pain, Nerve Pain, Cancer Pain, and Disorders Characterized by Pain, Such as Fibromyalgia, Shingles, Angina, Arthritis, and Headaches

Along with Information about Pain Medications and Management Techniques, Complementary and Alternative Pain Relief Options, Tips for People Living with Chronic Pain, a Glossary, and a Directory of Sources for Further Information

Edited by Karen Bellenir. 670 pages. 2002. 0-7808-0612-3. $78.

ALSO AVAILABLE: Pain Sourcebook, 1st Edition. Edited by Allan R. Cook. 667 pages. 1997. 0-7808-0213-6. $78.

"A source of valuable information. . . . This book offers help to nonmedical people who need information about pain and pain management. It is also an excellent reference for those who participate in patient education."
— Doody's Review Service, Sep '02

"The text is readable, easily understood, and well indexed. This excellent volume belongs in all patient education libraries, consumer health sections of public libraries, and many personal collections."
— American Reference Books Annual, 1999

"A beneficial reference." — Booklist Health Sciences Supplement, American Library Association, Oct '98

"The information is basic in terms of scholarship and is appropriate for general readers. Written in journalistic style . . . intended for non-professionals. Quite thorough in its coverage of different pain conditions and summarizes the latest clinical information regarding pain treatment." — Choice, Association of College and Research Libraries, Jun '98

"Recommended reference source."
— Booklist, American Library Association, Mar '98

Pediatric Cancer Sourcebook

Basic Consumer Health Information about Leukemias, Brain Tumors, Sarcomas, Lymphomas, and Other Cancers in Infants, Children, and Adolescents, Including Descriptions of Cancers, Treatments, and Coping Strategies

Along with Suggestions for Parents, Caregivers, and Concerned Relatives, a Glossary of Cancer Terms, and Resource Listings

Edited by Edward J. Prucha. 587 pages. 1999. 0-7808-0245-4. $78.

"An excellent source of information. Recommended for public, hospital, and health science libraries with consumer health collections." — E-Streams, Jun '00

"Recommended reference source."
— Booklist, American Library Association, Feb '00

"A valuable addition to all libraries specializing in health services and many public libraries."
— American Reference Books Annual, 2000

Physical & Mental Issues in Aging Sourcebook

Basic Consumer Health Information on Physical and Mental Disorders Associated with the Aging Process, Including Concerns about Cardiovascular Disease, Pulmonary Disease, Oral Health, Digestive Disorders, Musculoskeletal and Skin Disorders, Metabolic Changes, Sexual and Reproductive Issues, and Changes in Vision, Hearing, and Other Senses

Along with Data about Longevity and Causes of Death, Information on Acute and Chronic Pain,

Descriptions of Mental Concerns, a Glossary of Terms, and Resource Listings for Additional Help

Edited by Jenifer Swanson. 660 pages. 1999. 0-7808-0233-0. $78.

"This is a treasure of health information for the layperson."
— Choice Health Sciences Supplement, Association of College & Research Libraries, May 2000

"Recommended for public libraries."
— American Reference Books Annual, 2000

"Recommended reference source."
— Booklist, American Library Association, Oct '99

SEE ALSO Healthy Aging Sourcebook

■

Podiatry Sourcebook

Basic Consumer Health Information about Foot Conditions, Diseases, and Injuries, Including Bunions, Corns, Calluses, Athlete's Foot, Plantar Warts, Hammertoes and Clawtoes, Clubfoot, Heel Pain, Gout, and More

Along with Facts about Foot Care, Disease Prevention, Foot Safety, Choosing a Foot Care Specialist, a Glossary of Terms, and Resource Listings for Additional Information

Edited by M. Lisa Weatherford. 380 pages. 2001. 0-7808-0215-2. $78.

"Recommended reference source."
— Booklist, American Library Association, Feb '02

"There is a lot of information presented here on a topic that is usually only covered sparingly in most larger comprehensive medical encyclopedias."
— American Reference Books Annual 2002

■

Pregnancy & Birth Sourcebook, 2nd Edition

Basic Consumer Health Information about Conception and Pregnancy, Including Facts about Fertility, Infertility, Pregnancy Symptoms and Complications, Fetal Growth and Development, Labor, Delivery, and the Postpartum Period, as Well as Information about Maintaining Health and Wellness during Pregnancy and Caring for a Newborn

Along with Information about Public Health Assistance for Low-Income Pregnant Women, a Glossary, and Directories of Agencies and Organizations Providing Help and Support

Edited by Amy L. Sutton. 626 pages. 2004. 0-7808-0672-7. $78.

ALSO AVAILABLE: Pregnancy & Birth Sourcebook, 1st Edition. Edited by Heather E. Aldred. 737 pages. 1997. 0-7808-0216-0. $78.

"A well-organized handbook. Recommended."
— Choice, Association of College and Research Libraries, Apr '98

"Recommended reference source."
— Booklist, American Library Association, Mar '98

"Recommended for public libraries."
— American Reference Books Annual, 1998

SEE ALSO Congenital Disorders Sourcebook, Family Planning Sourcebook

■

Prostate Cancer Sourcebook

Basic Consumer Health Information about Prostate Cancer, Including Information about the Associated Risk Factors, Detection, Diagnosis, and Treatment of Prostate Cancer

Along with Information on Non-Malignant Prostate Conditions, and Featuring a Section Listing Support and Treatment Centers and a Glossary of Related Terms

Edited by Dawn D. Matthews. 358 pages. 2001. 0-7808-0324-8. $78.

"Recommended reference source."
— Booklist, American Library Association, Jan '02

"A valuable resource for health care consumers seeking information on the subject. . . .All text is written in a clear, easy-to-understand language that avoids technical jargon. Any library that collects consumer health resources would strengthen their collection with the addition of the Prostate Cancer Sourcebook."
— American Reference Books Annual 2002

■

Public Health Sourcebook

Basic Information about Government Health Agencies, Including National Health Statistics and Trends, Healthy People 2000 Program Goals and Objectives, the Centers for Disease Control and Prevention, the Food and Drug Administration, and the National Institutes of Health

Along with Full Contact Information for Each Agency

Edited by Wendy Wilcox. 698 pages. 1998. 0-7808-0220-9. $78.

"Recommended reference source."
— Booklist, American Library Association, Sep '98

"This consumer guide provides welcome assistance in navigating the maze of federal health agencies and their data on public health concerns."
— SciTech Book News, Sep '98

■

Reconstructive & Cosmetic Surgery Sourcebook

Basic Consumer Health Information on Cosmetic and Reconstructive Plastic Surgery, Including Statistical Information about Different Surgical Procedures, Things to Consider Prior to Surgery, Plastic Surgery Techniques and Tools, Emotional and Psychological Considerations, and Procedure-Specific Information

Along with a Glossary of Terms and a Listing of Resources for Additional Help and Information

Edited by M. Lisa Weatherford. 374 pages. 2001. 0-7808-0214-4. $78.

"An excellent reference that addresses cosmetic and medically necessary reconstructive surgeries. . . . The style of the prose is calm and reassuring, discussing the many positive outcomes now available due to advances in surgical techniques."
— *American Reference Books Annual 2002*

"Recommended for health science libraries that are open to the public, as well as hospital libraries that are open to the patients. This book is a good resource for the consumer interested in plastic surgery."
— *E-Streams, Dec '01*

"Recommended reference source."
— *Booklist, American Library Association, July '01*

■

Rehabilitation Sourcebook

Basic Consumer Health Information about Rehabilitation for People Recovering from Heart Surgery, Spinal Cord Injury, Stroke, Orthopedic Impairments, Amputation, Pulmonary Impairments, Traumatic Injury, and More, Including Physical Therapy, Occupational Therapy, Speech/ Language Therapy, Massage Therapy, Dance Therapy, Art Therapy, and Recreational Therapy

Along with Information on Assistive and Adaptive Devices, a Glossary, and Resources for Additional Help and Information

Edited by Dawn D. Matthews. 531 pages. 1999. 0-7808-0236-5. $78.

"This is an excellent resource for public library reference and health collections."
— *American Reference Books Annual, 2001*

"Recommended reference source."
— *Booklist, American Library Association, May '00*

■

Respiratory Diseases & Disorders Sourcebook

Basic Information about Respiratory Diseases and Disorders, Including Asthma, Cystic Fibrosis, Pneumonia, the Common Cold, Influenza, and Others, Featuring Facts about the Respiratory System, Statistical and Demographic Data, Treatments, Self-Help Management Suggestions, and Current Research Initiatives

Edited by Allan R. Cook and Peter D. Dresser. 771 pages. 1995. 0-7808-0037-0. $78.

"Designed for the layperson and for patients and their families coping with respiratory illness. . . . an extensive array of information on diagnosis, treatment, management, and prevention of respiratory illnesses for the general reader." — *Choice, Association of College and Research Libraries, Jun '96*

"A highly recommended text for all collections. It is a comforting reminder of the power of knowledge that good books carry between their covers."
— *Academic Library Book Review, Spring '96*

"A comprehensive collection of authoritative information presented in a nontechnical, humanitarian style for patients, families, and caregivers."
— *Association of Operating Room Nurses, Sep/Oct '95*

SEE ALSO *Lung Disorders Sourcebook*

■

Sexually Transmitted Diseases Sourcebook, 2nd Edition

Basic Consumer Health Information about Sexually Transmitted Diseases, Including Information on the Diagnosis and Treatment of Chlamydia, Gonorrhea, Hepatitis, Herpes, HIV, Mononucleosis, Syphilis, and Others

Along with Information on Prevention, Such as Condom Use, Vaccines, and STD Education; And Featuring a Section on Issues Related to Youth and Adolescents, a Glossary, and Resources for Additional Help and Information

Edited by Dawn D. Matthews. 538 pages. 2001. 0-7808-0249-7. $78.

ALSO AVAILABLE: *Sexually Transmitted Diseases Sourcebook, 1st Edition.* Edited by Linda M. Ross. 550 pages. 1997. 0-7808-0217-9. $78.

"Recommended for consumer health collections in public libraries, and secondary school and community college libraries."
— *American Reference Books Annual 2002*

"Every school and public library should have a copy of this comprehensive and user-friendly reference book."
— *Choice, Association of College & Research Libraries, Sep '01*

"This is a highly recommended book. This is an especially important book for all school and public libraries." — *AIDS Book Review Journal, Jul-Aug '01*

"Recommended reference source."
— *Booklist, American Library Association, Apr '01*

"Recommended pick both for specialty health library collections and any general consumer health reference collection." — *The Bookwatch, Apr '01*

■

Skin Disorders Sourcebook

Basic Information about Common Skin and Scalp Conditions Caused by Aging, Allergies, Immune Reactions, Sun Exposure, Infectious Organisms, Parasites, Cosmetics, and Skin Traumas, Including Abrasions, Cuts, and Pressure Sores

Along with Information on Prevention and Treatment

Edited by Allan R. Cook. 647 pages. 1997. 0-7808-0080-X. $78.

". . . comprehensive, easily read reference book."
— *Doody's Health Sciences Book Reviews, Oct '97*

SEE ALSO *Burns Sourcebook*

Sleep Disorders Sourcebook

Basic Consumer Health Information about Sleep and Its Disorders, Including Insomnia, Sleepwalking, Sleep Apnea, Restless Leg Syndrome, and Narcolepsy

Along with Data about Shiftwork and Its Effects, Information on the Societal Costs of Sleep Deprivation, Descriptions of Treatment Options, a Glossary of Terms, and Resource Listings for Additional Help

Edited by Jenifer Swanson. 439 pages. 1998. 0-7808-0234-9. $78.

"This text will complement any home or medical library. It is user-friendly and ideal for the adult reader."
— American Reference Books Annual, 2000

"A useful resource that provides accurate, relevant, and accessible information on sleep to the general public. Health care providers who deal with sleep disorders patients may also find it helpful in being prepared to answer some of the questions patients ask."
— Respiratory Care, Jul '99

"Recommended reference source."
— Booklist, American Library Association, Feb '99

■

Sports Injuries Sourcebook, 2nd Edition

Basic Consumer Health Information about the Diagnosis, Treatment, and Rehabilitation of Common Sports-Related Injuries in Children and Adults

Along with Suggestions for Conditioning and Training, Information and Prevention Tips for Injuries Frequently Associated with Specific Sports and Special Populations, a Glossary, and a Directory of Additional Resources

Edited by Joyce Brennfleck Shannon. 614 pages. 2002. 0-7808-0604-2. $78.

ALSO AVAILABLE: *Sports Injuries Sourcebook, 1st Edition.* Edited by Heather E. Aldred. 624 pages. 1999. 0-7808-0218-7. $78.

"This is an excellent reference for consumers and it is recommended for public, community college, and undergraduate libraries."
— American Reference Books Annual, 2003

"Recommended reference source."
— Booklist, American Library Association, Feb '03

■

Stress-Related Disorders Sourcebook

Basic Consumer Health Information about Stress and Stress-Related Disorders, Including Stress Origins and Signals, Environmental Stress at Work and Home, Mental and Emotional Stress Associated with Depression, Post-Traumatic Stress Disorder, Panic Disorder, Suicide, and the Physical Effects of Stress on the Cardiovascular, Immune, and Nervous Systems

Along with Stress Management Techniques, a Glossary, and a Listing of Additional Resources

Edited by Joyce Brennfleck Shannon. 610 pages. 2002. 0-7808-0560-7. $78.

"Well written for a general readership, the *Stress-Related Disorders Sourcebook* is a useful addition to the health reference literature."
— American Reference Books Annual, 2003

"I am impressed by the amount of information. It offers a thorough overview of the causes and consequences of stress for the layperson. . . . A well-done and thorough reference guide for professionals and nonprofessionals alike."
— Doody's Review Service, Dec '02

■

Stroke Sourcebook

Basic Consumer Health Information about Stroke, Including Ischemic, Hemorrhagic, Transient Ischemic Attack (TIA), and Pediatric Stroke, Stroke Triggers and Risks, Diagnostic Tests, Treatments, and Rehabilitation Information

Along with Stroke Prevention Guidelines, Legal and Financial Information, a Glossary, and a Directory of Additional Resources

Edited by Joyce Brennfleck Shannon. 606 pages. 2003. 0-7808-0630-1. $78.

■

Substance Abuse Sourcebook

Basic Health-Related Information about the Abuse of Legal and Illegal Substances Such as Alcohol, Tobacco, Prescription Drugs, Marijuana, Cocaine, and Heroin; and Including Facts about Substance Abuse Prevention Strategies, Intervention Methods, Treatment and Recovery Programs, and a Section Addressing the Special Problems Related to Substance Abuse during Pregnancy

Edited by Karen Bellenir. 573 pages. 1996. 0-7808-0038-9. $78.

"A valuable addition to any health reference section. Highly recommended."
— The Book Report, Mar/Apr '97

". . . a comprehensive collection of substance abuse information that's both highly readable and compact. Families and caregivers of substance abusers will find the information enlightening and helpful, while teachers, social workers and journalists should benefit from the concise format. Recommended."
— Drug Abuse Update, Winter '96/'97

SEE ALSO *Alcoholism Sourcebook, Drug Abuse Sourcebook*

■

Surgery Sourcebook

Basic Consumer Health Information about Inpatient and Outpatient Surgeries, Including Cardiac, Vascular, Orthopedic, Ocular, Reconstructive, Cosmetic, Gynecologic, and Ear, Nose, and Throat Procedures and More

Along with Information about Operating Room Policies and Instruments, Laser Surgery Techniques, Hospital Errors, Statistical Data, a Glossary, and Listings of Sources for Further Help and Information

Edited by Annemarie S. Muth and Karen Bellenir. 596 pages. 2002. 0-7808-0380-9. $78.

"Invaluable reference for public and school library collections alike." — *Library Bookwatch, Apr '03*

■

Transplantation Sourcebook

Basic Consumer Health Information about Organ and Tissue Transplantation, Including Physical and Financial Preparations, Procedures and Issues Relating to Specific Solid Organ and Tissue Transplants, Rehabilitation, Pediatric Transplant Information, the Future of Transplantation, and Organ and Tissue Donation

Along with a Glossary and Listings of Additional Resources

Edited by Joyce Brennfleck Shannon. 628 pages. 2002. 0-7808-0322-1. $78.

"Along with these advances [in transplantation technology] have come a number of daunting questions for potential transplant patients, their families, and their health care providers. This reference text is the best single tool to address many of these questions. . . . It will be a much-needed addition to the reference collections in health care, academic, and large public libraries."
— *American Reference Books Annual, 2003*

"Recommended for libraries with an interest in offering consumer health information." — *E-Streams, Jul '02*

"This is a unique and valuable resource for patients facing transplantation and their families."
— *Doody's Review Service, Jun '02*

■

Traveler's Health Sourcebook

Basic Consumer Health Information for Travelers, Including Physical and Medical Preparations, Transportation Health and Safety, Essential Information about Food and Water, Sun Exposure, Insect and Snake Bites, Camping and Wilderness Medicine, and Travel with Physical or Medical Disabilities

Along with International Travel Tips, Vaccination Recommendations, Geographical Health Issues, Disease Risks, a Glossary, and a Listing of Additional Resources

Edited by Joyce Brennfleck Shannon. 613 pages. 2000. 0-7808-0384-1. $78.

"Recommended reference source."
— *Booklist, American Library Association, Feb '01*

"This book is recommended for any public library, any travel collection, and especially any collection for the physically disabled."
— *American Reference Books Annual, 2001*

■

Vegetarian Sourcebook

Basic Consumer Health Information about Vegetarian Diets, Lifestyle, and Philosophy, Including Definitions of Vegetarianism and Veganism, Tips about Adopting Vegetarianism, Creating a Vegetarian Pantry, and Meeting Nutritional Needs of Vegetarians, with Facts Regarding Vegetarianism's Effect on Pregnant and Lactating Women, Children, Athletes, and Senior Citizens

Along with a Glossary of Commonly Used Vegetarian Terms and Resources for Additional Help and Information

Edited by Chad T. Kimball. 360 pages. 2002. 0-7808-0439-2. $78.

"Organizes into one concise volume the answers to the most common questions concerning vegetarian diets and lifestyles. This title is recommended for public and secondary school libraries." — *E-Streams, Apr '03*

"Invaluable reference for public and school library collections alike." — *Library Bookwatch, Apr '03*

"The articles in this volume are easy to read and come from authoritative sources. The book does not necessarily support the vegetarian diet but instead provides the pros and cons of this important decision. The *Vegetarian Sourcebook* is recommended for public libraries and consumer health libraries."
— *American Reference Books Annual, 2003*

■

Women's Health Concerns Sourcebook, 2nd Edition

Basic Consumer Health Information about the Medical and Mental Concerns of Women, Including Maintaining Health and Wellness, Gynecological Concerns, Breast Health, Sexuality and Reproductive Issues, Menopause, Cancer in Women, the Leading Causes of Death and Disability among Women, Physical Concerns of Special Significance to Women, and Women's Mental and Emotional Health

Along with a Glossary of Related Terms and Directories of Resources for Additional Help and Information

Edited by Amy L. Sutton. 748 pages. 2004. 0-7808-0673-5. $78.

ALSO AVAILABLE: Women's Health Concerns Sourcebook, 1st Edition. Edited by Heather E. Aldred. 567 pages. 1997. 0-7808-0219-5. $78.

"Handy compilation. There is an impressive range of diseases, devices, disorders, procedures, and other physical and emotional issues covered . . . well organized, illustrated, and indexed." — *Choice, Association of College and Research Libraries, Jan '98*

SEE ALSO Breast Cancer Sourcebook, Cancer Sourcebook for Women, Healthy Heart Sourcebook for Women, Osteoporosis Sourcebook

■

Workplace Health & Safety Sourcebook

Basic Consumer Health Information about Workplace Health and Safety, Including the Effect of Workplace Hazards on the Lungs, Skin, Heart, Ears, Eyes, Brain, Reproductive Organs, Musculoskeletal System, and Other Organs and Body Parts

Along with Information about Occupational Cancer, Personal Protective Equipment, Toxic and Hazardous Chemicals, Child Labor, Stress, and Workplace Violence

Edited by Chad T. Kimball. 626 pages. 2000. 0-7808-0231-4. $78.

"As a reference for the general public, this would be useful in any library." —*E-Streams, Jun '01*

"Provides helpful information for primary care physicians and other caregivers interested in occupational medicine. . . . General readers; professionals." — *Choice, Association of College & Research Libraries, May '01*

"Recommended reference source." —*Booklist, American Library Association, Feb '01*

"Highly recommended." — *The Bookwatch, Jan '01*

■

Worldwide Health Sourcebook

Basic Information about Global Health Issues, Including Malnutrition, Reproductive Health, Disease Dispersion and Prevention, Emerging Diseases, Risky Health Behaviors, and the Leading Causes of Death

Along with Global Health Concerns for Children, Women, and the Elderly, Mental Health Issues, Research and Technology Advancements, and Economic, Environmental, and Political Health Implications, a Glossary, and a Resource Listing for Additional Help and Information

Edited by Joyce Brennfleck Shannon. 614 pages. 2001. 0-7808-0330-2. $78.

"Named an Outstanding Academic Title." —*Choice, Association of College & Research Libraries, Jan '02*

"Yet another handy but also unique compilation in the extensive Health Reference Series, this is a useful work because many of the international publications reprinted or excerpted are not readily available. Highly recommended." —*Choice, Association of College & Research Libraries, Nov '01*

"Recommended reference source." —*Booklist, American Library Association, Oct '01*

Teen Health Series

Helping Young Adults Understand, Manage, and Avoid Serious Illness

Cancer Information for Teens

Health Tips about Cancer Awareness, Prevention, Diagnosis, and Treatment

Including Facts about Frequently Occurring Cancers, Cancer Risk Factors, and Coping Strategies for Teens Fighting Cancer or Dealing with Cancer in Friends or Family Members

Edited by Wilma R. Caldwell. 415 pages. 2004. 0-7808-0678-6. $58.

■

Diet Information for Teens

Health Tips about Diet and Nutrition

Including Facts about Nutrients, Dietary Guidelines, Breakfasts, School Lunches, Snacks, Party Food, Weight Control, Eating Disorders, and More

Edited by Karen Bellenir. 399 pages. 2001. 0-7808-0441-4. $58.

"Full of helpful insights and facts throughout the book. . . . An excellent resource to be placed in public libraries or even in personal collections."
—American Reference Books Annual 2002

"Recommended for middle and high school libraries and media centers as well as academic libraries that educate future teachers of teenagers. It is also a suitable addition to health science libraries that serve patrons who are interested in teen health promotion and education." —E-Streams, Oct '01

"This comprehensive book would be beneficial to collections that need information about nutrition, dietary guidelines, meal planning, and weight control. . . . This reference is so easy to use that its purchase is recommended." —The Book Report, Sep-Oct '01

"This book is written in an easy to understand format describing issues that many teens face every day, and then provides thoughtful explanations so that teens can make informed decisions. This is an interesting book that provides important facts and information for today's teens." —Doody's Health Sciences Book Review Journal, Jul-Aug '01

"A comprehensive compendium of diet and nutrition. The information is presented in a straightforward, plain-spoken manner. This title will be useful to those working on reports on a variety of topics, as well as to general readers concerned about their dietary health."
—School Library Journal, Jun '01

Drug Information for Teens

Health Tips about the Physical and Mental Effects of Substance Abuse

Including Facts about Alcohol, Anabolic Steroids, Club Drugs, Cocaine, Depressants, Hallucinogens, Herbal Products, Inhalants, Marijuana, Narcotics, Stimulants, Tobacco, and More

Edited by Karen Bellenir. 452 pages. 2002. 0-7808-0444-9. $58.

"The chapters are quick to make a connection to their teenage reading audience. The prose is straightforward and the book lends itself to spot reading. It should be useful both for practical information and for research, and it is suitable for public and school libraries."
—American Reference Books Annual, 2003

"Recommended reference source."
—Booklist, American Library Association, Feb '03

"This is an excellent resource for teens and their parents. Education about drugs and substances is key to discouraging teen drug abuse and this book provides this much needed information in a way that is interesting and factual." —Doody's Review Service, Dec '02

■

Fitness Information for Teens

Health Tips about Exercise, Physical Well-Being, and Health Maintenance

Including Facts about Aerobic and Anaerobic Conditioning, Stretching, Body Shape and Body Image, Sports Training, Nutrition, and Activities for Non-Athletes

Edited by Karen Bellenir. 426 pages. 2004. 0-7808-0679-4. $58.

■

Mental Health Information for Teens

Health Tips about Mental Health and Mental Illness

Including Facts about Anxiety, Depression, Suicide, Eating Disorders, Obsessive-Compulsive Disorders, Panic Attacks, Phobias, Schizophrenia, and More

Edited by Karen Bellenir. 406 pages. 2001. 0-7808-0442-2. $58.

"In both language and approach, this user-friendly entry in the Teen Health Series is on target for teens needing information on mental health concerns." —Booklist, American Library Association, Jan '02

Sexual Health Information for Teens

Health Tips about Sexual Development, Human Reproduction, and Sexually Transmitted Diseases

Including Facts about Puberty, Reproductive Health, Chlamydia, Human Papillomavirus, Pelvic Inflammatory Disease, Herpes, AIDS, Contraception, Pregnancy, and More

Edited by Deborah A. Stanley. 391 pages. 2003. 0-7808-0445-7. $58.

Skin Health Information For Teens

Health Tips about Dermatological Concerns and Skin Cancer Risks

Including Facts about Acne, Warts, Hives, and Other Conditions and Lifestyle Choices, Such as Tanning, Tattooing, and Piercing, That Affect the Skin, Nails, Scalp, and Hair

Edited by Robert Aquinas McNally. 430 pages. 2003. 0-7808-0446-5. $58.

Sports Injuries Information For Teens

Health Tips about Sports Injuries and Injury Protection

Including Facts about Specific Injuries, Emergency Treatment, Rehabilitation, Sports Safety, Competition Stress, Fitness, Sports Nutrition, Steroid Risks, and More

Edited by Joyce Brennfleck Shannon. 425 pages. 2003. 0-7808-0447-3. $58.

Health Reference Series

Adolescent Health Sourcebook

AIDS Sourcebook, 3rd Edition

Alcoholism Sourcebook

Allergies Sourcebook, 2nd Edition

Alternative Medicine Sourcebook, 2nd Edition

Alzheimer's Disease Sourcebook, 3rd Edition

Arthritis Sourcebook

Asthma Sourcebook

Attention Deficit Disorder Sourcebook

Back & Neck Disorders Sourcebook

Blood & Circulatory Disorders Sourcebook

Brain Disorders Sourcebook

Breast Cancer Sourcebook

Breastfeeding Sourcebook

Burns Sourcebook

Cancer Sourcebook, 4th Edition

Cancer Sourcebook for Women, 2nd Edition

Caregiving Sourcebook

Child Abuse Sourcebook

Childhood Diseases & Disorders Sourcebook

Colds, Flu & Other Common Ailments Sourcebook

Communication Disorders Sourcebook

Congenital Disorders Sourcebook

Consumer Issues in Health Care Sourcebook

Contagious & Non-Contagious Infectious Diseases Sourcebook

Death & Dying Sourcebook

Dental Care & Oral Health Sourcebook, 2nd Edition

Depression Sourcebook

Diabetes Sourcebook, 3rd Edition

Diet & Nutrition Sourcebook, 2nd Edition

Digestive Diseases & Disorder Sourcebook

Disabilities Sourcebook

Domestic Violence Sourcebook, 2nd Edition

Drug Abuse Sourcebook

Ear, Nose & Throat Disorders Sourcebook

Eating Disorders Sourcebook

Emergency Medical Services Sourcebook

Endocrine & Metabolic Disorders Sourcebook

Environmentally Health Sourcebook, 2nd Edition

Ethnic Diseases Sourcebook

Eye Care Sourcebook, 2nd Edition

Family Planning Sourcebook

Fitness & Exercise Sourcebook, 2nd Edition

Food & Animal Borne Diseases Sourcebook

Food Safety Sourcebook

Forensic Medicine Sourcebook

Gastrointestinal Diseases & Disorders Sourcebook

Genetic Disorders Sourcebook, 2nd Edition

Head Trauma Sourcebook

Headache Sourcebook

Health Insurance Sourcebook

Health Reference Series Cumulative Index 1999

Healthy Aging Sourcebook

Healthy Children Sourcebook